SIXTH EDITION

Basic
IMMUNOLOGY

FUNCTIONS AND DISORDERS OF THE IMMUNE SYSTEM

Abul K. Abbas, MBBS
Professor Emeritus, Pathology
University of California San Francisco
San Francisco, California

Andrew H. Lichtman, MD, PhD
Professor of Pathology
Harvard Medical School
Brigham and Women's Hospital
Boston, Massachusetts

Shiv Pillai, MBBS, PhD
Professor of Medicine and Health Sciences
    and Technology
Harvard Medical School
Massachusetts General Hospital
Boston, Massachusetts

Illustrations by David L. Baker, MA
DNA Illustrations, Inc.

ELSEVIER

Previous editions copyrighted 2016, 2014, 2011, 2009, 2006, 2004, and 2001.

International Standard Book Number: 978-0-323-54943-1

Executive Content Strategist: James Merritt
Senior Content Strategist: Jeremy Bowes
Director, Content Development: Rebecca Gruliow
Publishing Services Manager: Julie Eddy
Book Production Specialist: Clay S. Broeker
Design Direction: Brian Salisbury

Printed in China

Last digit is the print number: 9   8   7   6   5   4   3   2   1

ELSEVIER

1600 John F. Kennedy Blvd.
Ste. 1600
Philadelphia, PA 19103-2899

Working together
to grow libraries in
developing countries

www.elsevier.com • www.bookaid.org

To our students

The sixth edition of *Basic Immunology* has been revised to include recent important advances in our knowledge of the immune system. The original goals of this book, from the earliest edition, were to present current concepts in immunology cogently and also in sufficient detail that they would be understood by students of the discipline, as well as to emphasize clinical aspects, including disease pathogenesis and the development of novel therapies based on the basic science of immunology. These are the goals that we continue to strive for. With improving understanding of the normal immune response, we believe it is possible to present the fundamental knowledge in a concise way. In addition, there has been exciting progress in applying basic principles to understanding and treating human diseases, a topic that is of paramount interest for students of medicine and allied health sciences. Foremost among these recent advances is the development of cancer immunotherapy, which dramatically illustrates how foundational science can be translated into clinical practice.

More specifically, we have focused on the following objectives. First, we have presented the most important principles governing the function of the immune system by synthesizing key concepts from the vast amount of experimental data that have emerged in the field of immunology. Our judgment of what is most important is based largely on what is most clearly established by scientific investigation and is essential for understanding the major functions of the immune system. We have also prioritized content that is relevant to human health and disease. We have realized that in any concise discussion of complex phenomena, it is inevitable that exceptions and caveats cannot be considered in detail, so these have largely been omitted. Second, we have focused on immune responses against infectious microbes, and most of our discussions of the immune system are in this context. Third, we have made liberal use of illustrations to highlight important principles, but we have reduced factual details that may be found in more comprehensive textbooks. Fourth, we have

also discussed immunologic diseases from the perspective of principles, emphasizing their relation to normal immune responses and avoiding details of clinical syndromes and treatments. We have included selected clinical cases in an appendix to illustrate how the principles of immunology may be applied to common human diseases. Finally, in order to make each chapter readable on its own, we have repeated key ideas in different places in the book. We feel such repetition will help students to grasp the most important concepts.

We hope that students will find this new edition of *Basic Immunology* clear, cogent, manageable, and enjoyable to read. We hope the book will convey our sense of excitement about how the field has evolved and how it continues to grow in relevance to human health and disease. Finally, although we were spurred to tackle this project because of our associations with medical school courses, we hope the book will be valued by students of allied health and biology as well. We will have succeeded if the book can answer many of the questions these students have about the immune system and, at the same time, encourage them to delve even more deeply into immunology.

Several individuals played key roles in the writing of this book. Our editor, James Merritt, has been an enthusiastic source of encouragement and advice. Our talented illustrator, David Baker, continues to effectively convert our ideas into pictures that are informative and aesthetically pleasing. Our development editor, Rebecca Gruliow, has kept the project organized and on track despite pressures of time and logistics. Clay Broeker has moved the book through the production process in an efficient and professional manner. To all of them we owe our many thanks. Finally, we owe an enormous debt of gratitude to our families, whose support and encouragement have been unwavering.

Abul K. Abbas
Andrew H. Lichtman
Shiv Pillai

CONTENTS

Basic
IMMUNOLOGY
FUNCTIONS AND DISORDERS OF THE IMMUNE SYSTEM

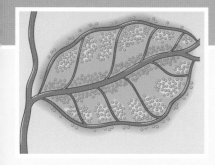

Introduction to the Immune System
Nomenclature, General Properties, and Components

The term "immunity" in a biologic context has historically referred to resistance to pathogens; however, reactions to some noninfectious substances including harmless environmental molecules, tumors, and even unaltered host components are also considered forms of immunity (allergy, tumor immunity, and autoimmunity, respectively). The collection of cells, tissues, and molecules that mediate these reactions is called the **immune system**, and the coordinated response of these cells and molecules to pathogens and other substances comprises an **immune response**.

The most important physiologic function of the immune system is to prevent or eradicate infections (Fig. 1.1), and this is the principal context in which immune responses are discussed throughout this book. In addition, it prevents the growth of some tumors, and some cancers can be treated by stimulating immune responses against tumor cells. The immune system also plays a major role in the repair of damaged tissues. Because the immune system can respond to microbial and nonmicrobial substances and also can cause disease under some circumstances,

a more inclusive definition of the immune response is a reaction to microbes, as well as to other molecules that are recognized as foreign, regardless of the physiologic or pathologic consequence of such a reaction. Immunology is the study of immune responses in this broader sense and of the cellular and molecular events that occur after an organism encounters microbes and other foreign molecules.

The importance of the immune system for health is dramatically illustrated by the frequent observation that individuals with defective immune responses are susceptible to serious, often life-threatening infections. Conversely, stimulating immune responses against microbes through vaccination is the most effective method for protecting individuals against infections; this approach has led to the worldwide eradication of smallpox, the only disease that has been eliminated from civilization by human intervention (Fig. 1.2). The appearance of acquired immunodeficiency syndrome (AIDS) in the 1980s tragically emphasized the importance of the immune system for defending individuals against infection.

Role of the immune system	Implications
Defense against infections	Deficient immunity results in increased susceptibility to infections; exemplified by AIDS
	Vaccination boosts immune defenses and protects against infections
Defense against tumors	Potential for immunotherapy of cancer
Control of tissue regeneration and scarring	Repair of damaged tissues
The immune system can injure cells and induce pathologic inflammation	Immune responses are the cause of allergic, autoimmune, and other inflammatory diseases
The immune system recognizes and responds to tissue grafts and newly introduced proteins	Immune responses are barriers to transplantation and gene therapy

Fig. 1.1 Importance of the immune system in health and disease. This table summarizes some of the physiologic functions of the immune system and its role in disease. *AIDS,* Acquired immunodeficiency syndrome.

In contrast to these beneficial roles, abnormal immune responses cause many inflammatory diseases with serious morbidity and mortality. The immune response is the major barrier to the success of organ transplantation, which is often used to treat organ failure. The products of immune cells can also be of great practical use. For example, antibodies, which are proteins made by certain cells of the immune system, are used in clinical laboratory testing and in research as highly specific reagents for detecting a wide variety of molecules in the circulation and in cells and tissues. Antibodies designed to block or eliminate potentially harmful molecules and cells are used widely for the treatment of immunologic diseases, cancers, and other types of disorders. For all these reasons, the field of immunology has captured the attention of clinicians, scientists, and the lay public.

This chapter introduces the nomenclature of immunology, important general properties of all immune responses, and the cells and tissues that are the principal components of the immune system. In particular, the following questions are addressed:
- What types of immune responses protect individuals from infections?
- What are the important characteristics of immunity, and what mechanisms are responsible for these characteristics?
- How are the cells and tissues of the immune system organized to find and respond to microbes in ways that lead to their elimination?

The basic principles introduced here set the stage for more detailed discussions of immune responses in later chapters. A Glossary of the important terms used in this book is provided near the end of the book.

INNATE AND ADAPTIVE IMMUNITY

Host defenses are grouped under innate immunity, which provides immediate protection against microbial invasion, and adaptive immunity, which develops more slowly and provides more specialized defense against infections (Fig. 1.3). Innate immunity, also called natural immunity or native immunity, is always present in healthy individuals (hence the term *innate*), prepared to block the entry of microbes and to rapidly eliminate microbes that do succeed in entering host tissues. Adaptive immunity, also called specific immunity or acquired immunity, requires proliferation and differentiation of lymphocytes in response to microbes before it can provide effective defense (i.e., it adapts to the presence of microbial invaders). Innate immunity is phylogenetically older, and the more specialized and powerful adaptive immune response evolved later.

Disease	Maximum number of cases (year)	Number of cases in 2014
Diptheria	206,939 (1921)	0
Measles	894,134 (1941)	72
Mumps	152,209 (1968)	40
Pertussis	265,269 (1934)	311
Polio (paralytic)	21,269 (1952)	0
Rubella	57,686 (1969)	0
Tetanus	1,560 (1923)	0
Hemophilus influenzae type B infection	~20,000 (1984)	134
Hepatitis B	26,611 (1985)	58

Fig. 1.2 **Effectiveness of vaccination for some common infectious diseases in the United States.** Many infectious diseases for which effective vaccines have been developed have been virtually eradicated in the United States and other developed countries. (Modified from Orenstein WA, Hinman AR, Bart KJ, Hadler SC. Immunization. In: Mandell GL, Bennett JE, Dolin R, editors: *Principles and practices of infectious diseases*, 4th ed. New York: Churchill Livingstone, 1995; and *MMWR* 66, No. 1, 2017.)

In innate immunity, the first line of defense is provided by epithelial barriers of the skin and mucosal tissues and by cells and natural antibiotics present in epithelia, all of which function to block the entry of microbes. If microbes do breach epithelia and enter the tissues or circulation, several other components of the innate immune system defend against them, including phagocytes and innate lymphoid cells, and several plasma proteins, such as the complement system. In addition to providing early defense against infections, innate immune responses are required to initiate adaptive immune responses against the infectious agents. The components and mechanisms of innate immunity are discussed in detail in Chapter 2.

The adaptive immune system consists of lymphocytes with highly diverse and variable receptors for foreign substances, and the products of these cells, such as antibodies. Adaptive immune responses are essential for defense against infectious microbes that are pathogenic for humans (i.e., capable of causing disease) and may have evolved to resist innate immunity. The cells and molecules of innate immunity recognize structures shared by classes of microbes, whereas the lymphocytes of adaptive immunity express receptors that specifically recognize a much wider variety of molecules produced by microbes, as well as noninfectious molecules. Any molecule that is specifically recognized by lymphocytes or antibodies is called an **antigen.** Adaptive immune responses often use the cells and molecules of the innate immune system to eliminate microbes. For example, antibodies (a component of adaptive immunity) bind to microbes, and these coated microbes avidly bind to and activate phagocytes (a component of innate immunity), which ingest and destroy the microbes. Examples of the cooperation between innate and adaptive immunity are discussed in later chapters.

By convention, the term *immune response* generally refers to adaptive immunity, and that is the focus of most of this chapter.

The cells of the immune system are located in different tissues and serve different roles in host defense. Most of these cells are derived from bone marrow precursors that circulate in the blood and are called leukocytes (white blood cells). Others are present in tissues at all times. Some of these cells function mainly in innate immunity, others in adaptive immunity, and some function in both types of responses. These cells are grouped into two broad categories—**lymphoid cells** (most of

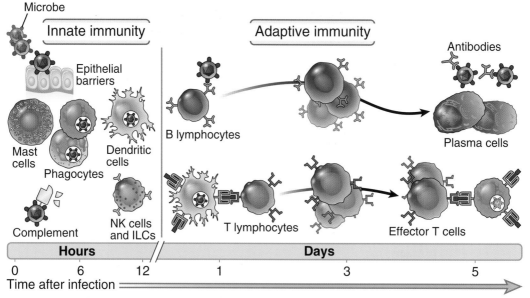

Fig. 1.3 Principal mechanisms of innate and adaptive immunity. The mechanisms of innate immunity provide the initial defense against infections. Some mechanisms (e.g., epithelial barriers) prevent infections, and other mechanisms (e.g., phagocytes, natural killer *[NK]* cells and other innate lymphoid cells *[ILCs]*, the complement system) eliminate microbes. Adaptive immune responses develop later and are mediated by lymphocytes and their products. Antibodies block infections and eliminate microbes, and T lymphocytes eradicate intracellular microbes. The kinetics of the innate and adaptive immune responses are approximations and may vary in different infections.

which are the mediators of adaptive immune responses) and nonlymphoid cells, also called **myeloid cells,** which play diverse roles, including in innate immune responses.

- Tissue-resident **dendritic cells, macrophages, and mast cells** serve as sentinels to detect the presence of microbes in tissues and initiate immune responses. Dendritic cells (DCs), so called because of their many protruding membrane extensions, also have the specialized function of capturing microbial antigens and displaying them to T lymphocytes to initiate adaptive immune responses and are therefore called **antigen-presenting cells** (APCs, discussed later).
- **Phagocytes** ingest and destroy microbes. They are myeloid cells and include neutrophils, which are recruited from the blood, and macrophages, which can develop from circulating monocytes and live in tissues much longer than neutrophils do. Macrophages are not only sentinels and destroyers of microbes, they also help to repair damaged tissues. Because the

sentinels and phagocytes are primarily cells of innate immunity, they are described in Chapter 2.

- **Lymphocytes,** including B and T cells, circulate through lymphoid organs and nonlymphoid tissues. They recognize foreign antigens and carry out adaptive immune responses. They are described further later in this chapter.

TYPES OF ADAPTIVE IMMUNITY

The two types of adaptive immunity, called humoral immunity and cell-mediated immunity, are mediated by different cells and molecules and provide defense against extracellular microbes and intracellular microbes, respectively (Fig. 1.4).

- **Humoral immunity** is mediated by proteins called **antibodies,** which are produced by cells called **B lymphocytes.** Secreted antibodies enter the circulation, extracellular tissue fluids, and the lumens of mucosal organs such as the gastrointestinal and respiratory tracts. The antibodies defend against microbes

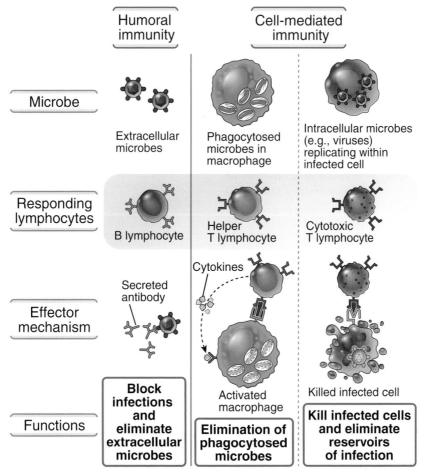

Humoral immunity

Cell-mediated immunity

Microbe

Extracellular microbes

Phagocytosed microbes in macrophage

Intracellular microbes (e.g., viruses) replicating within infected cell

Responding lymphocytes

B lymphocyte

Helper T lymphocyte

Cytotoxic T lymphocyte

Effector mechanism

Secreted antibody

Cytokines

Activated macrophage

Killed infected cell

Functions

Block infections and eliminate extracellular microbes

Elimination of phagocytosed microbes

Kill infected cells and eliminate reservoirs of infection

Fig. 1.4 Types of adaptive immunity. In humoral immunity, B lymphocytes secrete antibodies that eliminate extracellular microbes. In cell-mediated immunity, some T lymphocytes secrete soluble proteins called cytokines that recruit and activate phagocytes to destroy ingested microbes, and other T lymphocytes kill infected cells.

present in these locations by preventing them from invading tissue cells and by neutralizing toxins made by the microbes. Microbes that live and divide outside cells but are readily killed once ingested by phagocytes are called extracellular microbes, and antibodies can enhance the uptake of these microbes into phagocytes. However, many microbes, often called intracellular microbes, can live and divide inside infected cells, including phagocytes. Although antibodies can prevent such microbes from infecting tissue cells, they are not effective after the microbes have entered the cells.

• Defense against microbes that have already entered host cells is called **cell-mediated immunity** because

it is mediated by cells, which are called **T lymphocytes.** Cell-mediated immunity is especially important to defend against intracellular organisms that can survive and replicate inside cells. Some T lymphocytes activate phagocytes to destroy microbes that have been ingested and live within intracellular vesicles of these phagocytes. Other T lymphocytes kill any type of host cells (including non-phagocytic cells) that harbor infectious microbes in the cytoplasm or nucleus. In both cases, the T cells recognize microbial antigens that are displayed on host cell surfaces, which indicates there is a microbe inside the cell. Some T lymphocytes also help to defend against extracellular microbes by recruiting large numbers of phagocytes to sites of infection, and the phagocytes ingest and destroy the microbes.

The specificities of B and T lymphocytes differ in important respects. Most T cells recognize only peptide fragments of protein antigens presented on cell surfaces, whereas B cells and antibodies are able to recognize many different types of molecules, including proteins, carbohydrates, nucleic acids, and lipids. These and other differences are discussed in more detail later.

Immunity may be induced in an individual by infection or vaccination (active immunity) or conferred on an individual by transfer of antibodies or lymphocytes from an actively immunized individual (passive immunity).

- In **active immunity,** an individual exposed to the antigens of a microbe mounts a response to eradicate the infection and develops resistance to later infection by that microbe. Such an individual is said to be immune to that microbe, in contrast with a naive individual who has not previously been exposed to that microbe's antigens.

- In **passive immunity,** a naive individual receives antibodies or cells (e.g., lymphocytes) from another individual already immune to an infection or protective antibodies that have been synthesized using modern bioengineering techniques. The recipient acquires the ability to combat the infection for as long as the transferred antibodies or cells last. Passive immunity is therefore useful for rapidly conferring immunity even before the individual is able to mount an active response, but it does not induce long-lived resistance to the infection. The only physiologic example of passive immunity is seen in newborns, whose immune systems are not mature enough to respond to many pathogens but who are protected against infections by acquiring antibodies during fetal life from their mothers through the placenta and in the neonatal period from breast milk. Clinically, passive immunity is useful for treating some immunodeficiency diseases with antibodies pooled from multiple donors and for emergency treatment of some viral infections and snakebites using serum from immunized donors. Antibodies and T cells designed to recognize tumors are now widely used for passive immunotherapy of cancers.

PROPERTIES OF ADAPTIVE IMMUNE RESPONSES

Several properties of adaptive immune responses are crucial for the effectiveness of these responses in combating infections (Fig. 1.5).

Feature	Functional significance
Specificity	Ensures that immune responses are precisely targeted to microbial pathogens
Diversity	Enables immune system to respond to a large variety of antigens
Memory	Leads to enhanced responses to repeated exposures to the same antigens
Clonal expansion	Increases number of antigen-specific lymphocytes from a small number of naive lymphocytes
Specialization	Generates responses that are optimal for defense against different types of microbes
Contraction and homeostasis	Allows immune system to respond to newly encountered antigens
Nonreactivity to self	Prevents injury to the host during responses to foreign antigens

Fig. 1.5 Properties of adaptive immune responses. This table summarizes the important properties of adaptive immune responses and how each feature contributes to host defense against microbes.

Specificity and Diversity

The adaptive immune system is capable of distinguishing millions of different antigens or portions of antigens, a feature that is referred to as specificity. It implies that the total collection of lymphocyte specificities, sometimes called the lymphocyte repertoire, is extremely diverse. The total population of B and T lymphocytes consists of many different clones (each clone made up of cells all derived from one lymphocyte), and all the cells of one clone express identical antigen receptors, which are different from the receptors of all other clones. We now know the molecular basis for the generation of this remarkable diversity of lymphocytes (see Chapter 4). The **clonal selection hypothesis**, formulated in the 1950s, correctly predicted that clones of lymphocytes specific for different antigens develop before an encounter with these antigens, and each antigen elicits an immune response by selecting and activating the lymphocytes of a specific clone (Fig. 1.6).

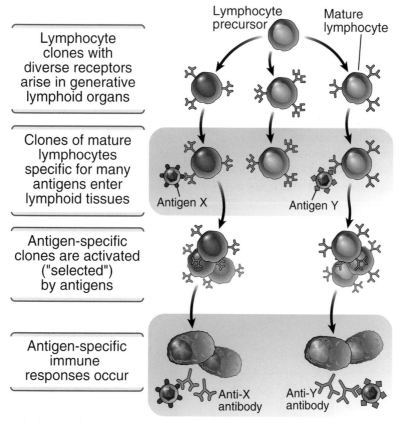

Fig. 1.6 Clonal selection. Mature lymphocytes with receptors for many antigens develop before encountering these antigens. A clone refers to a population of lymphocytes with identical antigen receptors and therefore specificities; all of these cells are presumably derived from one precursor cell. Each antigen (e.g., X and Y) selects a preexisting clone of specific lymphocytes and stimulates the proliferation and differentiation of that clone. The diagram shows only B lymphocytes giving rise to antibody-secreting cells, but the same principle applies to T lymphocytes. The antigens shown are surface molecules of microbes, but clonal selection is true for all extracellular and intracellular antigens.

The diversity of the lymphocyte repertoire, which enables the immune system to respond to a vast number and variety of antigens, also means that before exposure to any one antigen, very few cells, perhaps as few as 1 in 100,000 or 1 in 1,000,000 lymphocytes, are specific for that antigen. Thus, the total number of lymphocytes that can recognize and react against any one antigen ranges from approximately 1,000 to 10,000 cells. To mount an effective defense against microbes, these few cells have to give rise to a large number of lymphocytes capable of destroying the microbes. Each unique lymphocyte that recognizes a single antigen and its progeny constitute an antigen-specific clone. The effectiveness of immune responses is attributable to several features of adaptive immunity, including the marked expansion of the clone of lymphocytes specific for any antigen upon exposure to that antigen, the selection and preservation of the most potent lymphocytes, and numerous positive feedback loops that amplify immune responses. These characteristics of the adaptive immune system are described in later chapters.

Memory

The adaptive immune system mounts faster, larger and more effective responses to repeated exposure to the same antigen. This feature of adaptive immune responses implies that the immune system remembers every encounter with antigen, and this property of adaptive immunity is therefore called **immunologic memory**. The response to the first exposure to antigen, called the **primary immune response**, is initiated by lymphocytes called naive lymphocytes that are seeing antigen for the first time (Fig. 1.7). The term *naive* refers to these cells being immunologically inexperienced, not having previously responded to antigens. Subsequent encounters with the same antigen lead to responses called **secondary immune responses** that usually are more rapid, larger, and better able to eliminate the antigen than primary responses. Secondary responses are the result of the activation of memory lymphocytes, which are long-lived cells that were induced during the primary immune response. Immunologic memory optimizes the ability of the immune system to combat persistent and recurrent infections, because each exposure to a microbe generates more memory cells and activates previously generated memory cells. Immunologic memory is one mechanism by which vaccines confer long-lasting protection against infections.

Other Features of Adaptive Immunity

Adaptive immune responses have other characteristics that are important for their functions (see Fig. 1.5).
- When naive or memory lymphocytes are activated by antigens, they undergo proliferation, generating many thousands of cells, all with the same antigen receptors and specificity. This process, called **clonal expansion,** rapidly increases the number of cells specific for the antigen encountered and ensures that adaptive immunity keeps pace with rapidly proliferating microbes.
- Immune responses are specialized, and different responses are designed to defend best against different types of microbes.
- All immune responses are self-limited and decline as the infection is eliminated, allowing the system to return to a resting state (homeostasis), prepared to respond to another infection.

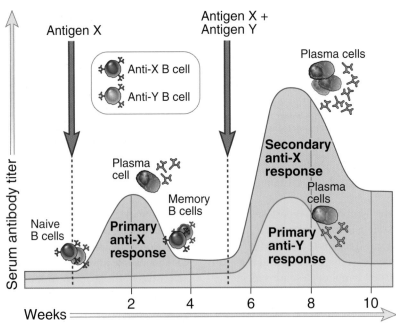

Fig. 1.7 Primary and secondary immune responses. The properties of memory and specificity can be demonstrated by repeated immunizations with defined antigens in animal experiments. Antigens *X* and *Y* induce the production of different antibodies (a reflection of specificity). The secondary response to antigen X is more rapid and larger than the primary response (illustrating memory) and is different from the primary response to antigen Y (again reflecting specificity). Antibody levels decline with time after each immunization. The level of antibody produced is shown as arbitrary values and varies with the type of antigen exposure. Only B cells are shown, but the same features are seen with T cell responses to antigens. The time after immunization may be 1 to 3 weeks for a primary response and 2 to 7 days for a secondary response, but the kinetics vary, depending on the antigen and the nature of immunization.

- The immune system is able to react against an enormous number and variety of microbes and other foreign antigens, but it normally does not react against the host's own potentially antigenic substances—so-called self antigens. This unresponsiveness to self is called **immunological tolerance,** referring to the ability of the immune system to coexist with (tolerate) potentially antigenic self molecules, cells, and tissues.

CELLS OF THE ADAPTIVE IMMUNE SYSTEM

This section of the chapter describes the important properties of the major cell populations of adaptive immunity—namely, lymphocytes and antigen-presenting cells (Fig. 1.8). Phagocytes and other cells of innate immunity are described in Chapter 2.

Lymphocytes

Lymphocytes are the only cells that produce clonally distributed receptors specific for diverse antigens and are the key mediators of adaptive immunity. A healthy adult contains 0.5 to 1×10^{12} lymphocytes. Although all lymphocytes are morphologically similar and rather unremarkable in appearance, they are heterogeneous in lineage, function, and phenotype and are capable of complex biologic responses and activities (Fig. 1.9). These cells often are distinguished by the expression of surface proteins that may be identified using panels of monoclonal antibodies. The standard nomenclature for these proteins is the CD (cluster of differentiation)

Cell type	Principal function(s)
Lymphocytes: B lymphocytes; T lymphocytes *Blood lymphocyte*	Specific recognition of antigens and generation of adaptive immune responses: • B lymphocytes: mediators of humoral immunity • T lymphocytes: mediators of cell-mediated immunity
Antigen-presenting cells: dendritic cells; macrophages; B cells; follicular dendritic cells *Dendritic cell*	Capture of antigens for display to lymphocytes: • Dendritic cells: initiation of T cell responses • Macrophages: effector phase of cell-mediated immunity • Follicular dendritic cells: display of antigens to B lymphocytes in humoral immune responses
Effector cells: T lymphocytes; macrophages; granulocytes *Macrophage*	Elimination of antigens: • T lymphocytes: activation of phagocytes, killing infected cells • Macrophages: phagocytosis and killing of microbes • Granulocytes: killing microbes

Fig. 1.8 Principal cells of the adaptive immune system. Micrographs illustrate the morphology of some cells of each type. The major functions of these cell types are listed.

Ⓐ

Fig. 1.9 **Classes of lymphocytes. A,** Different classes of lymphocytes in the adaptive immune system recognize distinct types of antigens and differentiate into effector cells whose function is to eliminate the antigens. B lymphocytes recognize soluble or microbial surface antigens and differentiate into antibody-secreting cells called plasma cells. Both helper T cells and cytotoxic T lymphocytes recognize peptides derived from intracellular microbial proteins displayed on the cell surface by MHC molecules, described in Chapter 3. Helper T cells recognize these peptides displayed on the surface of macrophages or other antigen presenting cells, and secrete cytokines that stimulate different mechanisms of immunity and inflammation. Cytotoxic T lymphocytes recognize peptides displayed by any type of infected cell type (or tumor cell), and kill these cells. Regulatory T cells limit the activation of other lymphocytes, especially of T cells, and prevent autoimmunity.

(B)

Class	Functions	Antigen receptor and specificity	Selected phenotypic markers	Percentage of total lymphocytes*		

αβ T Lymphocytes

Class	Functions	Antigen receptor and specificity	Selected phenotypic markers	Blood	Lymph node	Spleen
CD4+ helper T lymphocytes	B cell activation (humoral immunity) Macrophage activation (cell-mediated immunity) Stimulation of inflammation	αβ heterodimers Diverse specificities for peptide–class II MHC complexes	CD3+ CD4+ CD8−	35–60	50–60	50–60
CD8+ cytotoxic T lymphocytes	Killing of cells infected with intracellular microbes, tumor cells	αβ heterodimers Diverse specificities for peptide–class I MHC complexes	CD3+ CD4− CD8+	15–40	15–20	10–15
Regulatory T cells	Suppress function of other T cells (regulation of immune responses, maintenance of self-tolerance)	αβ heterodimers Specific for self and some foreign antigens (peptide–class II MHC complexes)	CD3+ CD4+ CD25+ FoxP3+ (most common)	0.5–2	5–10	5–10

B Lymphocytes

Class	Functions	Antigen receptor and specificity	Selected phenotypic markers	Blood	Lymph node	Spleen
B cells	Antibody production (humoral immunity)	Surface Ig Diverse specificities for many types of molecules	Fc receptors class II MHC CD19 CD23	5–20	20–25	40–45

Fig. 1.9, cont'd B, The table summarizes the major properties of the lymphocytes of the adaptive immune system. Not included are γδ T cells, natural killer cells and other innate lymphoid cells, which are discussed in Chapter 2. *The percentages are approximations, based on data from human peripheral blood and mouse lymphoid organs. *Ig*, Immunoglobulin; *MHC*, major histocompatibility complex.

numeric designation, which is used to delineate surface proteins that define a particular cell type or stage of cell differentiation and that are recognized by a cluster or group of antibodies. (A list of CD molecules mentioned in the book is provided in Appendix I.)

As alluded to earlier, B lymphocytes are the only cells capable of producing antibodies; therefore they are the cells that mediate humoral immunity. B cells express membrane-bound antibodies that serve as the receptors that recognize antigens and initiate the process of activation of the cells. Soluble antigens and antigens on the surface of microbes and other cells may bind to these B lymphocyte antigen receptors, resulting in the proliferation and differentiation of the antigen-specific B cells. This leads to the secretion of soluble forms of antibodies with the same antigen specificity as the membrane receptors.

T lymphocytes are responsible for cell-mediated immunity. The antigen receptors of most T lymphocytes recognize only peptide fragments of protein antigens that are bound to specialized peptide display molecules, called major histocompatibility complex (MHC) molecules, on the surface of specialized cells, called antigen-presenting cells (see Chapter 3). Among T lymphocytes, CD4+ T cells are called **helper T cells** because they help B lymphocytes to produce antibodies and help phagocytes to destroy ingested microbes. CD8+ T lymphocytes are called **cytotoxic T lymphocytes** (CTLs) because they kill cells harboring intracellular microbes. Some CD4+ T cells belong to a special subset that functions to prevent or limit immune responses; these are called **regulatory T lymphocytes.**

All lymphocytes arise from common lymphoid precursor cells in the bone marrow (Fig. 1.10). **B lymphocytes mature in the bone marrow, and T lymphocytes mature in an organ called the thymus.** These sites in which mature lymphocytes are produced (generated) are called the **generative** (or **central**) **lymphoid organs.** Mature lymphocytes leave the generative lymphoid organs and enter the circulation and **peripheral (secondary) lymphoid organs**, which are the major site of immune responses where lymphocytes encounter antigens and are activated.

When naive lymphocytes recognize microbial antigens and also receive additional signals induced by microbes, the antigen-specific lymphocytes proliferate and then differentiate into effector cells and memory cells (Fig. 1.11).
- **Naive lymphocytes** express receptors for antigens but do not perform the functions that are required to eliminate antigens. These cells reside in and circulate between peripheral lymphoid organs and survive for several months up to a few years, waiting to find and respond to antigen. If they are not activated by antigen, naive lymphocytes die by the process of apoptosis and are replaced by new cells that have arisen in the generative lymphoid organs. The differentiation of naive lymphocytes into effector cells and memory cells is initiated by antigen recognition, thus ensuring that the immune response that develops is specific for the antigen that is recognized.
- **Effector lymphocytes** are the differentiated progeny of naive cells that have the ability to produce molecules that function to eliminate antigens. The effector cells in the B lymphocyte lineage are antibody-secreting cells, called **plasma cells.** Plasma cells develop in response to antigenic stimulation in the peripheral

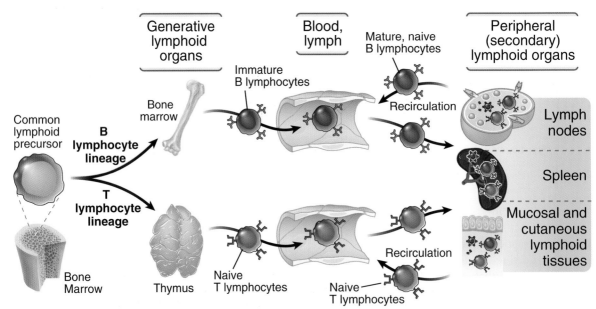

Fig. 1.10 Maturation and tissue distribution of lymphocytes. Lymphocytes develop from precursors in the generative lymphoid organs (bone marrow and thymus). Mature lymphocytes enter the peripheral lymphoid organs, where they respond to foreign antigens and recirculate in the blood and lymph. Some immature B cells leave the bone marrow and complete their maturation in the spleen (not shown).

Ⓐ

Cell type	Stage		
	Naive cell	Activated or effector lymphocyte	Memory lymphocyte
B lymphocytes	**Antigen recognition**	**Proliferation**	**Differentiation**
T lymphocytes	**Antigen recognition**	**Proliferation**	**Differentiation**

Ⓑ

	Naive cell	Activated or effector lymphocyte	Memory lymphocyte
T lymphocytes			
Migration	Preferentially to peripheral lymph nodes	Preferentially to inflamed tissues	Heterogenous: different subsets to lymph nodes, mucosa and other tissues
Frequency of cells responsive to particular antigen	Very low	High	Low
Effector functions	None	Cytokine secretion; cytotoxic activity	None
B lymphocytes			
Membrane immunoglobulin (Ig) isotype	IgM and IgD	Frequently IgG, IgA, and IgE (low level in plasma cells)	Frequently IgG, IgA, and IgE
Affinity of Ig produced	Relatively low	Increases during immune response	Relatively high
Effector functions	None	Antibody secretion	None

Fig. 1.11 Stages in the life history of lymphocytes. A, Naive lymphocytes recognize foreign antigens to initiate adaptive immune responses. Naive lymphocytes need signals in addition to antigens to proliferate and differentiate into effector cells; these additional signals are not shown. Effector cells, which develop from naive cells, function to eliminate antigens. The effector cells of the B lymphocyte lineage are antibody-secreting plasma cells (some of which are long lived). The effector cells of the CD4 T lymphocyte lineage produce cytokines. (The effector cells of the CD8 lineage are CTLs; these are not shown.) Other progeny of the antigen-stimulated lymphocytes differentiate into long-lived memory cells. **B,** The important characteristics of naive, effector, and memory cells in the B and T lymphocyte lineages are summarized. The generation and functions of effector cells, including changes in migration patterns and types of immunoglobulin produced, are described in later chapters.

lymphoid organs, where they may stay and produce antibodies. Small numbers of antibody-secreting cells are also found in the blood; these are called plasmablasts. Some of these migrate to the bone marrow, where they mature into long-lived plasma cells and continue to produce antibody years after the infection is eradicated, providing immediate protection in case the infection recurs.

Effector CD4$^+$ T cells (helper T cells) produce proteins called **cytokines** that activate B cells, macrophages, and other cell types, thereby mediating the helper function of this lineage. The properties of cytokines are listed in Appendix II and will be discussed in later chapters. Effector CD8$^+$ T cells (CTLs) have the machinery to kill infected host cells. The development and functions of these effector cells are also discussed in later chapters. Effector T lymphocytes are short lived and die as the antigen is eliminated.

- **Memory cells,** also generated from the progeny of antigen-stimulated lymphocytes, can survive for long periods in the absence of antigen. Therefore the frequency of memory cells increases with age, presumably because of exposure to environmental microbes. In fact, memory cells make up less than 5% of peripheral blood T cells in a newborn but 50% or more in an adult (Fig. 1.12). As individuals age, the gradual accumulation of memory cells compensates for the reduced output of new, naive T cells from the thymus,

Fig. 1.12 Change in proportions of naive and memory T cells with age. The proportions of naive and memory T cells are based on data from multiple healthy individuals. The estimate of thymic output is an approximation. (Courtesy Dr. Donna L. Farber, Columbia University College of Physicians and Surgeons, New York, NY.)

which involutes after puberty (see Chapter 4). Memory cells are functionally inactive; they do not perform effector functions unless stimulated by antigen. When memory cells encounter the same antigen that induced their development, the cells rapidly respond to initiate secondary immune responses. The signals that generate and maintain memory cells are not well understood but include cytokines.

Antigen-Presenting Cells

The common portals of entry for microbes—the skin and gastrointestinal, respiratory, and genitourinary tracts—contain specialized cells located in the epithelium that capture antigens, transport them to peripheral lymphoid tissues, and display (present) them to lymphocytes. These are the first steps in the development of adaptive immune responses against antigens. This function of antigen capture and presentation is best understood for dendritic cells, the most specialized antigen-presenting cells (APCs) in the immune system. Dendritic cells capture protein antigens of microbes that cross epithelial barriers and transport these antigens to regional lymph nodes, where they display fragments of the proteins for recognition by T lymphocytes. If a microbe has invaded through the epithelium, it may be phagocytosed and presented by tissue macrophages. Microbes or their antigens that enter lymphoid organs may be captured by dendritic cells or macrophages that reside in these organs and presented to lymphocytes. The process of antigen presentation to T cells is described in Chapter 3.

Dendritic cells have another important feature that gives them the ability to stimulate T cell responses. These specialized cells respond to microbes by producing surface proteins, called costimulators, which are required, together with antigen, to activate naive T lymphocytes to proliferate and differentiate into effector cells. Dendritic cells express higher levels of these costimulatory proteins than do other cell types and are thus the most potent stimulators of naive T cells and the most efficient initiators of T cell responses. Other antigen-presentingcells, such as macrophages and B cells, present antigens to differentiated effector T cells in various immune responses.

B lymphocytes may directly recognize the antigens of microbes (either released or on the surface of the microbes), and macrophages and dendritic cells in peripheral lymphoid organs may also capture antigens and display them to B cells. A distinct type of cell called the **follicular dendritic cell** (FDC) resides in the germinal centers of lymphoid follicles in the peripheral lymphoid organs and displays antigens that stimulate the differentiation of B cells in the follicles (see Chapter 7). FDCs do not present antigens to T cells and differ from the dendritic cells described earlier that function as APCs for T lymphocytes.

TISSUES OF THE IMMUNE SYSTEM

The tissues of the immune system consist of the generative lymphoid organs, in which T and B lymphocytes mature and become competent to respond to antigens, and the peripheral lymphoid organs, in which adaptive immune responses to microbes are initiated (see Fig. 1.10). Most of the lymphocytes in a healthy human are found in lymphoid organs and other tissues (Fig. 1.13). However, as we discuss later, lymphocytes are unique among the cells of the body because of their ability to recirculate, repeatedly going through the blood to visit every secondary lymphoid organ in the body. The generative (also called primary or central) lymphoid organs are described in Chapter 4, when we discuss the process of lymphocyte maturation. The following section highlights some of the features of peripheral (or secondary) lymphoid organs that are important for the development of adaptive immunity.

Tissue	Number of lymphocytes
Spleen	70×10^9
Lymph nodes	190×10^9
Bone marrow	50×10^9
Blood	10×10^9
Skin	20×10^9
Intestines	50×10^9
Liver	10×10^9
Lungs	30×10^9

Fig. 1.13 Distribution of lymphocytes in lymphoid organs and other tissues. Approximate numbers of lymphocytes in different organs of healthy adults are shown.

Peripheral (Secondary) Lymphoid Organs and Tissues

The peripheral lymphoid organs and tissues, which consist of the lymph nodes, the spleen, and the mucosal and cutaneous immune systems, are organized in a way that promotes the development of adaptive immune responses. T and B lymphocytes must locate microbes that enter at any site in the body, then respond to these microbes and eliminate them. The anatomic organization of peripheral lymphoid organs enables APCs to concentrate antigens in these organs and lymphocytes to locate and respond to the antigens. This organization is complemented by a remarkable ability of lymphocytes to circulate throughout the body in such a way that naive lymphocytes preferentially go to the peripheral lymphoid organs and tissues, in which antigen is concentrated, whereas most effector cells go to sites of infection where microbes must be eliminated. Furthermore, different types of lymphocytes often need to communicate to generate effective immune responses. For example, within peripheral lymphoid organs, helper T cells specific for an antigen interact with and help B lymphocytes specific for the same antigen, resulting in antibody production. An important function of lymphoid organs is to bring these rare cells together after stimulation by antigen so they interact when they need to.

The major peripheral lymphoid organs share many characteristics but also have some unique features.

- **Lymph nodes** are encapsulated nodular aggregates of lymphoid tissues located along lymphatic channels throughout the body (Fig. 1.14). Fluid constantly leaks out of small blood vessels in all epithelia and connective tissues and most parenchymal organs. This fluid, called **lymph,** is drained by lymphatic vessels from the tissues to the lymph nodes and eventually back into the blood circulation. Therefore the lymph contains a mixture of substances absorbed from epithelia and tissues. As the lymph passes through lymph nodes, APCs in the nodes are able to sample the antigens of microbes that may enter through epithelia into tissues. In addition, dendritic cells pick up antigens of microbes from epithelia and other tissues and transport these antigens to the lymph nodes. The net result of these processes of antigen capture and transport is that the antigens of microbes entering through epithelia or colonizing tissues become concentrated in draining lymph nodes.

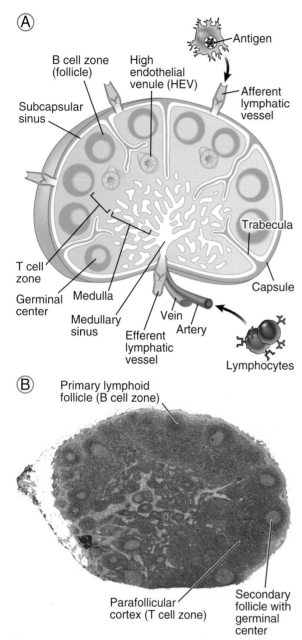

Fig. 1.14 Morphology of lymph nodes. A, Schematic diagram shows the structural organization of a lymph node. B, Light micrograph shows a cross section of a lymph node with numerous follicles in the cortex, some of which contain lightly stained central areas (germinal centers).

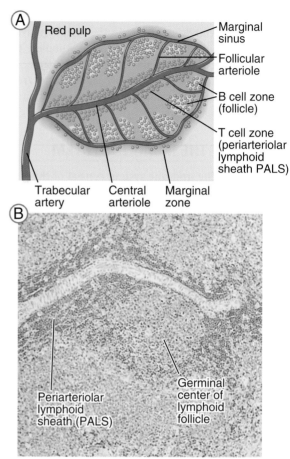

Fig. 1.15 Morphology of the spleen. A, Schematic diagram shows a splenic arteriole surrounded by the periarteriolar lymphoid sheath (PALS) and attached follicles. The PALS and lymphoid follicles together constitute the white pulp. The marginal zone with its sinus is the indistinct boundary between the white pulp and the red pulp. B, Light micrograph of a section of spleen shows an arteriole with the PALS and a follicle with a prominent germinal center. These are surrounded by the red pulp, which is rich in vascular sinusoids.

- The **spleen** is a highly vascularized abdominal organ that serves the same role in immune responses to blood-borne antigens as that of lymph nodes in responses to lymph-borne antigens (Fig. 1.15). Blood entering the spleen flows through a network of channels (sinusoids). Blood-borne antigens are captured and concentrated by dendritic cells and macrophages in the spleen. The spleen contains abundant phagocytes that line the sinusoids, which ingest and destroy microbes in the blood. These macrophages also ingest and destroy old red blood cells.

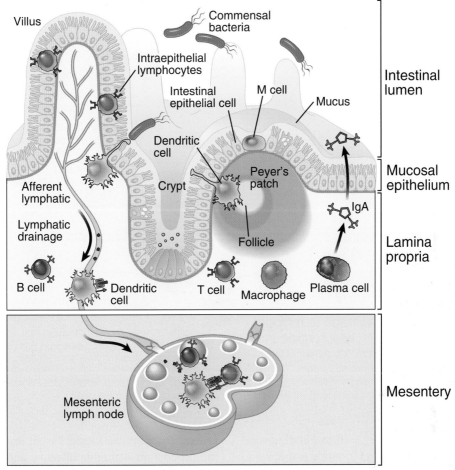

Fig. 1.16 Mucosal immune system. Schematic diagram of the mucosal immune system uses the small bowel as an example. Many commensal bacteria are present in the lumen. The mucus-secreting epithelium provides an innate barrier to microbial invasion (discussed in Chapter 2). Specialized epithelial cells, such as M cells, promote the transport of antigens from the lumen into underlying tissues. Cells in the lamina propria, including dendritic cells, T lymphocytes, and macrophages, provide innate and adaptive immune defense against invading microbes; some of these cells are organized into specialized structures, such as Peyer patches in the small intestine. Immunoglobulin A *(IgA)* is a type of antibody abundantly produced in mucosal tissues that is transported into the lumen, where it binds and neutralizes microbes (see Chapter 8).

- The **cutaneous immune system** and **mucosal immune system** are specialized collections of lymphoid tissues and APCs located in and under the epithelia of the skin and the gastrointestinal and respiratory tracts, respectively. Although most of the immune cells in these tissues are diffusely scattered beneath the epithelial barriers, there are discrete collections of lymphocytes and APCs organized in a similar way as in lymph nodes. For example, tonsils in the pharynx and Peyer patches in the intestine are two anatomically defined mucosal lymphoid tissues (Fig. 1.16). The immune system of the skin consists of most of the cells of innate and adaptive immunity, but without any anatomically defined structures (Fig. 1.17). At any time, at least a quarter of the body's lymphocytes are in the mucosal tissues and skin (reflecting the large size of these tissues) (see Fig. 1.13), and many

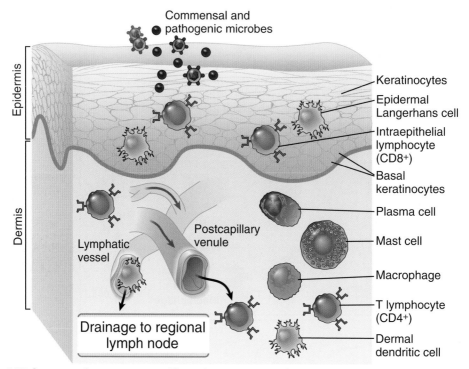

Fig. 1.17 Cutaneous immune system. The major components of the cutaneous immune system shown in this schematic diagram include keratinocytes, Langerhans cells, and intraepithelial lymphocytes, all located in the epidermis, and T lymphocytes, dendritic cells, and macrophages, located in the dermis.

of these are memory cells. Cutaneous and mucosal lymphoid tissues are sites of immune responses to antigens that breach epithelia. A remarkable property of the cutaneous and mucosal immune systems is that they are able to respond to pathogens but do not react to the enormous numbers of usually harmless commensal microbes present at the epithelial barriers. This is accomplished by several mechanisms, including the action of regulatory T cells and other cells that suppress rather than activate T lymphocytes.

Within the peripheral lymphoid organs, T lymphocytes and B lymphocytes are segregated into different anatomic compartments (Fig. 1.18). In lymph nodes, the B cells are concentrated in discrete structures, called **follicles**, located around the periphery, or cortex, of each node. If the B cells in a follicle have recently responded to a protein antigen and received signals from helper T cells, this follicle may contain a central lightly staining region called a **germinal center**. The germinal center has an important role in the production of highly effective antibodies and is described in Chapter 7. The T lymphocytes are concentrated outside but adjacent to the follicles, in the paracortex. The follicles contain the FDCs described earlier that are involved in the activation of B cells, and the paracortex contains dendritic cells that present antigens to T lymphocytes. In the spleen, T lymphocytes are concentrated in periarteriolar lymphoid sheaths surrounding small arterioles, and B cells reside in the follicles.

The anatomic organization of peripheral lymphoid organs is tightly regulated to allow immune responses to develop after stimulation by antigens. B lymphocytes are attracted to and retained in the follicles because of the action of a class of cytokines called **chemokines** (chemoattractant cytokines; chemokines and other cytokines are discussed in more detail in later chapters). FDCs in the follicles secrete a particular chemokine for which naive B cells express a receptor, called CXCR5.

Fig. 1.18 Segregation of T and B lymphocytes in different regions of peripheral lymphoid organs.
A, Schematic diagram illustrates the path by which naive T and B lymphocytes migrate to different areas of a lymph node. Naive B and T lymphocytes enter through a high endothelial venule (HEV), shown in cross section, and are drawn to different areas of the node by chemokines that are produced in these areas and bind selectively to either cell type. Also shown is the migration of dendritic cells, which pick up antigens from epithelia, enter through afferent lymphatic vessels, and migrate to the T cell–rich areas of the node (see Chapter 3). **B,** In this histologic section of a lymph node, the B lymphocytes, located in the follicles, are stained green, and the T cells, in the parafollicular cortex, are stained red using immunofluorescence. In this technique, a section of the tissue is stained with antibodies specific for T or B cells coupled to fluorochromes that emit different colors when excited at the appropriate wavelengths. The anatomic segregation of T and B cells also occurs in the spleen (not shown). (Courtesy Drs. Kathryn Pape and Jennifer Walter, University of Minnesota Medical School, Minneapolis, MN.)

The chemokine that binds to CXCR5 attracts B cells from the blood into the follicles of lymphoid organs. Similarly, T cells are segregated in the paracortex of lymph nodes and the periarteriolar lymphoid sheaths of the spleen because naive T lymphocytes express a receptor, called CCR7, which recognizes chemokines that are produced in these regions of the lymph nodes and spleen. When the lymphocytes are activated by antigens, they alter their expression of chemokine receptors. As a result, the antigen-activated B cells and T cells migrate toward each other and meet at the edge of follicles, where helper T cells interact with and help B cells to dif-

ferentiate into antibody-producing cells (see Chapter 7). Thus, these lymphocyte populations are kept apart from each other until it is useful for them to interact, after exposure to an antigen. This is an excellent example of how the structure of lymphoid organs ensures that the cells that have recognized and responded to an antigen interact and communicate with one another only when necessary.

Many of the effector T cells exit the node through efferent lymphatic vessels and leave the spleen through veins. These activated lymphocytes end up in the circulation and can go to distant sites of infection.

Some activated T cells remain in the lymphoid organ where they were generated and migrate into lymphoid follicles, where they help B cells to make high-affinity antibodies.

Lymphocyte Recirculation and Migration into Tissues

Naive lymphocytes constantly recirculate between the blood and peripheral lymphoid organs, where they may be activated by antigens to become effector cells, and the effector lymphocytes migrate from lymphoid tissues to sites of infection, where microbes are eliminated (Fig. 1.19). Thus, lymphocytes at distinct stages of their lives migrate to the different sites where they are needed for their functions. Migration of effector lymphocytes to sites of infection is most relevant for T cells because effector T cells have to locate and eliminate microbes at these sites. By contrast, plasma cells do not need to migrate to sites of infection; instead, they secrete antibodies, and the antibodies enter the blood. These antibodies bind pathogens or toxins in the blood, or in tissues into which the antibodies enter. Plasma cells in mucosal organs secrete antibodies that enter the lumens of these organs, where they bind to and combat ingested and inhaled microbes.

The migration of different lymphocyte populations has distinct features and is controlled by different molecular interactions.

- Naive T lymphocytes that have matured in the thymus and entered the circulation migrate to lymph nodes, where they can find antigens that are brought to the lymph nodes through lymphatic vessels that drain epithelia and parenchymal organs. These naive T cells enter lymph nodes through specialized postcapillary venules, called **high endothelial venules** (HEVs). The adhesion molecules used by the T cells to bind to the endothelium are described in Chapter 5. Chemokines produced in the T cell zones of the lymph nodes and displayed on HEV surfaces bind to the chemokine receptor CCR7 expressed on naive T cells, which causes the T cells to bind tightly to HEVs. The naive T cells then migrate into the T cell zone, where antigens are displayed by dendritic cells. Naive B cells also enter lymphoid tissues but then migrate to follicles in response to chemokines that bind CXCR5, the chemokine receptor expressed on these B cells.
- In the lymph node, T cells move around rapidly, scanning the surfaces of dendritic cells for antigens. If a T cell specifically recognizes an antigen on a dendritic cell, that T cell forms stable conjugates with

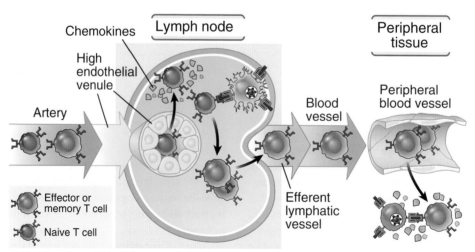

Fig. 1.19 Migration of T lymphocytes. Naive T lymphocytes migrate from the blood through high endothelial venules into the T cell zones of lymph nodes, where the cells are activated by antigens. Activated T cells exit the nodes, enter the bloodstream, and migrate preferentially to peripheral tissues at sites of infection and inflammation. The adhesion molecules involved in the attachment of T cells to endothelial cells are described in Chapters 5 and 6.

the dendritic cell and is activated. Such an encounter between an antigen and a specific lymphocyte is likely to be a random event, but most T cells in the body circulate through some lymph nodes at least once a day. As mentioned earlier and described further in Chapter 3, the likelihood of the correct T cell finding its antigen is increased in peripheral lymphoid organs, particularly lymph nodes, because microbial antigens are concentrated in the same regions of these organs through which naive T cells circulate. Thus, T cells find the antigen they can recognize, and these T cells are activated to proliferate and differentiate. Naive cells that have not encountered specific antigens leave the lymph nodes and reenter the circulation.

- The effector cells that are generated upon T cell activation preferentially migrate into the tissues infected by microbes, where the T lymphocytes perform their function of eradicating the infection. Specific signals control these precise patterns of migration of naive and activated T cells (see Chapter 6).

- B lymphocytes that recognize and respond to antigen in lymph node follicles differentiate into antibody-secreting plasma cells, most of which migrate to the bone marrow or mucosal tissues (see Chapter 7).

- Memory T cells consist of different populations (see Chapter 6); some cells recirculate through lymph nodes, where they can mount secondary responses to captured antigens, and other cells migrate to sites of infection, where they can respond rapidly to eliminate the infection. Yet other memory cells permanently reside in epithelial tissues, such as mucosal tissues and the skin.

We know less about lymphocyte circulation through the spleen or other lymphoid tissues. The spleen does not contain HEVs, but the general pattern of naive lymphocyte migration through this organ probably is similar to migration through lymph nodes.

SUMMARY

- The physiologic function of the immune system is to protect individuals against infections and cancers.
- Innate immunity is the early line of defense, mediated by cells and molecules that are always present and ready to eliminate infectious microbes.
- Adaptive immunity is mediated by lymphocytes stimulated by microbial antigens, which leads to the proliferation and differentiation of the lymphocytes and generation of effector cells, and responds more effectively against each successive exposure to a microbe.
- Lymphocytes are the cells of adaptive immunity and are the only cells with clonally distributed receptors specific for different antigens.
- Adaptive immunity consists of humoral immunity, in which antibodies neutralize and eradicate extracellular microbes and toxins, and cell-mediated immunity, in which T lymphocytes eradicate intracellular microbes.
- Adaptive immune responses consist of sequential phases: antigen recognition by lymphocytes, activation of the lymphocytes to proliferate and to differentiate into effector and memory cells, elimination of the microbes, decline of the immune response, and long-lived memory.
- Different populations of lymphocytes serve distinct functions and may be distinguished by the surface expression of particular membrane molecules.

- B lymphocytes are the only cells that produce antibodies. B lymphocytes express membrane antibodies that recognize antigens, and the progeny of activated B cells, called plasma cells, secrete the antibodies that neutralize and eliminate the antigen.
- T lymphocytes recognize peptide fragments of protein antigens displayed on other cells. Helper T lymphocytes produce cytokines that activate phagocytes to destroy ingested microbes, recruit leukocytes, and activate B lymphocytes to produce antibodies. Cytotoxic T lymphocytes (CTLs) kill infected cells harboring microbes in the cytoplasm.
- Antigen-presenting cells (APCs) capture antigens of microbes that enter through epithelia, concentrate these antigens in lymphoid organs, and display the antigens for recognition by T cells.
- Lymphocytes and APCs are organized in peripheral (secondary) lymphoid organs, where immune responses are initiated and develop.
- Naive lymphocytes circulate through peripheral lymphoid organs, searching for foreign antigens. Effector T lymphocytes migrate to peripheral sites of infection, where they function to eliminate infectious microbes. Plasma cells remain in lymphoid organs and the bone marrow, where they secrete antibodies that enter the circulation and find and eliminate microbes.

REVIEW QUESTIONS

1. What are the two types of adaptive immunity, and what types of microbes do these adaptive immune responses combat?
2. What are the principal classes of lymphocytes, and how do they differ in function?
3. What are the important differences among naive, effector, and memory T and B lymphocytes?
4. Where are T and B lymphocytes located in lymph nodes, and how is their anatomic separation maintained?
5. How do naive and effector T lymphocytes differ in their patterns of migration?

Answers to and discussion of the Review Questions are available at Student Consult.

Innate Immunity
The Early Defense Against Infections

The survival of multicellular organisms requires mechanisms for defense against microbial infections and the elimination of damaged and necrotic cells. The mechanisms that evolved first in invertebrates and persist in all higher vertebrates are always present and functional within the organism, ready to recognize and eliminate microbes and dead cells. Therefore, this type of host defense is known as **innate immunity**, also called natural immunity or native immunity. The cells and molecules that are responsible for innate immunity make up the **innate immune system**.

Innate immunity is the first line of host defense against infections. It blocks microbial invasion through epithelial barriers, destroys many microbes that do enter the body, and is capable of controlling and even eradicating infections. The innate immune response is able to combat microbes immediately upon infection; in contrast, to defend against a microbe not previously encountered, the adaptive immune response needs to be stimulated by antigen to undergo cell proliferation and differentiation steps and therefore is delayed. Innate immunity provides essential protection against infections during this delay. The innate immune response also instructs the adaptive immune system to respond to different microbes in ways that are effective for combating these microbes. In addition, innate immunity is a key participant in the clearance of dead tissues and the initiation of repair after tissue damage.

Before we consider adaptive immunity, the main topic of this book, we discuss the early defense reactions of innate immunity in this chapter. The discussion focuses on the following three questions:

1. How does the innate immune system recognize microbes and damaged cells?
2. How do the different components of innate immunity function to combat different types of microbes?
3. How do innate immune reactions stimulate adaptive immune responses?

GENERAL FEATURES AND SPECIFICITY OF INNATE IMMUNE RESPONSES

The innate immune system performs its defensive functions with a small set of reactions, which are more limited than the varied and specialized responses of adaptive immunity. The specificity of innate immunity is also different in several respects from the specificity of lymphocytes, the antigen-recognizing cells of adaptive immunity (Fig. 2.1).

The two principal types of reactions of the innate immune system are inflammation and antiviral defense. Inflammation consists of the accumulation and activation of leukocytes and plasma proteins at sites of infection or tissue injury. These cells and proteins act together to kill mainly extracellular microbes and to eliminate damaged tissues. Innate immune defense against intracellular viruses, even in the absence of inflammation, is mediated by natural killer (NK) cells, which kill virus-infected cells, and by cytokines called type I interferons (IFNs), which block viral replication within host cells.

The innate immune system responds in essentially the same way to repeat encounters with a microbe, whereas the adaptive immune system mounts stronger, more rapid and thus more effective responses on successive encounters with a microbe. In other words, for the most part, the innate immune system does not remember prior encounters with microbes and resets to baseline after each such encounter, whereas memory is a cardinal feature of the adaptive immune response. There is emerging evidence that some cells of innate immunity (such as macrophages and natural killer cells) are altered by encounters with microbes such that they respond better upon repeat encounters. But it is not clear if this process results in improved protection against recurrent infections or is specific for different microbes.

The innate immune system recognizes structures that are shared by various classes of microbes and are not present on normal host cells. The cells and molecules of innate immunity recognize and respond to a limited number of microbial structures, much less than the almost unlimited number of microbial and nonmicrobial antigens that can be recognized by the adaptive immune system. Each component of innate immunity may recognize many bacteria, viruses, or fungi. For example, phagocytes express receptors for bacterial endotoxin, also called lipopolysaccharide (LPS), and other receptors for peptidoglycans, each of which is present in the outer membranes or cell walls of many bacterial species but is not produced by mammalian cells. Other receptors of phagocytes recognize terminal mannose residues, which are typical of bacterial and fungal but not mammalian glycoconjugates. Receptors in mammalian cells recognize and respond to double-stranded ribonucleic acid (dsRNA), which is produced during replication of many viruses but is not produced in mammalian cells, and to unmethylated CG-rich (CpG) oligonucleotides, which are common in microbial DNA but are not abundant in mammalian DNA. The microbial molecules that stimulate innate immunity are often called **pathogen-associated molecular patterns (PAMPs)** to indicate that they are present in infectious agents (pathogens) and shared by microbes of the same type (i.e., they are molecular patterns). The receptors of innate immunity that recognize these shared structures are called **pattern recognition receptors.**

Innate immune receptors are specific for structures of microbes that are often essential for the survival and infectivity of these microbes. This characteristic of innate immunity makes it a highly effective defense mechanism because a microbe cannot evade innate immunity simply by mutating or not expressing the targets of innate immune recognition. Microbes that do not express functional forms of these structures lose their ability to infect and colonize the host. In contrast, microbes frequently evade adaptive immunity by mutating the antigens that are recognized by lymphocytes, because these antigens are usually not required for the life of the microbes.

The innate immune system also recognizes molecules that are released from damaged or necrotic host cells. Such molecules are called **damage-associated molecular patterns (DAMPs)**. Examples include high mobility group box protein 1 (HMGB1), a histone protein that is released from cells with damaged nuclei, and extracellular ATP, which is released from damaged mitochondria. The subsequent responses to DAMPs serve to eliminate the damaged cells and to initiate the process of tissue repair. Thus, innate responses occur even following sterile injury, such as infarction, the death of tissue due to loss of its blood supply.

Feature	Innate immunity	Adaptive immunity
Specificity	For structures shared by classes of microbes (pathogen-associated molecular patterns)	For structural detail of microbial molecules (antigens); may recognize nonmicrobial antigens
Number of microbial molecules recognized	About 1000 molecular patterns (estimated)	>10^7 antigens
Receptors	Encoded in germline; limited diversity (pattern recognition receptors)	Encoded by genes produced by somatic recombination of gene segments; greater diversity
Number and types of receptors	<100 different types of invariant receptors	Only 2 types of receptors (Ig and TCR), with millions of variations of each
Distribution of receptors	Nonclonal: Identical receptors on all cells of the same lineage	Clonal: clones of lymphocytes with distinct specificities express different receptors
Genes encoding receptors	Germline encoded, in all cells	Formed by somatic recombination of gene segments only in B and T cells
Discrimination of self and nonself	Yes; healthy host cells are not recognized or they may express molecules that prevent innate immune reactions	Yes; based on elimination or inactivation of self-reactive lymphocytes; may be imperfect (hence the possibility of autoimmunity)

Fig. 2.1 Specificity and receptors of innate immunity and adaptive immunity. This figure summarizes the important features of the specificity and receptors of innate and adaptive immunity, with select examples illustrated. *Ig,* Immunoglobulin (antibody); *TCR,* T cell receptor.

The receptors of the innate immune system are encoded by inherited genes that are identical in all cells. The pattern recognition receptors of the innate immune system are nonclonally distributed; that is, identical receptors are expressed on all the cells of a particular type, such as macrophages. Therefore, many cells of innate immunity may recognize and respond to the same microbe. This is in contrast to the antigen receptors of the adaptive immune system, which are encoded by genes formed by rearrangement of gene segments during lymphocyte development, resulting in many clones of B and T lymphocytes, each expressing a unique receptor. It is estimated that there are about 100 types of innate immune receptors that are capable of recognizing about 1000 PAMPs and DAMPs. In striking contrast, there are only two kinds of specific receptors in the adaptive immune system (immuno-globulin [Ig] and T cell receptors [TCRs]), but because of their diversity they are able to recognize millions of different antigens.

The innate immune system does not react against healthy cells. Several features of the innate immune system account for its inability to react against an individual's own cells and molecules. First, the receptors of innate immunity have evolved to be specific for microbial structures (and products of damaged cells) but not for substances in healthy cells. Second, some pattern recognition receptors can recognize substances such as nucleic acids that are present in normal cells, but these receptors are located in cellular compartments (such as endosomes; see below) from where components of healthy cells are excluded. Third, normal mammalian cells express regulatory molecules that prevent innate immune reactions. The adaptive immune system also discriminates between self and nonself; in the adaptive immune system, lymphocytes capable of recognizing self antigens are produced, but they die or are inactivated on encounter with self antigens.

The innate immune response can be considered as a series of reactions that provide defense at every stage of microbial infections:

- At the portals of entry for microbes: Most microbial infections are acquired through the epithelial barrier of the skin and gastrointestinal, respiratory and genitourinary systems. The earliest defense mechanisms active at these sites are epithelia, providing physical barriers and antimicrobial molecules, and lymphoid cells.
- In the tissues: Microbes that breach epithelia, as well as dead cells in tissues, are detected by resident macrophages, dendritic cells, and mast cells. Some of these cells react by secreting cytokines, which initiate the process of inflammation, and phagocytes residing in the tissues or recruited from the blood destroy the microbes and eliminate the damaged cells.
- In the blood: Plasma proteins, including proteins of the complement system, react against microbes that enter the circulation and promote their destruction.

We will return to a more detailed discussion of these components of innate immunity and their reactions later in the chapter. We start with a consideration of how microbes, damaged cells, and other foreign substances are detected and how innate immune responses are triggered.

CELLULAR RECEPTORS FOR MICROBES AND DAMAGED CELLS

The pattern recognition receptors used by the innate immune system to detect microbes and damaged cells are expressed on phagocytes, dendritic cells, and many other cell types and are located in different cellular compartments where microbes or their products may be found. These receptors are present on the cell surface, where they detect extracellular microbes; in vesicles (endosomes) into which microbial products are ingested; and in the cytosol, where they function as sensors of cytoplasmic microbes and products of cell damage (Fig. 2.2). These receptors for PAMPs and DAMPs belong to several protein families.

Toll-Like Receptors

Toll-like receptors (**TLRs**) are homologous to a Drosophila protein called Toll, which was discovered for its role in the development of the fly and later shown to be essential for protecting flies against fungal infections. In vertebrates, there are 10 different TLRs specific for different components of microbes (Fig. 2.3). TLR-2 recognizes several glycolipids and peptidoglycans that are made by gram-positive bacteria and some parasites; TLR-3 is specific for double-stranded RNA, and TLR-7 and TLR-8 are specific for single-stranded RNA; TLR-4 is specific for bacterial LPS (endotoxin), made by gram-negative bacteria; TLR-5 is specific for a bacterial flagellar protein called flagellin; and TLR-9 recognizes unmethylated CpG DNA, which is abundant in microbial genomes. TLRs specific for microbial proteins, lipids, and polysaccharides (many of which are present in bacterial cell walls) are located on cell surfaces, where they recognize these products of extracellular microbes. TLRs that recognize nucleic acids are in endosomes, into which microbes are ingested and where they are digested and their nucleic acids are released.

Signals generated by TLRs activate transcription factors that stimulate expression of cytokines and other proteins involved in the inflammatory response and in the antimicrobial functions of activated phagocytes and other cells (Fig. 2.4). Among the most important transcription factors activated by TLR signals are members of the nuclear factor κB (NF-κB) family, which promote expression of various cytokines and endothelial adhesion molecules that play important roles in inflammation, and interferon regulatory factors (IRFs), which stimulate production of the antiviral cytokines, type I interferons.

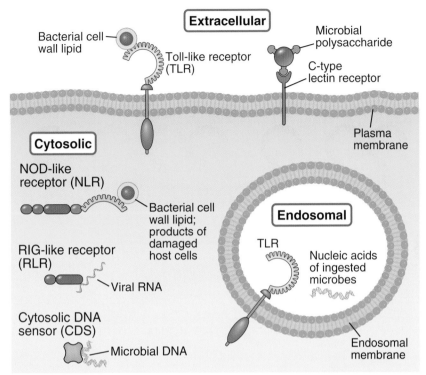

Fig. 2.2 Cellular locations of receptors of the innate immune system. Some receptors, such as certain Toll-like receptors (TLRs) and lectins, are located on cell surfaces; other TLRs are in endosomes. Some receptors for viral nucleic acids, bacterial peptides, and products of damaged cells are in the cytoplasm. NOD and RIG refer to the founding members of families of structurally homologous cytosolic receptors for bacterial and viral products, respectively. (Their full names are complex and do not reflect their functions.) There are five major families of cellular receptors in innate immunity: TLRs, CLRs (C-type lectin receptors), NLRs (NOD-like receptors), RLRs (RIG-like receptors), and CDSs (cytosolic DNA sensors). Formylpeptide receptors (not shown) are involved in migration of leukocytes in response to bacteria.

Rare autosomal recessive diseases characterized by recurrent infections are caused by mutations affecting TLRs or their signaling molecules, highlighting the importance of these pathways in host defense against microbes. For example, individuals with mutations affecting TLR-3 are susceptible to herpes simplex virus infections, particularly encephalitis, and mutations in MyD88, the adaptor protein downstream of several TLRs, make individuals susceptible to bacterial pneumonias.

NOD-Like Receptors

The NOD-like receptors (NLRs) are a large family of innate receptors that sense DAMPs and PAMPs in the cytosol of cells and initiate signaling events that promote inflammation. All NLRs contain a nucleotide oligomerization domain (NOD, named because of the activity it was originally associated with) but different NLRs have different N-terminal domains. Two important NLRs, NOD1 and

NOD2, have N-terminal caspase related domains (CARDs), and are expressed in several cell types including mucosal barrier epithelial cells and phagocytes. NOD1 and NOD2 both recognize peptides derived from bacterial cell wall peptidoglycans, and in response, they generate signals that activate the NF-κB transcription factor, which promotes expression of genes encoding inflammatory proteins. NOD2 is highly expressed in intestinal Paneth cells in the small bowel, where it stimulates expression of antimicrobial substances called defensins in response to pathogens. Some polymorphisms of the *NOD2* gene are associated with inflammatory bowel disease, perhaps because these variants have reduced function and allow luminal microbes to penetrate the intestinal wall and trigger inflammation.

Inflammasomes

Inflammasomes are multiprotein complexes that assemble in the cytosol of cells in response to microbes or

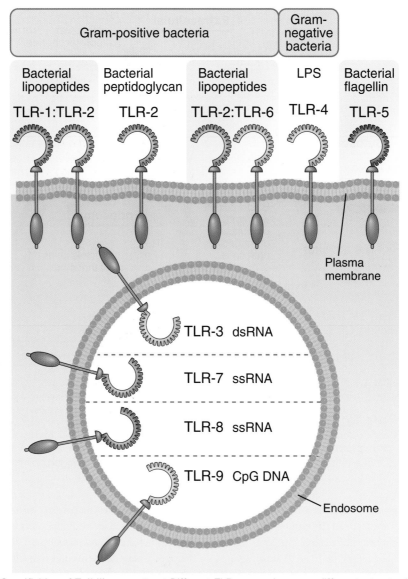

Fig. 2.3 Specificities of Toll-like receptors. Different TLRs recognize many different, structurally diverse products of microbes. Plasma membrane TLRs are specific for cell wall components of bacteria, and endosomal TLRs recognize nucleic acids. All TLRs contain a ligand-binding domain composed of leucine-rich motifs and a cytoplasmic signaling, Toll-like interleukin-1 (IL-1) receptor (TIR) domain. *ds,* Double-stranded; *LPS,* lipopolysaccharide; *ss,* single-stranded.

changes associated with cell injury, and proteolytically generate active forms of the inflammatory cytokines IL-1β and IL-18. IL-1β and IL-18 are synthesized as inactive precursors, which must be cleaved by the enzyme caspase-1 to become active cytokines that are released from the cell and promote inflammation. Inflammasomes are composed of oligomers of a sensor, caspase-1, and an adaptor that links the two. There are many different types of inflammasomes, most of which use 1 of 10 different NLR-family proteins as sensors. These sensors directly recognize microbial products in the cytosol or sense changes in the amount of endogenous molecules or ions in the cytosol that indirectly indicate the presence of infection or cell damage. Some inflammasomes use sensors that are not in the NLR family, such as AIM-family DNA sensors and a protein called pyrin. After recognition of microbial or endogenous ligands, the

Fig. 2.4 Signaling functions of toll-like receptors. TLRs activate similar signaling mechanisms, which involve adaptor proteins and lead to the activation of transcription factors. These transcription factors stimulate the production of proteins that mediate inflammation and antiviral defense. *NF-κB,* Nuclear factor κB.

NLR sensors oligomerize with an adaptor protein and an inactive (pro) form of the enzyme caspase-1 to form the inflammasome, resulting in generation of the active form of caspase-1 (Fig. 2.5). Active caspase-1 cleaves the precursor form of the cytokine interleukin-1β (IL-1β), pro-IL-1β, to generate biologically active IL-1β. As discussed later, IL-1 induces acute inflammation and causes fever.

One of the best characterized inflammasomes uses NLRP3 (NOD-like receptor family, pyrin domain containing 3) as a sensor. The NLRP3 inflammasome is expressed in innate immune cells including macrophages and neutrophils, as well as keratinocytes in the

skin and other cells. A wide variety of stimuli induce formation of the NLRP3 inflammasome, including crystalline substances such as uric acid (a by-product of DNA breakdown, indicating nuclear damage) and cholesterol crystals, extracellular adenosine triphosphate (ATP) (an indicator of mitochondrial damage) binding to cell surface purinoceptors, reduced intracellular potassium ion (K^+) concentration (which indicates plasma membrane damage), and reactive oxygen species. Thus, the inflammasome reacts to injury affecting various cellular components. How NLRP3 recognizes such diverse types of cellular stress or damage is not clearly understood. Inflammasome activation is tightly controlled by posttranslational modifications such as ubiquitination and phosphorylation, which block inflammasome assembly or activation, and some micro-RNAs, which inhibit NLRP3 messenger RNA.

Inflammasome activation also causes an inflammatory form of programmed cell death of macrophages and DCs called **pyroptosis**, characterized by swelling of cells, loss of plasma membrane integrity, and release of inflammatory cytokines. Activated caspase-1 cleaves a protein called gasdermin D. The N-terminal fragment of gasdermin D oligomerizes and forms a channel in the plasma membrane that initially allows the egress of mature IL-1β, and eventually permits the influx of ions, followed by cell swelling and pyroptosis.

The inflammasome is important not only for host defense but also because of its role in several diseases. Gain-of-function mutations in NLRP3, and less frequently, loss-of-function mutations in regulators of inflammasome activation, are the cause of **autoinflammatory syndromes**, characterized by uncontrolled and spontaneous inflammation. IL-1 antagonists are effective treatments for these diseases. The common joint disease **gout** is caused by deposition of urate crystals and subsequent inflammation mediated by inflammasome recognition of the crystals and IL-1β production. The inflammasome may also contribute to atherosclerosis, in which inflammation caused by cholesterol crystals may play a role.

Cytosolic RNA and DNA Sensors

The innate immune system includes several cytosolic proteins that recognize microbial RNA or DNA and respond by generating signals that lead to the production of inflammatory and antiviral cytokines.

- The RIG-like receptors (RLRs) are cytosolic proteins that sense viral RNA and induce the production of the antiviral type I IFNs. RLRs recognize features of viral

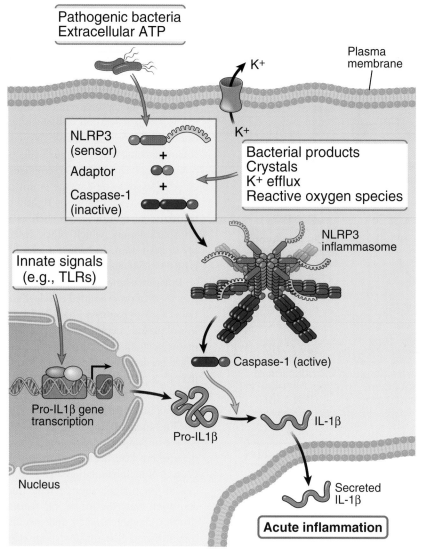

Fig. 2.5 The inflammasome. Shown is the activation of the NLRP3 inflammasome, which processes pro–interleukin-1β (pro–IL-1β) to active IL-1. The synthesis of pro–IL-1β is induced by various PAMPs or DAMPs through pattern recognition receptor signaling. Subsequent production of biologically active IL-1β is mediated by the inflammasome. The inflammasome also stimulates production of active IL-18, which is closely related to IL-1 (not shown). Other forms of the inflammasome exist which contain sensors other than NLRP3, including NLRP1, NLRC4, or AIM2. *ATP*, Adenosine triphosphate; *NLRP3*, NOD-like receptor family, pyrin domain containing 3; *TLRs*, Toll-like receptors.

RNAs not typical of mammalian RNA, such as dsRNA that is longer than dsRNA that may be formed transiently in normal cells, or RNA with a 5′ triphosphate moiety not present in mammalian host cell cytosolic RNA. (Host RNAs are modified and have a 5′ 7methyl-guanosine "cap.") RLRs are expressed in many cell types that are susceptible to infection by RNA viruses. After binding viral RNAs, RLRs interact with a mitochondrial membrane protein called mitochondrial antiviral-signaling (MAVS), which is required to initiate signaling events that activate transcription factors that induce the production of type I IFNs.

Fig. 2.6 Cytosolic DNA sensors and the STING pathway. Cytoplasmic microbial dsDNA activates the enzyme cGAS, which catalyzes the synthesis of cyclic GMP-AMP (cGAMP) from ATP and GTP. cGAMP binds to STING in the endoplasmic reticulum membrane, and then STING recruits and activates the kinase TBK1, which phosphorylates IRF3. Phospo-IRF3 moves to the nucleus, where it induces type I IFN gene expression. The bacterial second messenger molecules cyclic di-GMP (c-di-GMP) and cyclic di-AMP (c-di-AMP) are directly sensed by STING. STING also stimulates autophagy and lysosomal degradation of pathogens associated with cytoplasmic organelles. *cGAS*, Cyclic GMP-AMP synthase; *IFN*, interferon; *IRF3*, interferon regulatory factor 3.

- Cytosolic DNA sensors (CDSs) include several structurally related proteins that recognize microbial double-stranded (ds) DNA in the cytosol and activate signaling pathways that initiate antimicrobial responses, including type 1 IFN production and autophagy. DNA may be released into the cytosol from various intracellular microbes. Since mammalian DNA is not normally in the cytosol, the innate cytosolic DNA sensors will see only microbial DNA.

Most innate cytosolic DNA sensors engage the stimulator of IFN genes (**STING**) pathway to induce type 1 IFN production (Fig. 2.6). In this pathway, cytosolic dsDNA binds to the enzyme cyclic GMP-AMP synthase (cGAS), which activates the production of a cyclic dinucleotide signaling molecule called cyclic GMP-AMP (cGAMP), which binds to an endoplasmic reticulum membrane adaptor protein called stimulator of interferon gene (STING). In addition, bacteria themselves produce other cyclic dinucleotides that also bind to STING. Upon binding these cyclic dinucleotides, STING initiates signaling events that lead to transcriptional activation and expression of type I IFN genes. STING also stimulates autophagy, a mechanism by which cells degrade their own organelles in lysosomes. Autophagy is used in innate immunity to deliver cytosolic microbes to the lysosome, where they are killed by proteolytic enzymes. Other cytosolic DNA sensors besides cGAS can also activate STING.

Other Cellular Receptors of Innate Immunity

Many other receptor types are involved in innate immune responses to microbes (see Fig. 2.2).

Some lectins (carbohydrate-recognizing proteins) in the plasma membrane are receptors specific for fungal glucans (these receptors are called dectins) or for terminal mannose residues (called mannose receptors); they are involved in the phagocytosis of fungi and bacteria and in inflammatory responses to these pathogens. A cell surface receptor expressed mainly on phagocytes, called formyl peptide receptor 1, recognizes polypeptides with an N-terminal formylmethionine, which is a specific feature of bacterial proteins. Signaling by this receptor promotes the migration as well as the antimicrobial activities of the phagocytes.

Although our emphasis thus far has been on cellular receptors, the innate immune system also contains several circulating molecules that recognize and provide defense against microbes, as discussed later.

COMPONENTS OF INNATE IMMUNITY

The components of the innate immune system include epithelial cells; sentinel cells in tissues (resident macrophages, dendritic cells, mast cells, and others); circulating and recruited phagocytes (monocytes and neutrophils); innate lymphoid cells; NK cells; and a number of plasma proteins. We next discuss the properties of these cells and soluble proteins and their roles in innate immune responses.

Epithelial Barriers

The major interfaces between the body and the external environment—the skin, gastrointestinal tract, respiratory tract, and genitourinary tract—are protected by layers of epithelial cells that provide physical and chemical barriers against infection (Fig. 2.7). Microbes come into contact with vertebrate hosts mainly at these interfaces by external physical contact,

ingestion, inhalation, and sexual activity. All these portals of entry are lined by continuous epithelia consisting of tightly adherent cells that form a mechanical barrier against microbes. Keratin on the surface of the skin and mucus secreted by mucosal epithelial cells prevent most microbes from interacting with and infecting or getting through the epithelia. Epithelial cells also produce antimicrobial peptides including defensins and cathelicidins, which kill bacteria and some viruses by disrupting their outer membranes. Thus, antimicrobial peptides provide a chemical barrier against infection. In addition, epithelia contain lymphocytes called intraepithelial T lymphocytes that belong to the T cell lineage but express antigen receptors of limited diversity. Some of these T cells express receptors composed of two chains, γ and δ, that are similar but not identical to the αβ T cell receptors expressed on the majority of T lymphocytes (see Chapters 4 and 5). Intraepithelial lymphocytes often recognize microbial lipids and other structures. Intraepithelial T lymphocytes presumably react against infectious agents that attempt to breach the epithelia, but the specificity and functions of these cells are poorly understood.

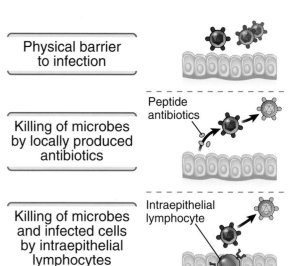

Fig. 2.7 Functions of epithelia in innate immunity. Epithelia present at the portals of entry of microbes provide physical barriers formed by keratin (in the skin) or secreted mucus (in the gastrointestinal, bronchopulmonary, and genitourinary systems) and by tight junctions between epithelial cells. Epithelia also produce antimicrobial substances (e.g., defensins) and harbor lymphocytes that kill microbes and infected cells.

Phagocytes: Neutrophils and Monocytes/Macrophages

The two types of circulating phagocytes, neutrophils and monocytes, are blood cells that are recruited to sites of infection, where they recognize and ingest microbes for intracellular killing (Fig. 2.8).

- **Neutrophils**, also called polymorphonuclear leukocytes (PMNs), are the most abundant leukocytes in the blood, numbering 4,000 to 10,000 per μL (Fig. 2.9A). In response to certain bacterial and fungal infections, the production of neutrophils from the bone marrow increases rapidly, and their numbers in the blood may rise up to 10 times the normal. The production of neutrophils is stimulated by cytokines, known as colony-stimulating factors (CSFs), which are secreted by many cell types in response to infections and act on hematopoietic cells to stimulate proliferation and maturation of neutrophil precursors. Neutrophils are the first and most numerous cell type to respond to most infections, particularly bacterial and fungal infections, and thus are the dominant cells of acute inflammation, as discussed later. Neutrophils ingest microbes in the circulation, and they rapidly enter extravascular tissues at sites of infection, where they also phagocytose (ingest) and destroy microbes. Neutrophils express receptors for products of complement activation and for antibodies that coat microbes. These receptors enhance phagocytosis of antibody- and complement-coated microbes and also transduce activating signals that enhance the ability of the neutrophils to kill ingested microbes. The process of phagocytosis and intracellular destruction of microbes is described later. Neutrophils are also recruited to sites of tissue damage in the absence of infection, where they initiate the clearance of cell

Feature	Neutrophils	Macrophages
Origin	HSCs in bone marrow	HSCs in bone marrow (in inflammatory reactions) Many tissue-resident macrophages: stem cells in yolk sac of fetal liver (early in development)
Life span in tissues	1–2 days	Inflammatory macrophages: days or weeks Tissue-resident macrophages: years
Responses to activating stimuli	Rapid, short lived, enzymatic activity	More prolonged, slower, often dependent on new gene transcription
Phagocytosis	Rapid ingestion of microbes	Prolonged ability to ingest microbes, apoptotic cells, tissue debris, foreign material
Reactive oxygen species	Rapidly induced by assembly of phagocyte oxidase (respiratory burst)	Less prominent
Nitric oxide	Low levels or none	Induced following transcriptional activation of iNOS
Degranulation	Major response; induced by cytoskeletal rearrangement	Not prominent
Cytokine production	Low levels per cell	Major functional activity, large amounts per cell, requires transcriptional activation of cytokine genes
Extracellular traps	Rapidly induced, by extrusion of nuclear contents	Little
Secretion of lysosomal enzymes	Prominent	Less

Fig. 2.8 Distinguishing properties of neutrophils and monocytes. This table lists the major differences between neutrophils and macrophages. These two cell types share many features, such as phagocytosis, chemotaxis, and ability to migrate through blood vessels into tissues. *HSC,* Hematopoietic stem cell; *iNOS,* inducible nitric oxide synthase; *NET,* neutrophil extracellular traps.

Fig. 2.9 Morphology of neutrophils and monocytes. A, Light micrograph of blood neutrophil shows the multilobed nucleus, which is why these cells are also called polymorphonuclear leukocytes, and the faint cytoplasmic granules, most of which are lysosomes. B, Light micrograph of blood monocyte shows the typical horseshoe-shaped nucleus.

debris. Neutrophils live for only several hours in tissues, so they are the early responders, but they do not provide prolonged defense.

• **Monocytes** are less abundant in the blood than neutrophils, numbering 500 to 1000 per μL (see Fig. 2.9B). They also ingest microbes in the blood and in tissues. During inflammatory reactions, monocytes enter extravascular tissues and differentiate into cells called **macrophages**, which, unlike neutrophils, survive in these sites for long periods. Thus, blood monocytes and tissue macrophages are two stages of the same cell lineage, which often is called the mononuclear phagocyte system (Fig. 2.10). Some macrophages that are resident in different tissues, such as

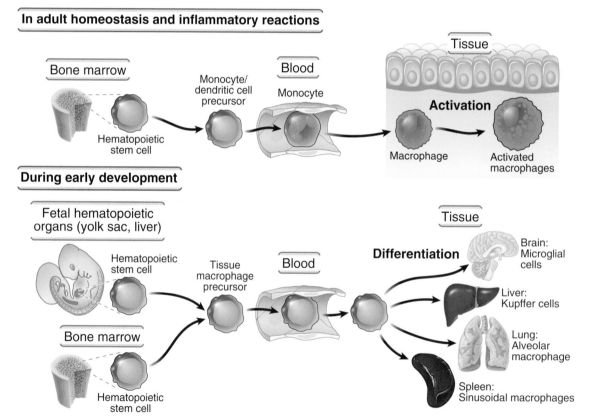

Fig. 2.10 Maturation of mononuclear phagocytes. In the steady state in adults, and during inflammatory reactions, precursors in the bone marrow give rise to circulating monocytes, which enter peripheral tissues, mature to form macrophages, and are activated locally. In fetal life, precursors in the yolk sac and liver give rise to cells that seed tissues to generate specialized tissue-resident macrophages.

the brain, liver, and lungs, are derived not from circulating monocytes but from progenitors in the yolk sac or fetal liver early during the development of the organism. Macrophages are also found in all connective tissues and organs of the body.

Macrophages serve several important roles in host defense: they ingest and destroy microbes, they clear dead tissues and initiate the process of tissue repair, and they produce cytokines that induce and regulate inflammation (Fig. 2.11). A number of receptor families are expressed in macrophages and involved in the activation and functions of these cells. Pattern recognition receptors discussed earlier, including TLRs and NLRs, recognize products of microbes and damaged cells and activate the macrophages. Phagocytosis is mediated by cell surface receptors, such as mannose receptors

and scavenger receptors, which directly bind microbes (and other particles), and receptors for antibodies or products of complement activation that are bound to microbes. These antibody and complement receptors are also expressed by neutrophils. Some of these phagocytic receptors activate the microbial killing functions of macrophages as well. In addition, macrophages respond to various cytokines.

Macrophages may be activated by two different pathways that serve distinct functions (see Fig. 6.9 in Chapter 6). These pathways of activation have been called classical and alternative. **Classical macrophage activation** is induced by innate immune signals, such as from TLRs, and by the cytokine IFN-γ, which may be produced in both innate and adaptive immune responses. Classically activated macrophages, also called M1, are involved

Fig. 2.11 Activation and functions of macrophages. In innate immune responses, macrophages are activated by microbial products binding to TLRs and by cytokines, such as NK cell–derived interferon-γ (IFN-γ), which lead to the production of proteins that mediate inflammatory and microbicidal functions of these cells. Cell surface complement receptors promote the phagocytosis of complement-coated microbes as well as activation of the macrophages. (Macrophage Fc receptors for IgG [not shown] bind antibody-coated microbes and perform similar functions as the complement receptors.) *IL,* Interleukin; *iNOS,* inducible nitric oxide synthase; *TNF,* tumor necrosis factor.

in destroying microbes and in triggering inflammation. **Alternative macrophage activation** occurs in the absence of strong TLR signals and is induced by the cytokines IL-4 and IL-13; these macrophages, called M2, appear to be more important for tissue repair and to terminate inflammation. The relative abundance of these two forms of activated macrophages may influence the outcome of host reactions and contribute to various disorders. We will return to the functions of these macrophage populations in Chapter 6, when we discuss cell-mediated immunity.

Although our discussion has been limited to the role of phagocytes in innate immunity, macrophages are also important effector cells in both the cell-mediated arm and the humoral arm of adaptive immunity, as discussed in Chapters 6 and 8, respectively.

Dendritic Cells

Dendritic cells function as sentinels in tissues that respond to microbes by producing numerous cytokines, which serve two main functions: they initiate inflammation and they stimulate adaptive immune responses. They also capture protein antigens and display fragments of these antigens to T cells. By sensing microbes and interacting with lymphocytes, especially T cells, dendritic cells constitute an important bridge between innate and adaptive immunity. We discuss the properties and functions of dendritic cells further in Chapter 3 in the context of antigen presentation.

Mast Cells

Mast cells are bone marrow–derived cells with abundant cytoplasmic granules that are present throughout the skin and mucosal barriers. Mast cells can be activated by microbial products binding to TLRs and by components of the complement system as part of innate immunity or by an antibody-dependent mechanism in adaptive immunity. Mast cell granules contain vasoactive amines such as histamine that cause vasodilation and increased capillary permeability, as well as proteolytic enzymes that can kill bacteria or inactivate microbial toxins. Mast cells also synthesize and secrete lipid mediators (e.g., prostaglandins and leukotrienes) and cytokines (e.g., tumor necrosis factor [TNF]), which stimulate inflammation. Mast cell products provide defense against helminths and other pathogens, as well as protection against snake and insect venoms, and they are responsible for symptoms of allergic diseases (see Chapter 11).

Innate Lymphoid Cells

Innate lymphoid cells (ILCs) are tissue-resident cells that produce cytokines similar to those secreted by helper T lymphocytes but do not express T cell antigen receptors (TCRs). ILCs have been divided into three major groups based on their secreted cytokines; these groups correspond to the Th1, Th2, and Th17 subsets of CD4$^+$ T cells that we describe in Chapter 6. The responses of ILCs are often stimulated by cytokines produced by damaged epithelial and other cells at sites of infection. ILCs likely provide early defense against infections in tissues, but their essential roles in host defense or immunological diseases, especially in humans, are not clear.

Natural Killer Cells

NK cells recognize infected and stressed cells and respond by killing these cells and by secreting the macrophage-activating cytokine IFN-γ (Fig. 2.12). NK cells are developmentally related to group 1 ILCs and

Fig. 2.12 Functions of natural killer *(NK)* cells. **A,** NK cells kill host cells infected by intracellular microbes, thus eliminating reservoirs of infection. **B,** NK cells respond to interleukin-12 *(IL-12)* produced by macrophages and secrete interferon-γ *(IFN-γ)*, which activates the macrophages to kill phagocytosed microbes.

make up approximately 10% of the cells with lymphocyte morphology in the blood and peripheral lymphoid organs. NK cells contain cytoplasmic granules and express some unique surface proteins but do not express immunoglobulins or T cell receptors, the antigen receptors of B and T lymphocytes, respectively.

On activation by infected cells, NK cells empty the contents of their cytoplasmic granules into the extracellular space at the point of contact with the infected cell. The granule proteins then enter infected cells and activate enzymes that induce apoptosis. The cytotoxic mechanisms of NK cells, which are the same as the mechanisms used by cytotoxic T lymphocytes (CTLs; see Chapter 6), result in the death of infected cells. Thus, as with CTLs, NK cells function to eliminate cellular reservoirs of infection and eradicate infections by obligate intracellular microbes, such as viruses. In addition, NK cells may contribute to the destruction of tumors.

Activated NK cells also synthesize and secrete the cytokine interferon-γ (IFN-γ), which activates macrophages to become more effective at killing phagocytosed microbes. Cytokines secreted by macrophages and dendritic cells that have encountered microbes enhance the ability of NK cells to protect against infections. Three of these NK cell–activating cytokines are interleukin-15 (IL-15), type I IFNs, and interleukin-12 (IL-12). IL-15 is important for the development and maturation of NK cells, and type I IFNs and IL-12 enhance the killing functions of NK cells. Thus, NK cells and macrophages are examples of two cell types that function cooperatively to eliminate intracellular microbes: macrophages ingest microbes and produce IL-12, IL-12 activates NK cells to secrete IFN-γ, and IFN-γ in turn activates the macrophages to kill the ingested microbes. As discussed in Chapter 6, essentially the same sequence of reactions involving macrophages and T lymphocytes is central to the cell-mediated arm of adaptive immunity.

The activation of NK cells is determined by a balance between engagement of activating and inhibitory receptors (Fig. 2.13). The activating receptors recognize cell surface molecules typically expressed on cells infected with viruses and intracellular bacteria, some cancer cells, and cells stressed by DNA damage. These receptors enable NK cells to eliminate

Fig. 2.13 Activating and inhibitory receptors of natural killer *(NK)* cells. **A,** Healthy host cells express self class I major histocompatibility complex *(MHC)* molecules, which are recognized by inhibitory receptors, thus ensuring that NK cells do not attack normal host cells. Note that healthy cells may express ligands for activating receptors (as shown) or may not express such ligands, but they are not attacked by NK cells because they engage the inhibitory receptors. **B,** NK cells are activated by infected cells in which ligands for activating receptors are expressed (often at high levels) and class I MHC expression is reduced so that the inhibitory receptors are not engaged. The result is that the infected cells are killed.

cells infected with intracellular microbes, as well as irreparably injured cells and tumor cells. One of the well-defined activating receptors of NK cells is called NKG2D; it recognizes molecules that resemble class I major histocompatibility complex (MHC) proteins and are expressed in response to many types of cellular stress. Another activating receptor, called CD16, is specific for immunoglobulin G (IgG) antibodies bound to cells. The recognition of antibody-coated cells results in killing of these cells, a phenomenon called **antibody-dependent cellular cytotoxicity** (ADCC). NK cells are the principal mediators of ADCC. The role of this reaction in antibody-mediated immunity is described in Chapter 8. Activating receptors on NK cells have signaling subunits that contain immunoreceptor tyrosine-based activation motifs (ITAMs) in their cytoplasmic tails. ITAMs, which also are present in subunits of lymphocyte antigen receptor–associated signaling molecules, become phosphorylated on tyrosine residues when the receptors recognize their activating ligands. The phosphorylated ITAMs bind and promote the activation of cytosolic protein tyrosine kinases, and these enzymes phosphorylate, and thereby activate, other substrates in several different downstream signal transduction pathways, eventually leading to cytotoxic granule exocytosis and production of IFN-γ.

The inhibitory receptors of NK cells block signaling by activating receptors and are specific for self class I MHC molecules, which are expressed on all healthy nucleated cells. Therefore, class I MHC expression protects healthy cells from destruction by NK cells. (In Chapter 3, we describe the important function of MHC molecules in displaying peptide antigens to T lymphocytes.) Two major families of NK cell inhibitory receptors in humans are the killer cell immunoglobulin-like receptors (KIRs), so called because they share structural homology with Ig molecules (see Chapter 4), and receptors consisting of a protein called CD94 and a lectin subunit called NKG2. Both families of inhibitory receptors contain in their cytoplasmic tails structural motifs called immunoreceptor tyrosine-based inhibitory motifs (ITIMs), which become phosphorylated on tyrosine residues when the receptors bind class I MHC molecules. The phosphorylated ITIMs bind and promote activation of cytosolic protein tyrosine phosphatases. These enzymes remove phosphate groups from the tyrosine residues of various signaling molecules, thereby counteracting the function of the ITAMs and blocking the activation of

NK cells through activating receptors. Therefore, when the inhibitory receptors of NK cells encounter self MHC molecules on normal host cells, the NK cells are shut off (see Fig. 2.13). Many viruses have developed mechanisms to block expression of class I molecules in infected cells, which allows them to evade killing by virus-specific CD8+ CTLs. When this happens, the NK cell inhibitory receptors are not engaged, and if the virus induces expression of activating ligands at the same time, the NK cells become activated and eliminate the virus-infected cells.

The role of NK cells and CTLs in defense illustrates how hosts and microbes are engaged in a constant struggle for survival. The host uses CTLs to recognize MHC-displayed viral antigens, viruses inhibit MHC expression to evade killing of the infected cells by CTLs, and NK cells can compensate for the defective CTL response because the NK cells are more effective in the absence of MHC molecules. The winner of this struggle, the host or the microbe, determines the outcome of the infection. The same principles may apply to the functions of NK cells in eradication of tumors, many of which also attempt to escape from CTL-mediated killing by reducing expression of class I MHC molecules (see Chapter 10).

Lymphocytes with Limited Diversity

Several types of lymphocytes that have some features of T and B lymphocytes also function in the early defense against microbes and may be considered part of the innate immune system. A unifying characteristic of these lymphocytes is that they express somatically rearranged antigen receptors (as do classical T and B cells), but the receptors have limited diversity.

- As mentioned earlier, **γδ T cells** are present in epithelia.
- **NK-T cells** express TCRs with limited diversity and surface molecules typically found on NK cells. They are present in epithelia and lymphoid organs. They recognize microbial lipids bound to a class I MHC–related molecule called CD1.
- **Mucosal associated invariant T (MAIT) cells** express TCRs with limited diversity but do not express CD4 or CD8. They are present in mucosal tissues and are most abundant in the human liver, accounting for 20% to 40% of all T cells in that organ. Many MAIT cells are specific for bacterial vitamin B metabolites and likely contribute to innate defense against intestinal bacteria that transgress the mucosal barrier and enter the portal circulation.

- **B-1 cells** are a population of B lymphocytes that are found mostly in the peritoneal cavity and mucosal tissues, where they produce antibodies in response to microbes and microbial toxins that pass through the walls of the intestine. Circulating IgM antibodies found in the blood of normal individuals, even without specific immunization, are called **natural antibodies.** They are the products of B-1 cells, and many of these antibodies are specific for carbohydrates that are present in the cell walls of many bacteria and for ABO blood group antigens found on red blood cells (discussed in Chapter 10).
- Another type of B lymphocyte, **marginal-zone B cells,** is present at the edges of lymphoid follicles in the spleen and other organs and also is involved in rapid antibody responses to blood-borne polysaccharide-rich microbes.

NK-T cells, MAIT cells, $\gamma\delta$ T cells, B-1 cells, and marginal-zone B lymphocytes all respond to infections in ways that are characteristic of adaptive immunity (e.g., cytokine secretion or antibody production) but have features of innate immunity (rapid responses, limited diversity of antigen recognition).

Complement System

The complement system is a collection of circulating and membrane-associated proteins that are important in defense against microbes. Many complement proteins are proteolytic enzymes, and complement activation involves the sequential activation of these enzymes. The complement cascade may be initiated by any of three pathways (Fig. 2.14):

- The **alternative pathway** is triggered when some complement proteins are activated on microbial surfaces and cannot be controlled, because complement regulatory proteins are not present on microbes (but are present on host cells). The alternative pathway is a component of innate immunity.
- The **classical pathway** is most often triggered by antibodies that bind to microbes or other antigens and is thus a component of the humoral arm of adaptive immunity.
- The **lectin pathway** is activated when a carbohydrate-binding plasma protein, mannose-binding lectin (MBL), binds to its carbohydrate ligands on microbes. This lectin activates proteins of the classical pathway, but because it is initiated by a microbial product in the absence of antibody, it is a component of innate immunity.

Activated complement proteins function as proteolytic enzymes to cleave other complement proteins. Such an enzymatic cascade can be rapidly amplified because each proteolytic step generates many products that are themselves enzymes in the cascade. The central component of all three complement pathways is a plasma protein called C3, which is cleaved by enzymes generated in the early steps. The major proteolytic fragment of C3, called C3b, becomes covalently attached to microbes and is able to recruit and activate downstream complement proteins on the microbial surface. The three pathways of complement activation differ in how they are initiated, but they share the late steps and perform the same effector functions.

The complement system serves three main functions in host defense:

- **Opsonization and phagocytosis.** C3b coats microbes and promotes the binding of these microbes to phagocytes by virtue of receptors for C3b that are expressed on the phagocytes. Thus, microbes that are coated with complement proteins are rapidly ingested and destroyed by phagocytes. This process of coating a microbe with molecules that are recognized by receptors on phagocytes is called **opsonization.**
- **Inflammation.** Some proteolytic fragments of complement proteins, especially C5a and C3a, are chemoattractants for leukocytes (mainly neutrophils and monocytes), and they also are activators of endothelial cells and mast cells. Thus, they promote movement of leukocytes and plasma proteins into tissues (inflammation) at the site of complement activation.
- **Cell lysis.** Complement activation culminates in the formation of a polymeric protein complex that inserts into the microbial cell membrane, disturbing the permeability barrier and causing osmotic lysis.

A more detailed discussion of the activation and functions of complement is presented in Chapter 8, where we consider the effector mechanisms of humoral immunity.

Other Plasma Proteins of Innate Immunity

Several circulating proteins in addition to complement proteins are involved in innate immune defense against infections. Plasma MBL recognizes microbial carbohydrates and can coat microbes for phagocytosis or activate the complement cascade by the lectin pathway, as discussed earlier. MBL belongs to a family of proteins called the collectins, because they are structurally similar

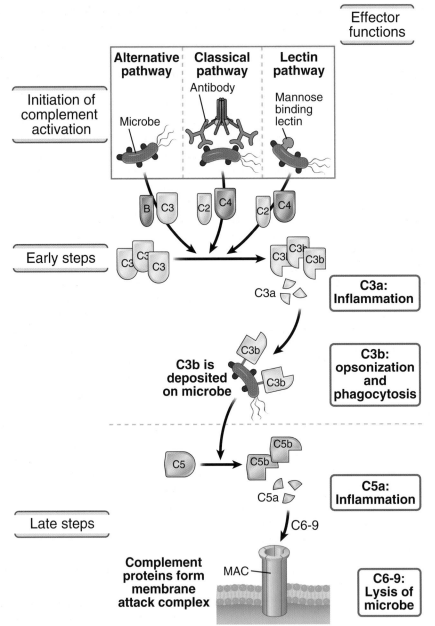

Fig. 2.14 Pathways of complement activation. The activation of the complement system (the early steps) may be initiated by three distinct pathways, all of which lead to the production of C3b. C3b initiates the late steps of complement activation, culminating in the formation of a multiprotein complex called the membrane attack complex *(MAC),* which is a transmembrane channel composed of polymerized C9 molecules that causes lysis of thin-walled microbes. Peptide by-products released during complement activation are the inflammation-inducing C3a and C5a. The principal functions of proteins produced at different steps are shown. The activation, functions, and regulation of the complement system are discussed in more detail in Chapter 8.

to collagen and contain a carbohydrate-binding (lectin) domain. Surfactant proteins in the lung also belong to the collectin family and protect the airways from infection. C-reactive protein (CRP) is a pentraxin (five-headed molecule) that binds to phosphorylcholine on microbes and opsonizes the microbes for phagocytosis by macrophages, which express a receptor for CRP. CRP also can activate proteins of the classical complement pathway.

The circulating levels of many of these plasma proteins increase rapidly after infection. This protective response is called the **acute-phase response** to infection.

Cytokines of Innate Immunity

In response to microbes, dendritic cells, macrophages, mast cells and other cells secrete cytokines that mediate many of the cellular reactions of innate immunity (Fig. 2.15). As mentioned earlier, cytokines are soluble proteins that mediate immune and inflammatory reactions and are responsible for communications between leukocytes and between leukocytes and other cells. Most of the molecularly defined cytokines are called interleukins with a number, for example interleukin-1, but several have other names, for example tumor necrosis factor, for historical reasons related to how they were discovered. In innate immunity, the principal sources of cytokines are dendritic cells, macrophages, and mast cells that are activated by recognition of microbes, although epithelial cells and other cell types also secrete cytokines. Recognition of bacterial cell wall components such as LPS and peptidoglycan by TLRs and recognition of microbial nucleic acids by TLRs, RLRs, and CDSs are powerful stimuli for cytokine secretion by macrophages, dendritic cells, and many tissue cells. In adaptive immunity, helper T lymphocytes are a major source of cytokines (see Chapters 5 and 6).

Cytokines are secreted in small amounts in response to an external stimulus and bind to high-affinity receptors on target cells. Most cytokines act on nearby cells (paracrine actions), and some act on the cells that produce them (autocrine actions). In innate immune reactions against infections, enough dendritic cells and macrophages may be activated that large amounts of cytokines are produced, and they may be active distant from their site of secretion (endocrine actions).

The cytokines of innate immunity serve various functions in host defense. Tumor necrosis factor (TNF), interleukin-1 (IL-1), and chemokines (chemoattractant cytokines) are the principal cytokines involved in recruiting blood neutrophils and monocytes to sites of infection (described later). TNF and IL-1 also have systemic effects, including inducing fever by acting on the hypothalamus, and these cytokines as well as IL-6 stimulate liver cells to produce various proteins of the acute phase response, such as C-reactive protein and fibrinogen, which contribute to microbial killing and walling off infectious sites. At high concentrations, TNF promotes thrombus formation on the endothelium and reduces blood pressure by a combination of reduced myocardial contractility and vascular dilation and leakiness. Severe, disseminated bacterial infections sometimes lead to a potentially lethal clinical syndrome called **septic shock**, which is characterized by low blood pressure (the defining feature of shock), disseminated intravascular coagulation, and metabolic disturbances. The early clinical and pathologic manifestations of septic shock may be caused by high levels of TNF, which is produced in response to the bacteria. Dendritic cells and macrophages also produce IL-12 in response to LPS and other microbial molecules. The role of IL-12 in activating NK cells, ultimately leading to increased killing activity and macrophage activation, was mentioned previously. NK cells produce IFN-γ, whose function as a macrophage-activating cytokine was also described earlier. Because IFN-γ is produced by T cells as well, it is considered a cytokine of both innate immunity and adaptive immunity. In viral infections, a subset of dendritic cells, and to a lesser extent other infected cells, produce type I IFNs, which inhibit viral replication and prevent spread of the infection to uninfected cells.

INNATE IMMUNE REACTIONS

The innate immune system eliminates microbes mainly by inducing the acute inflammatory response and by antiviral defense mechanisms. Different microbes may elicit different types of innate immune reactions, each type of response being particularly effective in eliminating a particular kind of microbe. The major protective innate immune responses to different microbes are the following:

- Extracellular bacteria and fungi are defended against mainly by the acute inflammatory response, in which neutrophils and monocytes are recruited to the site of infection, aided by the complement system.

A, Activation of dendritic cells, macrophages, and NK cells

Microbes

Inflammation

IL-12

IFN-γ

Natural killer cell

Dendritic cell

Macrophage

TNF, IL-1, chemokines

Neutrophil

Blood vessel

B,

Cytokine	Principal cell source(s)	Principal cellular targets and biologic effects
Tumor necrosis factor (TNF)	Macrophages, T cells, mast cells	Endothelial cells: activation (inflammation, coagulation) Neutrophils: activation Hypothalamus: fever Liver: synthesis of acute-phase proteins Muscle, fat: catabolism (cachexia) Many cell types: apoptosis
Interleukin-1 (IL-1)	Macrophages, dendritic cells, endothelial cells, some epithelial cells, mast cells	Endothelial cells: activation (inflammation, coagulation) Hypothalamus: fever Liver: synthesis of acute-phase proteins T cells: Th17 differentiation
Chemokines	Macrophages, dendritic cells, endothelial cells, T lymphocytes, fibroblasts, platelets	Leukocytes: increased integrin affinity, chemotaxis, activation
Interleukin-12 (IL-12)	Dendritic cells, macrophages,	Natural killer (NK) cells and T cells: IFN-γ production, increased cytotoxic activity T cells: Th1 differentiation
Interferon-γ (IFN-γ)	NK cells, T lymphocytes	Activation of macrophages Stimulation of some antibody responses
Type I IFNs (IFN-α, IFN-β)	IFN-α: Dendritic cells, macrophages IFN-β: Fibroblasts, epithelial cells	All cells: antiviral state, increased class I major histocompatibility complex (MHC) expression NK cells: activation
Interleukin-10 (IL-10)	Macrophages, dendritic cells, T cells	Macrophages, dendritic cells: inhibition of cytokine and chemokine production, reduced expression of costimulators and class II MHC molecules
Interleukin-6 (IL-6)	Macrophages, endothelial cells, T cells	Liver: synthesis of acute-phase proteins B cells: proliferation of antibody-producing cells
Interleukin-15 (IL-15)	Macrophages, others	NK cells: proliferation T cells: proliferation
Interleukin-18 (IL-18)	Macrophages	NK cells and T cells: IFN-γ synthesis
TGF-β	Many cell types	Inhibition of inflammation T cells: differentiation of Th17, regulatory T cells

Fig. 2.15 Cytokines of innate immunity. A, Dendritic cells, macrophages, and other cells (such as mast cells and ILCs, not shown) respond to microbes by producing cytokines that stimulate inflammation (leukocyte recruitment) and activate natural killer *(NK)* cells to produce the macrophage-activating cytokine interferon-γ *(IFN-γ)*. **B,** Some important characteristics of the major cytokines of innate immunity are listed. Note that IFN-γ and transforming growth factor beta *(TGF-β)* are cytokines of both innate and adaptive immunity (see Chapters 5 and 6). More information about these cytokines and their receptors is provided in Appendix II. *MHC,* Major histocompatibility complex.

- Intracellular bacteria, which can survive inside phagocytes, are eliminated by phagocytes that are activated by Toll-like receptors and other innate sensors as well as by cytokines.
- Protection against viruses is provided by type I interferons and natural killer cells.

Inflammation

Inflammation is a tissue reaction that delivers mediators of host defense—circulating cells and proteins—to sites of infection and tissue damage (Fig. 2.16). The process of inflammation consists of recruitment of cells and leakage of plasma proteins through blood vessels and activation of these cells and proteins in the extravascular tissues. The initial release of histamine, TNF, prostaglandins, and other mediators by mast cells and macrophages causes an increase in local blood flow and exudation of plasma proteins. These contribute to redness, warmth, and swelling, which are characteristic features of inflammation. This is often followed by a local accumulation in the tissue of phagocytes, mainly neutrophils and blood monocyte-derived macrophages, in response to cytokines, discussed below. Activated phagocytes engulf microbes and necrotic material and destroy these potentially harmful substances. We next describe the cellular events in a typical inflammatory response.

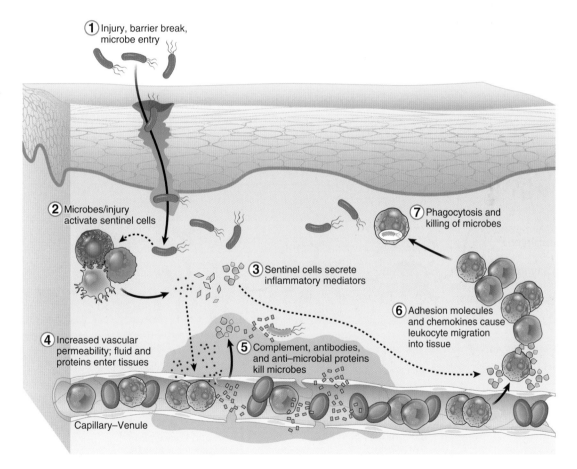

Fig. 2.16 Acute inflammatory response. Cytokines and other mediators are produced by macrophages, dendritic cells, mast cells, and other cells in tissues in response to microbial products and damaged host cells. Some of these mediators (e.g., histamine, prostaglandins) increase the permeability of blood vessels, leading to the entry of plasma proteins (e.g., complement proteins) into the tissues, and others (IL-1, TNF) increase expression of endothelial adhesion molecules and chemokines that promote the movement of leukocytes from the blood into the tissues, where the leukocytes destroy microbes, clear damaged cells, and promote more inflammation and repair.

Recruitment of Phagocytes to Sites of Infection and Tissue Damage

Neutrophils and monocytes migrate to extravascular sites of infection or tissue damage by binding to venular endothelial adhesion molecules and in response to chemoattractants produced by tissue cells reacting to infection or injury. Leukocyte migration from the blood into tissues is a multistep process in which initial weak adhesive interactions of the leukocytes with endothelial cells are followed by firm adhesion and then transmigration through the endothelium (Fig. 2.17).

If an infectious microbe breaches an epithelium and enters the subepithelial tissue, resident dendritic cells, macrophages, and other cells recognize the microbe and respond by producing cytokines. Two of these cytokines, TNF and IL-1, act on the endothelium of venules near the site of infection and initiate the sequence of events in leukocyte migration into tissues.

- **Rolling of leukocytes.** In response to TNF and IL-1, venular endothelial cells express an adhesion molecule of the **selectin** family called E-selectin. Other stimuli, including thrombin, cause rapid translocation of P-selectin to the endothelial surface. (The term *selectin* refers to the carbohydrate-binding, or lectin, property of these molecules.) Circulating neutrophils and monocytes express surface carbohydrates that bind specifically to the selectins. The neutrophils become tethered to the endothelium, flowing blood disrupts this binding, the bonds reform downstream, and this repetitive process results in the rolling of the leukocytes along the endothelial surface.

- **Firm adhesion.** Leukocytes express another set of adhesion molecules that are called **integrins** because they integrate extrinsic signals into cytoskeletal alterations. Leukocyte integrins, such as LFA-1 and

Fig. 2.17 Sequence of events in migration of blood leukocytes to sites of infection. At sites of infection, macrophages, dendritic cells, and other cells that have encountered microbes produce cytokines such as tumor necrosis factor *(TNF)* and interleukin-1 *(IL-1)* that activate the endothelial cells of nearby venules to express selectins and ligands for integrins and to secrete chemokines. Selectins mediate weak tethering and rolling of blood neutrophils on the endothelium, integrins mediate firm adhesion of neutrophils, and chemokines activate the neutrophils and stimulate their migration through the endothelium to the site of infection. Blood monocytes and activated T lymphocytes use the same mechanisms to migrate to sites of infection.

VLA-4, are present in a low-affinity state on unactivated cells. Within a site of infection, tissue macrophages and endothelial cells produce **chemokines**, which bind to proteoglycans on the luminal surface of endothelial cells and are thus displayed at a high concentration to the leukocytes that are rolling on the endothelium. These immobilized chemokines bind to chemokine receptors on the leukocytes and stimulate a rapid increase in the affinity of the leukocyte integrins for their ligands on the endothelium. Concurrently, TNF and IL-1 act on the endothelium to stimulate expression of ligands for integrins, including ICAM-1 and VCAM-1. The firm binding of integrins to their ligands arrests the rolling leukocytes on the endothelium. The cytoskeleton of the leukocytes is reorganized, and the cells spread out on the endothelial surface.

- **Leukocyte migration.** Leukocytes adherent to the endothelium crawl to and then through the junctions between endothelial cells, exiting the blood vessels. Within the tissue, leukocytes migrate along extracellular matrix fibers, directed by concentration gradients of chemoattractants, including chemokines, bacterial formyl peptides, and complement fragments C5a and C3a. The concentrations of these chemoattractants are highest where the microbes are located, and leukocytes have receptors for these molecules that stimulate migration toward their source.

The sequence of selectin-mediated rolling, integrin-mediated firm adhesion, and chemokine-mediated motility leads to the migration of blood leukocytes to an extravascular site of infection within minutes after the infection. (As discussed in Chapters 5 and 6, the same sequence of events is responsible for the migration of activated T lymphocytes into infected tissues.) Inherited deficiencies in integrins and selectin ligands lead to defective leukocyte recruitment to sites of infection and increased susceptibility to infections. These disorders are called **leukocyte adhesion deficiencies** (LADs).

The phagocytes work together with plasma proteins that have entered the site of inflammation, such as complement proteins, to destroy the offending agents. In some infections, blood leukocytes other than neutrophils and macrophages, such as eosinophils, may be recruited to sites of infection and provide defense against the pathogens.

Phagocytosis and Destruction of Microbes

Neutrophils and macrophages ingest (phagocytose) microbes and destroy the ingested microbes in intracellular vesicles (Fig. 2.18). Phagocytosis is a process of ingestion of particles larger than 0.5 µm in diameter. It begins with membrane receptors binding to the microbe. The principal phagocytic receptors are some pattern recognition receptors, such as mannose receptors and other lectins, and receptors for antibodies and complement. Microbes opsonized with antibodies and complement fragments can bind avidly to specific receptors on phagocytes, resulting in greatly enhanced internalization (see Chapter 8). Binding of the microbe to the cell is followed by extension of the phagocyte plasma membrane around the particle. The membrane then closes up and pinches off, and the microbe is internalized in a membrane-bound vesicle, called a phagosome. The phagosomes fuse with lysosomes to form phagolysosomes.

At the same time that the microbe is being bound by the phagocyte's receptors and ingested, the phagocyte receives signals from various receptors that activate several enzymes. One of these enzymes, called phagocyte oxidase, rapidly assembles in the phagolysosomal membrane, mainly in neutrophils, and converts molecular oxygen into superoxide anion and free radicals, a process called the oxidative burst (or respiratory burst). These free radicals are called **reactive oxygen species** (ROS) and are toxic to the ingested microbes. A second enzyme, inducible nitric oxide synthase (iNOS), is produced mainly in macrophages and catalyzes the conversion of arginine to **nitric oxide** (NO), also a microbicidal substance. A third set of enzymes, the lysosomal proteases, break down microbial proteins. All these microbicidal substances are produced mainly within lysosomes and phagolysosomes, where they act on the ingested microbes but do not damage the phagocytes.

In addition to intracellular killing, neutrophils use additional mechanisms to destroy microbes. They can release microbicidal granule contents into the extracellular environment. In response to pathogens and inflammatory mediators, neutrophils die, and during this process they extrude their nuclear contents to form networks of chromatin called neutrophil extracellular traps (NETs), which contain antimicrobial substances that are normally sequestered in neutrophil granules. These NETs trap bacteria and fungi and kill the organisms. In some cases, the enzymes and ROS that are liberated into the extracellular space may injure host tissues. This is the reason why inflammation, normally a protective host response to infections, may cause tissue injury as well.

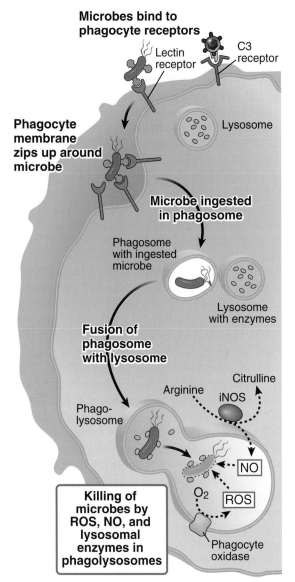

Microbes bind to phagocyte receptors

Lectin receptor

C3 receptor

Lysosome

Phagocyte membrane zips up around microbe

Microbe ingested in phagosome

Phagosome with ingested microbe

Lysosome with enzymes

Fusion of phagosome with lysosome

Citrulline

Arginine   iNOS

Phago-lysosome

NO

O₂   ROS

Killing of microbes by ROS, NO, and lysosomal enzymes in phagolysosomes

Phagocyte oxidase

Fig. 2.18 Phagocytosis and intracellular killing of microbes. Macrophages and neutrophils express many surface receptors that may bind microbes for subsequent phagocytosis; select examples of such receptors are shown. Microbes are ingested into phagosomes, which fuse with lysosomes, and the microbes are killed by enzymes and several toxic substances produced in the phagolysosomes. The same substances may be released from the phagocytes and may kill extracellular microbes (not shown). *iNOS*, Inducible nitric oxide synthase; *NO*, nitric oxide; *ROS*, reactive oxygen species.

Inherited deficiency of the phagocyte oxidase enzyme is the cause of an immunodeficiency disorder called **chronic granulomatous disease** (CGD). In CGD,

neutrophils are unable to eradicate intracellular microbes, and the host tries to contain the infection by calling in more macrophages, resulting in collections of activated macrophages around the microbes called granulomas.

Tissue Repair

In addition to eliminating pathogenic microbes and damaged cells, cells of the immune system initiate the process of tissue repair. Macrophages, especially of the alternatively activated type, produce growth factors that stimulate the proliferation of residual tissue cells and fibroblasts, resulting in regeneration of the tissue and scarring of what cannot be replaced. Other immune cells, such as helper T cells and ILCs, may serve similar roles.

Antiviral Defense

Defense against viruses is a special type of host response that involves interferons, NK cells, and other mechanisms, which may occur concomitantly with, but are distinct from, inflammation.

Type I interferons inhibit viral replication and induce an antiviral state, in which cells become resistant to infection. Type I IFNs, which include several forms of IFN-α and one of IFN-β, are secreted by many cell types infected by viruses. A major source of these cytokines is a type of dendritic cell called the plasmacytoid dendritic cell (so named because these cells morphologically resemble plasma cells), which secretes type I IFNs in response to recognition of viral nucleic acids by TLRs and other pattern recognition receptors. When type I IFNs secreted from dendritic cells or other infected cells bind to the type I IFN receptor on the infected or adjacent uninfected cells, signaling pathways are activated that inhibit viral replication and destroy viral genomes (Fig. 2.19). This action is the basis for the use of IFN-α to treat some forms of chronic viral hepatitis.

Virus-infected cells may be destroyed by NK cells, as described earlier. Type I IFNs enhance the ability of NK cells to kill infected cells. Recognition of viral DNA by CDSs also induces autophagy, by which cellular organelles containing viruses are engulfed by lysosomes and proteolytically destroyed (see Fig. 2.6). In addition, part of the innate response to viral infections includes increased apoptosis of infected cells, which also helps to eliminate the reservoir of infection.

Regulation of Innate Immune Responses

Innate immune responses are regulated by a variety of mechanisms that are designed to prevent

Fig. 2.19 Antiviral actions of type I interferons. Type I interferons (IFN-α, IFN-β) are produced by plasmacytoid dendritic cells and virus-infected cells in response to intracellular TLR signaling and other sensors of viral nucleic acids. Type I interferons bind to receptors on the infected and uninfected cells and activate signaling pathways that induce expression of enzymes that interfere with viral replication at different steps, including inhibition of viral protein translation, increasing viral RNA degradation, and inhibition of viral gene expression and virion assembly. Type I IFNs also increase the infected cell's susceptibility to CTL-mediated killing (not shown).

excessive damage to tissues. These regulatory mechanisms include the production of antiinflammatory cytokines by macrophages and dendritic cells, including interleukin-10 (IL-10), which inhibits the microbicidal and proinflammatory functions of macrophages (classical pathway of macrophage activation), and IL-1 receptor antagonist, which blocks the actions of IL-1. There are also many feedback mechanisms in which signals that induce proinflammatory cytokine production also induce expression of inhibitors of cytokine signaling. For example, TLR signaling stimulates expression of proteins called suppressors of cytokine signaling (SOCS), which block the responses of cells to various cytokines, including IFNs. Intracellular regulators of inflammasome activation were mentioned earlier.

Microbial Evasion of Innate Immunity

Pathogenic microbes have evolved to resist the mechanisms of innate immunity and are thus able to enter and colonize their hosts (Fig. 2.20). Some intracellular bacteria resist destruction inside phagocytes. *Listeria monocytogenes* produces a protein that enables it to escape from phagocytic vesicles and enter the cytoplasm of infected cells, where it is no longer susceptible to ROS or NO (which are produced mainly in phagolysosomes). The cell walls of mycobacteria contain a lipid that inhibits fusion of phagosomes containing ingested bacteria with lysosomes. Other microbes have cell walls that are resistant to the actions of complement proteins. As discussed in Chapters 6 and 8, these mechanisms also enable microbes to resist the effector mechanisms of cell-mediated and humoral immunity, the two arms of adaptive immunity.

ROLE OF INNATE IMMUNITY IN STIMULATING ADAPTIVE IMMUNE RESPONSES

So far we have focused on how the innate immune system recognizes microbes and combats infections. We mentioned at the beginning of this chapter that, in addition to its roles in host defense, the innate immune response to microbes serves an important warning function by alerting the adaptive immune system that an effective immune response is needed. In this final section, we summarize some of the mechanisms by which innate immune responses stimulate adaptive immune responses.

Innate immune responses generate molecules that provide signals, in addition to antigens, that are required to activate naive T and B lymphocytes. In Chapter 1, we introduced the concept that full

Mechanism of immune evasion	Organism (example)	Mechanism
Resistance to phagocytosis	Pneumococci	Capsular polysaccharide inhibits phagocytosis
Resistance to reactive oxygen intermediates in phagocytes	Staphylococci	Production of catalase, which breaks down reactive oxygen intermediates
Resistance to complement activation (alternative pathway)	Neisseria meningitidis	Sialic acid expression inhibits C3 and C5 convertases
	Streptococci	M protein blocks C3 binding to organism, and C3b binding to complement receptors
Resistance to antimicrobial peptide antibiotics	Pseudomonas	Synthesis of modified LPS that resists action of anti-bacterial peptides

Fig. 2.20 Evasion of innate immunity by microbes. Selected examples of the mechanisms by which microbes may evade or resist innate immunity. *LPS,* Lipopolysaccharide.

activation of antigen-specific lymphocytes requires two signals. Antigen may be referred to as signal 1, and innate immune responses to microbes and to host cells damaged by microbes may provide signal 2 (Fig. 2.21). The stimuli that warn the adaptive immune system that it needs to respond have also been called danger signals. This requirement for microbe-dependent second signals ensures that lymphocytes respond to infectious agents and not to harmless, noninfectious substances. In experimental situations or for vaccination, adaptive immune responses may be induced by antigens without microbes. In all such instances, the antigens need to be administered with substances called **adjuvants** that elicit the same innate immune reactions as microbes do. In fact, many potent adjuvants are the products of microbes. The nature and mechanisms of action of second signals are described in the discussion of the activation of T and B lymphocytes in Chapters 5 and 7, respectively. Here we describe two illustrative examples of second signals that are generated during innate immune reactions.

In infected tissues, microbes (or IFN-γ produced by NK cells in response to microbes) stimulate dendritic cells and macrophages to produce two types of second signals that can activate T lymphocytes. First, dendritic cells increase their expression of surface molecules called **costimulators**, which bind to receptors on

Fig. 2.21 Two-signal requirement for lymphocyte activation. Antigen recognition by lymphocytes provides signal 1 for activation of the lymphocytes, and substances produced during innate immune responses to microbes (or components of microbes) provide signal 2. In this illustration, the lymphocytes could be T cells or B cells. By convention, the major second signals for T cells are called costimulators because they function together with antigens to stimulate the cells. The nature of second signals for T and B lymphocytes is described further in later chapters.

naive T cells and function together with antigen recognition to activate the T cells. Second, the dendritic cells and macrophages secrete cytokines such as IL-12, IL-1, and IL-6, which stimulate the differentiation of naive T cells into effector cells of cell-mediated adaptive immunity.

Blood-borne microbes activate the complement system by the alternative pathway. One of the proteins produced during complement activation by proteolysis of C3b, called C3d, becomes covalently attached to the microbe. At the same time that B lymphocytes recognize microbial antigens by their antigen receptors, the B cells recognize the C3d bound to the microbe by a receptor for C3d. The combination of antigen recognition and C3d recognition initiates the process of B cell differentiation into antibody-secreting cells. Thus, a complement product serves as the second signal for humoral immune responses.

These examples illustrate an important feature of second signals: these signals not only stimulate adaptive immunity, but they also guide the nature of the adaptive immune response. Intracellular and phagocytosed microbes need to be eliminated by cell-mediated immunity, the adaptive response mediated by T lymphocytes. Microbes that are encountered and ingested by dendritic cells or macrophages induce the second signals—that is, costimulators and cytokines—that stimulate T cell responses. By contrast, blood-borne microbes need to be combated by antibodies, which are produced by B lymphocytes during humoral immune responses. Blood-borne microbes activate the plasma complement system, which in turn stimulates B cell activation and antibody production. Thus, different types of microbes induce innate immune responses that stimulate the types of adaptive immunity that are best able to combat different infectious pathogens.

▮ SUMMARY

- All multicellular organisms have intrinsic mechanisms of defense against infections, which constitute innate immunity.
- The innate immune system uses germline-encoded receptors to respond to structures that are characteristic of various classes of microbes and also recognizes products of dead cells. Innate immune reactions usually are not enhanced by repeat exposures to microbes.
- Toll-like receptors (TLRs), expressed on plasma membranes and endosomal membranes of many cell types, are a major class of innate immune system receptors that recognize different microbial products, including bacterial cell wall constituents and microbial nucleic acids. Some cytosolic receptors of the NOD-like receptor (NLR) family recognize microbial cell wall lipoproteins, while other NLRs respond to products of damaged cells and cytosolic changes typical of infection or cell injury, forming a multiprotein complex, the inflammasome, that generates the active form the proinflammatory cytokine interleukin-1 (IL-1).
- The principal components of innate immunity are: epithelial barrier cells in skin, gastrointestinal tract, and respiratory tract; phagocytes; dendritic cells; mast cells; natural killer cells; cytokines; and plasma proteins, including the proteins of the complement system.

- Epithelia provide physical barriers against microbes; produce antimicrobial peptides, including defensins and cathelicidins; and contain lymphocytes that may prevent infections.
- The principal phagocytes—neutrophils and monocytes/macrophages—are blood cells that are recruited to sites of infection, where they are activated by engagement of different receptors. Some activated macrophages destroy microbes and dead cells, and other macrophages limit inflammation and initiate tissue repair.
- Innate lymphoid cells (ILCs) secrete various cytokines that induce inflammation. Natural killer (NK) cells kill host cells infected by intracellular microbes and produce the cytokine interferon-γ, which activates macrophages to kill phagocytosed microbes.
- The complement system is a family of proteins that are activated on encounter with some microbes (in innate immunity) and by antibodies (in the humoral arm of adaptive immunity). Complement proteins coat (opsonize) microbes for phagocytosis, stimulate inflammation, and lyse microbes.
- Cytokines of innate immunity function to stimulate inflammation (TNF, IL-1, IL-6, chemokines), activate NK cells (IL-12), activate macrophages (IFN-γ), and prevent viral infections (type I IFNs).

- In inflammation, phagocytes are recruited from the circulation to sites of infection and tissue damage. The cells bind to endothelial adhesion molecules that are induced by the cytokines TNF and IL-1 and migrate in response to soluble chemoattractants, including chemokines, complement fragments, and bacterial peptides. The leukocytes are activated, and they ingest and destroy microbes and damaged cells.

- Antiviral defense is mediated by type I interferons, which inhibit viral replication, and by NK cells, which kill infected cells.
- In addition to providing early defense against infections, innate immune responses provide signals that work together with antigens to activate B and T lymphocytes. The requirement for these second signals ensures that adaptive immunity is elicited by microbes (the most potent inducers of innate immune reactions) and not by nonmicrobial substances.

REVIEW QUESTIONS

1. How does the specificity of innate immunity differ from that of adaptive immunity?
2. What are examples of microbial substances recognized by the innate immune system, and what are the receptors for these substances?
3. What is the inflammasome, and how is it stimulated?
4. What are the mechanisms by which the epithelium of the skin prevents the entry of microbes?
5. How do phagocytes ingest and kill microbes?
6. What is the role of MHC molecules in the recognition of infected cells by NK cells, and what is the physiologic significance of this recognition?
7. What are the roles of the cytokines TNF, IL-12, and type I interferons in defense against infections?
8. How do innate immune responses enhance adaptive immunity?

Answers to and discussion of the Review Questions are available at Student Consult.

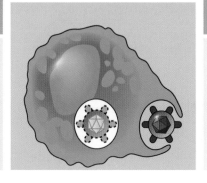

Antigen Capture and Presentation to Lymphocytes
What Lymphocytes See

Adaptive immune responses are initiated by the recognition of antigens by antigen receptors of lymphocytes. B and T lymphocytes differ in the types of antigens they recognize. The antigen receptors of B lymphocytes—namely, membrane-bound antibodies—can recognize a variety of macromolecules (proteins, polysaccharides, lipids, nucleic acids), in soluble form or cell surface–associated form, as well as small chemicals. Therefore, B cell–mediated humoral immune responses may be generated against many types of microbial cell wall and soluble antigens. The antigen receptors of most T lymphocytes, on the other hand, can see only peptide fragments of protein antigens, and only when these peptides

are displayed on host cell surfaces bound to specialized proteins called major histocompatibility complex (MHC) molecules. Because the association of antigenic peptides and MHC molecules occurs inside cells, T cell–mediated immune responses may be generated only against protein antigens that are either produced in or taken up by host cells. This chapter focuses on the nature of the antigens that are recognized by lymphocytes. Chapter 4 describes the receptors used by lymphocytes to detect these antigens.

The induction of immune responses by antigens is a highly orchestrated process with a number of remarkable features. The first is that very few naive lymphocytes are specific for any one antigen, as few as 1 in 10^5 or 10^6 circulating lymphocytes, and this small fraction of the body's lymphocytes needs to locate and react rapidly to the antigen, wherever it is introduced. Second, different types of adaptive immune responses are required to defend against different types of microbes. In fact, the immune system has to react in different ways even to the same microbe at different stages of the microbe's life cycle. For example, defense against a microbe (e.g., a virus) that has entered the bloodstream depends on antibodies that bind the microbe, prevent it from infecting host cells, and help to eliminate it. The production of potent antibodies requires the activation of CD4+ helper T cells. After it has infected host cells, however, the microbe is safe from antibodies, which cannot enter the cells. As a result, activation of CD8+ cytotoxic T lymphocytes (CTLs) may be necessary to kill the infected cells and eliminate the reservoir of infection. Thus, we are faced with two important questions:

- How do the rare naive lymphocytes specific for any microbial antigen find that microbe, especially considering that microbes may enter anywhere in the body?
- How do different types of T cells recognize microbes in different cellular compartments? Specifically, helper T cells recognize and respond to both extracellular and intracellular microbes that can be internalized into vesicular compartments in host cells, whereas CTLs kill infected cells that harbor microbial antigens in the cytosol and nucleus outside vesicular compartments. As we shall see in this chapter, MHC molecules play a central role in this segregation of antigen recognition by T cells.

The answer to both questions is that the immune system has developed a highly specialized system for capturing and displaying antigens to lymphocytes. Research by immunologists, cell biologists, and biochemists has led to a sophisticated understanding of how protein antigens are captured, broken down, and displayed for recognition by T lymphocytes. This is the major topic of discussion in this chapter.

ANTIGENS RECOGNIZED BY T LYMPHOCYTES

The majority of T lymphocytes recognize peptide antigens that are bound to and displayed by the MHC molecules of antigen-presenting cells (APCs). The MHC is a genetic locus whose principal protein products function as the peptide display molecules of the immune system. CD4+ and CD8+ T cells can see peptides only when these

Fig. 3.1 Model showing how a T cell receptor recognizes a complex of peptide antigen displayed by an MHC molecule. Major histocompatibility complex (MHC) molecules are expressed on antigen-presenting cells and function to display peptides derived from protein antigens. Peptides bind to the MHC molecules by anchor residues, which attach the peptides to pockets in the MHC molecules. The antigen receptor of every T cell recognizes some amino acid residues of the peptide and some (polymorphic) residues of the MHC molecule.

peptides are displayed by that individual's MHC molecules. This property of T cells is called **MHC restriction**. The T cell receptor (TCR) recognizes some amino acid residues of the peptide antigen and simultaneously also recognizes residues of the MHC molecule that is displaying that peptide (Fig. 3.1). Each TCR, and hence each clone of CD4+ or CD8+ T cells, recognizes one peptide displayed by one of the many MHC molecules in every individual. The properties of MHC molecules and the significance of MHC restriction are described later in this chapter. How we generate T cells that recognize peptides presented only by self MHC molecules is described in Chapter 4. Also, some small populations of T cells recognize lipid and other nonpeptide antigens either presented by nonpolymorphic class I MHC–like molecules or without a requirement for a specialized antigen display system.

The cells that capture microbial antigens and display them for recognition by T lymphocytes are called **antigen-presenting cells** (APCs). Naive T lymphocytes must see protein antigens presented by dendritic cells to initiate clonal expansion and differentiation of the T cells into effector and memory cells. Differentiated effector T cells again need to see antigens, which may be presented by various kinds of APCs besides dendritic cells, to activate the effector functions of the T cells in both humoral and cell-mediated immune responses. We first describe how APCs capture and present antigens to trigger immune responses and then examine the role of MHC molecules in antigen presentation to T cells.

Fig. 3.2 Capture and display of microbial antigens. Microbes enter through an epithelial barrier and are captured by antigen-presenting cells resident in the tissue or microbes enter lymphatic vessels or blood vessels. The microbes and their antigens are transported to peripheral lymphoid organs, the lymph nodes and the spleen, where peptide fragments of protein antigens are displayed by dendritic cell (MHC) molecules for recognition by T lymphocytes.

CAPTURE OF PROTEIN ANTIGENS BY ANTIGEN-PRESENTING CELLS

Protein antigens of microbes that enter the body are captured mainly by dendritic cells and concentrated in the peripheral (secondary) lymphoid organs, where immune responses are initiated (Fig. 3.2). Microbes usually enter the body through the skin (by contact), the gastrointestinal tract (by ingestion), the respiratory tract (by inhalation), and the genitourinary tract (by sexual contact). Some microbes may enter the bloodstream. Microbial antigens can also be produced in any infected tissue. Because of the vast surface area of the epithelial barriers and the large volume of blood, connective tissues, and internal organs, it would be impossible for lymphocytes of all possible specificities to efficiently patrol all these sites searching for foreign invaders; instead, antigens are taken to the lymphoid organs through which lymphocytes recirculate.

Fig. 3.3 Dendritic cells. A, Immature dendritic cells reside in tissues including epithelia, such as the skin, and form a network of cells with interdigitating processes, seen as blue cells on the section of skin stained with an antibody that recognizes dendritic cells. **B,** Mature dendritic cells reside in the T cell–rich areas of lymph nodes (and spleen, not shown) and are seen in the section of a lymph node stained with fluorochrome-conjugated antibodies against dendritic cells *(red)* and B cells in follicles *(green)*. Note that the dendritic cells are in the same regions of the lymph node as T cells (see Fig. 1.18B). (**A,** Micrograph of skin courtesy Dr. Y.-J. Liu, MD, Anderson Cancer Center, Houston, TX. **B,** Courtesy Drs. Kathryn Pape and Jennifer Walter, University of Minnesota Medical School, Minneapolis, MN.)

Antigens are taken to peripheral lymphoid organs in two ways.

- Microbes or their antigens may enter the lymph or blood and circulate to lymph nodes or spleen, respectively, where they are captured by resident dendritic cells and presented to T cells. Other APCs may also capture antigens and display them to B cells in these organs.
- Dendritic cells in epithelia, connective tissues, and organs transport microbial antigens to lymphoid organs. This process involves a series of events following the encounter of dendritic cells with microbes—capture of antigens, activation of the dendritic cells, migration of the antigen-carrying cells to lymph nodes, and display of the antigen to T cells. These steps are described next.

All the interfaces between the body and the external environment are lined by continuous epithelia, which provide barriers to infection. The epithelia and subepithelial tissues contain a network of cells with long processes, called **dendritic cells**; these cells are also present in the T cell–rich areas of peripheral lymphoid organs and, in smaller numbers, in most other organs (Fig. 3.3). There are two major populations of dendritic cells, called conventional (or classical) and plasmacytoid, which differ in their locations and responses (Fig. 3.4). The majority of dendritic cells in tissues and lymphoid organs belong to the classical subset. In the skin, the epidermal dendritic cells are called Langerhans cells. Plasmacytoid dendritic cells are named because of their morphologic resemblance to plasma cells; they are present in the blood and tissues. Plasmacytoid dendritic cells are also the major source of type I interferons in innate immune responses to viral infections (see Chapter 2).

Dendritic cells use various membrane receptors to bind microbes, such as cell surface lectins that recognize carbohydrate structures typical of microbial but not mammalian glycoproteins. These microbes or their antigens are taken up by dendritic cells by phagocytosis or receptor-mediated endocytosis. At the same time

Feature	Classical dendritic cells	Plasmacytoid dendritic cells
Selected surface markers (human)	CD11c high BDCA1 (CD1c) Dectin	BDCA2 (CD303), others
Major location	Tissues	Blood and tissues
Expression of Toll-like receptors	TLRs 4, 5, 8 high	TLRs 7, 9 high
Major cytokines produced	TNF, IL-6, IL-12, IL-23	Type I interferons
Postulated major functions	Induction of T cell responses against most antigens	Antiviral innate immunity and induction of T cell responses against viruses

Fig. 3.4 **Populations of dendritic cells.** This figure lists the properties of two major classes of dendritic cells: classical (or conventional) and plasmacytoid. Many subsets of classical dendritic cells have been described (not shown) that may perform specialized functions in different tissues. Dectin is a receptor for carbohydrates. *IL,* Interleukin; *TLRs,* toll-like receptors; *TNF,* tumor necrosis factor.

that the dendritic cells are capturing antigens, products of the microbes stimulate innate immune reactions by binding to Toll-like receptors (TLRs) and to other innate pattern-recognition receptors in the dendritic cells, tissue epithelial cells, and resident macrophages (see Chapter 2). This results in the production of inflammatory cytokines such as tumor necrosis factor (TNF) and interleukin-1 (IL-1). The combination of innate receptor signaling and cytokines activates the dendritic cells, resulting in several changes in their phenotype, migration, and function.

Upon activation, classical dendritic cells lose their adhesiveness for epithelia and begin to express the chemokine receptor CCR7, which is specific for chemoattracting cytokines (chemokines) produced by lymphatic endothelium and by stromal cells in the T cell zones of lymph nodes. These chemokines direct the dendritic cells to exit the epithelium and migrate through lymphatic vessels to the lymph nodes draining that epithelium (Fig. 3.5). During the process of migration, the dendritic cells mature from cells designed to capture antigens into APCs capable of stimulating T lymphocytes. This maturation is reflected by increased synthesis and stable expression of MHC molecules, which display antigens to T cells, and of costimulators, which were introduced in Chapter 2 as molecules required for full T cell responses.

The net result of this sequence of events is that the protein antigens of microbes that enter the body are transported to and concentrated in the regions of the lymph nodes (and spleen) where the antigens are most likely to encounter T lymphocytes. Recall that naive T lymphocytes continuously recirculate through lymph nodes and also express CCR7, which promotes their entry into the T cell zones of lymph nodes (see Chapter 1). Therefore, dendritic cells bearing captured antigen and naive T cells poised to recognize antigens come together in lymph nodes. This process is remarkably efficient; it is estimated that if a microbial antigen is introduced at any site in the body, a T cell response to the antigen begins in the lymph nodes draining that site within 12 to 18 hours.

Different types of APC serve distinct functions in T cell–dependent immune responses (Fig. 3.6).
- Dendritic cells are the principal inducers of T-dependent responses, because these cells are located at sites of microbe entry and are the most potent APCs for activating naive T lymphocytes.
- One important type of APC for effector T cells, especially of the helper T cell lineage, is the macrophage, which is abundant in all tissues. In cell-mediated immune reactions, macrophages phagocytose microbes and display the antigens of these microbes to effector T cells, which then are reactivated and induce the macrophages to kill these ingested microbes (see Chapter 6).

Fig. 3.5 Capture, transport, and presentation of protein antigens by dendritic cells. Immature dendritic cells in epithelial barrier tissues, such as the epithelium or dermis of the skin, shown here, capture microbial antigens, are activated, and leave the epithelium. The dendritic cells migrate to draining lymph nodes, being attracted there by chemokines produced in the lymphatic vessels and nodes. In response to signals induced by the microbe, such as Toll-like receptor (TLR) signals and cytokines, the dendritic cells mature and acquire the ability to present antigens to naive T lymphocytes in the lymph nodes. Dendritic cells at different stages of their maturation may express different membrane proteins. Immature dendritic cells express surface receptors that capture microbial antigens, whereas mature dendritic cells express high levels of major histocompatibility complex molecules and costimulators, which function to stimulate T cells.

- B lymphocytes endocytose protein antigens and display them to helper T cells within lymphoid tissues; this process is important for the development of humoral immune responses to protein antigens (see Chapter 7).
- As discussed later in this chapter, any nucleated cell containing foreign (microbial or tumor) protein antigens in the cytosol can present peptides derived from these antigens to CD8+ T cells.

Now that we know how protein antigens are captured, transported to, and concentrated in peripheral lymphoid organs, we next ask, how are these antigens displayed to T lymphocytes? To answer this question, we first need to appreciate the structure of MHC

Cell type	Expression of		Principal function
	Class II MHC	Costimulators	
Dendritic cells	Constitutive; increases with maturation; increased by IFN-γ	Constitutive; increased with maturation; induced by TLR ligands, IFN-γ, and T cells (CD40-CD40L interactions)	Antigen presentation to naive T cells in the initiation of T cell responses to protein antigens (priming)
Macrophages	Low or negative; inducible by IFN-γ	Low; induced by TLR ligands, IFN-γ, and T cells (CD40-CD40L interactions)	Antigen presentation to CD4+ effector T cells in the effector phase of cell-mediated immune responses
B lymphocytes	Constitutive; increased by cytokines (e.g., IL-4)	Induced by T cells (CD40-CD40L interactions), antigen receptor cross-linking	Antigen presentation to CD4+ helper T cells in humoral immune responses (T cell–B cell interactions)

Fig. 3.6 Major antigen-presenting cells (APCs). The properties of the principal class II major histocompatibility complex (MHC)–expressing APCs, which present antigens to CD4+ helper T cells, are summarized. Other cell types, such as vascular endothelial cells, also express class II MHC, but their roles in initiating immune responses to microbes are not established. In the thymus, epithelial cells express class II MHC molecules and play a role in the maturation and selection of T cells. All nucleated cells can present class I MHC–associated peptides to CD8+ T cells. *IFN-γ*, Interferon-γ; *IL-4*, interleukin-4; *TLR*, Toll-like receptor.

molecules and examine how they function in immune responses.

STRUCTURE AND FUNCTION OF MAJOR HISTOCOMPATIBILITY COMPLEX MOLECULES

MHC molecules are membrane proteins on APCs that display peptide antigens for recognition by T lymphocytes. The MHC was discovered as the genetic locus that is the principal determinant of acceptance or rejection of tissue grafts exchanged between individuals (tissue, or histo, compatibility). In other words, individuals who are identical at their MHC locus (inbred animals and identical twins) will accept grafts from one another, and individuals who differ at their MHC loci will reject such grafts. Because graft rejection is not a natural biologic phenomenon, MHC genes and the molecules they encode must have evolved to perform other functions. We now know that the physiologic role of MHC molecules is to display peptides derived from microbial protein antigens to antigen-specific T lymphocytes as a first step in protective T cell–mediated immune responses to microbes. This function of MHC molecules explains the

phenomenon of MHC restriction of T cells, mentioned earlier.

All vertebrates possess maternally and paternally inherited MHC loci, which include genes encoding the MHC proteins (and other proteins involved in immune responses) (Fig. 3.7). MHC molecules were first discovered as proteins encoded by the murine MHC locus involved in graft rejection. They were rediscovered in humans when it was found that women who had multiple pregnancies, or recipients of multiple blood transfusions, made antibodies that recognized proteins on the white blood cells (leukocytes) of paternal or donor origin, respectively. These proteins were called **human leukocyte antigens** (HLAs) and were soon shown to be analogous to the MHC molecules identified in mice. (Pregnancy and transfusions expose individuals to cellular antigens of other individuals, so antibodies produced against these cells reflect histoincompatibility, as in the mouse grafting experiments.) In all vertebrates, the MHC contains two sets of highly polymorphic genes, called the class I and class II MHC genes. (As discussed later, polymorphism refers to the presence of many variants of these genes in the population.)

Fig. 3.7 Genes of the major histocompatibility complex (MHC). Schematic maps show the human MHC, called the human leukocyte antigen *(HLA)* complex, and the mouse MHC, called the H-2 complex, illustrating the major genes that code for molecules involved in immune responses. Sizes of genes and intervening DNA segments are not drawn to scale. Class II genes are shown as single blocks, but each consists of two genes encoding the α and β chains, respectively. The products of some of the genes (DM, proteasome components, TAP) are involved in antigen processing. The MHC also contains genes that encode molecules other than peptide display molecules, including some complement proteins and cytokines. *LT,* Lymphotoxin; *TAP,* transporter associated with antigen processing; *TNF,* tumor necrosis factor.

These genes encode the class I and class II MHC molecules that display peptides to T cells. In addition to the polymorphic genes, the MHC contains many nonpolymorphic genes, some of which code for proteins involved in antigen presentation.

Structure of MHC Molecules

Class I and class II MHC molecules are membrane proteins that each contains an extracellular peptide-binding cleft. Although the two classes of molecules differ in subunit composition, they are very similar in overall structure (Fig. 3.8).

Class I MHC Molecules

Each **class I MHC molecule** consists of an α chain noncovalently associated with a protein called β_2-microglobulin that is encoded by a gene outside the MHC. The α chain consists of three extracellular domains followed by transmembrane and cytoplasmic domains.

- The amino-terminal α1 and α2 domains of the α chain form two walls and a peptide-binding cleft, or groove, that can accommodate peptides typically 8 to 9 amino acids long. The floor of the peptide-binding cleft contains amino acid residues that bind peptides for display to T lymphocytes, and the tops of the cleft

walls make contact with the T cell receptor (which also contacts part of the displayed peptide; see Fig. 3.1). The polymorphic residues of class I molecules—that is, the amino acids that differ among different individuals' MHC molecules—are located in the α1 and α2 domains of the α chain. Most of these polymorphic residues contribute to variations in the floor of the peptide-binding cleft and thus influence the ability of different MHC molecules to bind distinct sets of peptides.

- The α3 domain is invariant and contains a site that binds the CD8 T cell coreceptor but not CD4. As discussed in Chapter 5, T cell activation requires recognition of MHC-associated peptide antigen by the TCR and simultaneous recognition of the MHC molecule by the coreceptor. Therefore, CD8+ T cells can only respond to peptides displayed by class I MHC molecules, the MHC molecules to which the CD8 coreceptor binds.

Class II MHC Molecules

Each **class II MHC molecule** consists of two transmembrane chains, called α and β. Each chain has two extracellular domains, followed by the transmembrane and cytoplasmic regions.

Class I MHC

Class II MHC

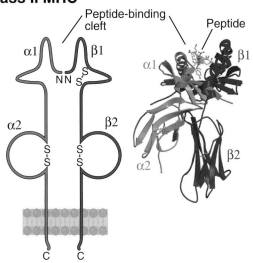

Fig. 3.8 Structure of class I and class II major histocompatibility complex (MHC) molecules. Schematic diagrams *(at left)* and models of the crystal structures *(at right)* of class I MHC and class II MHC molecules illustrate the domains of the molecules and the fundamental similarities between them. Both types of MHC molecules contain peptide-binding clefts and invariant portions that bind CD8 (the α3 domain of class I) or CD4 (the α2 and β2 domains of class II). *Ig,* Immunoglobulin; *β2m,* β_2-microglobulin. (Crystal structures courtesy Dr. P. Bjorkman, California Institute of Technology, Pasadena, CA.)

- The amino-terminal regions of both chains, called the α1 and β1 domains, contain polymorphic residues and form a cleft that is large enough to accommodate peptides of 10 to 30 residues.

- The nonpolymorphic α2 and β2 domains contain the binding site for the CD4 T cell coreceptor. Because CD4 binds to class II MHC molecules but not to class I, CD4+ T cells can only respond to peptides presented by class II MHC molecules.

Properties of MHC Genes and Proteins

Several features of MHC genes and proteins are important for the normal function of these molecules (Fig. 3.9):

- **MHC genes are highly polymorphic**, meaning that many different alleles (variants) are present among the different individuals in the population. The total number of different HLA proteins in the population is estimated to be more than 14,000, with about 10,500 class I and 3500 class II molecules, making MHC molecules the most polymorphic of all proteins in mammals. The polymorphism of MHC proteins is so great that any two individuals in an outbred population are extremely unlikely to have exactly the same MHC molecules. These different polymorphic variants are inherited and not generated de novo in individuals by somatic gene recombination, as are antigen receptors (see Chapter 4). Any one individual inherits and expresses only two alleles of each MHC gene (one from each parent), which represent very few of the many variants in the population. Because the polymorphic residues determine which peptides are presented by specific MHC molecules, the existence of multiple alleles ensures that there are always some members of the population who will be able to present some peptide from any particular microbial protein antigen. Therefore, MHC polymorphism ensures that a population will be able to deal with the diversity of microbes, and at least some individuals will be able to mount effective immune responses to the peptide antigens of these microbes. Thus, everyone will not succumb to a newly encountered or mutated microbe.

- **MHC genes are codominantly expressed, meaning that the alleles inherited from both parents are expressed equally.** Codominant expression maximizes the number of HLA proteins expressed by each individual and thus enables each individual to display a large number of peptides.

- **Class I molecules are expressed on all nucleated cells, but class II molecules are expressed mainly on dendritic cells, macrophages, and B lymphocytes.** The physiologic significance of this strikingly different expression pattern is described later. Class II molecules also are expressed on thymic epithelial

Feature	Significance	
Polymorphic genes: Many different alleles are present in the population	Different individuals are able to present and respond to different microbial peptides	
Co-dominant expression: Both parental alleles of each MHC gene are expressed	Increases number of different MHC molecules that can present peptides to T cells	T cells MHC molecules Parental chromosomes
MHC-expressing cell types: Class I: All nucleated cells	CD8+ CTLs can kill any type of virus-infected cell	Leukocytes Epithelial cells Mesenchymal cells
Class II: Dendritic cells, macrophages, B cells	CD4+ helper T lymphocytes interact with dendritic cells, macrophages, B lymphocytes	Dendritic cell Macrophage B cell

Fig. 3.9 Properties of major histocompatibility complex (MHC) molecules and genes. Some of the important features of MHC molecules and their significance for immune responses. *CTLs,* Cytotoxic T lymphocytes.

cells and endothelial cells and can be induced on other cell types by the cytokine interferon-γ.

Inheritance Patterns and Nomenclature of HLA Genes

Three polymorphic class I genes, called HLA-A, HLA-B, and HLA-C, exist in humans, and each person inherits one of these genes from each parent, so any cell can express six different class I molecules. In the class II locus, every individual inherits from each parent two separate genes encoding the α chain and the β chain of HLA-DP, two encoding DQα and DQβ, one or two for DRβ (HLA-DRB1 always and sometimes HLA-DRB3, HLA-DR4, or HLA-DR5), and one for DRα. The polymorphism resides mainly in the β chains for class II genes and exclusively in the α chain for class I genes.

Because of several reasons, including the extra DRβ genes in some individuals (not everyone has the extra HLADRB3/4/5 locus), and the fact that some α chains encoded on one chromosome can associate with β chains encoded from the other chromosome, the total number of expressed class II molecules may be considerably more than six.

The set of MHC genes present on each chromosome is called an **MHC haplotype**. The genes in an MHC haplotype are tightly linked and inherited together in a Mendelian fashion. Therefore, the chance that two siblings will inherit identical sets of HLA alleles is 25%. This is why siblings are often tested before unrelated individuals for their suitability as donors for transplantation—the chance of finding an HLA match with the recipient is much greater for siblings. In humans, each HLA allele is given a numeric designation. For example, an HLA haplotype of an individual could be HLA-A2, B5, DR3, and so on. In the modern terminology, based on molecular typing, individual alleles may be called HLA-A*0201, referring to the 01 subtype of HLA-A2, or HLA-DRB1*0401, referring to the 01 subtype of the DR4B1 gene, and so on.

Peptide Binding to MHC Molecules

The peptide-binding clefts of MHC molecules bind peptides derived from protein antigens and display these peptides for recognition by T cells (Fig. 3.10). There are pockets in the floors of the peptide-binding clefts of most MHC molecules. Some of the amino acids in the peptide antigens fit into these MHC pockets and anchor the peptides in the cleft of the MHC molecule; these amino acids are called anchor residues. Other residues of the bound peptide project upward and are recognized by the antigen receptors of T cells.

Several features of the interaction of peptide antigens with MHC molecules are important for understanding the peptide display function of MHC molecules (Fig. 3.11):

- Each MHC molecule can present only one peptide at a time, because there is only one binding cleft, but each MHC molecule is capable of presenting many different peptides. As long as the pockets of the MHC molecule can accommodate the anchor residues of the peptide, that peptide can be displayed by the MHC molecule. Therefore, only one or two residues in a peptide determine if that peptide will bind to the cleft of a particular MHC molecule. Thus, MHC

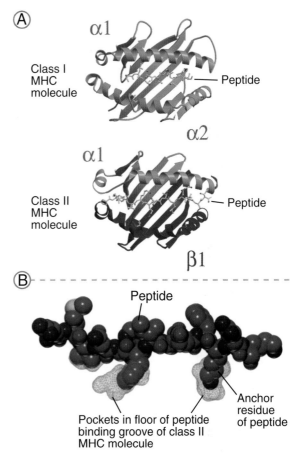

Fig. 3.10 Binding of peptides to major histocompatibility complex (MHC) molecules. **A,** The top views of the crystal structures of MHC molecules show how peptides (in *yellow*) lie on the floors of the peptide-binding clefts and are available for recognition by T cells. **B,** The side view of a cutout of a peptide bound to a class II MHC molecule shows how anchor residues of the peptide hold it in the pockets in the cleft of the MHC molecule. (**A,** Courtesy Dr. P. Bjorkman, California Institute of Technology, Pasadena, CA. **B,** From Scott CA, Peterson PA, Teyton L, Wilson IA: Crystal structures of two I-A^d-peptide complexes reveal that high affinity can be achieved without large anchor residues, *Immunity* 8:319–329, 1998. Copyright Cell Press; with permission.)

molecules are said to have a broad specificity for peptide binding; each MHC molecule can bind many peptides as long as they have the optimal length and amino acid sequence. This broad specificity is essential for the antigen display function of MHC molecules, because each individual has only a few different MHC molecules that must be able to present peptides derived from a vast number and variety of protein antigens.

Feature	Significance	
Broad specificity	Many different peptides can bind to the same MHC molecule	
Each MHC molecule displays one peptide at a time	Each T cell responds to a single peptide bound to an MHC molecule	
MHC molecules bind only peptides	MHC-restricted T cells respond mainly to protein antigens*	Proteins → Peptides → ... Lipids → Carbohydrate sugars → Nucleic acids →
Class I and class II MHC molecules display peptides from different cellular compartments	Class I and class II MHC molecules provide immune surveillance for microbes in different locations	Peptides from proteins in cytosol. Cytosolic protein — Proteasome — Class I MHC. Endosome/lysosome — Peptides from internalized proteins in endocytic vesicles. Endocytosis of extracellular protein — Class II MHC
Stable surface expression of MHC molecule requires bound peptide	Only peptide-loaded MHC molecules are expressed on the cell surface for recognition by T cells	MHC molecule with bound peptide. "Empty" MHC molecule
Very slow off-rate	MHC molecule displays bound peptide for long enough to be located by T cell	β2-microglobulin + α + Peptide → → Days

Fig. 3.11 Features of peptide binding to MHC molecules. Some of the important features of peptide binding to MHC molecules, with their significance for immune responses. *ER,* Endoplasmic reticulum; *I,* invariant chain. *Some small chemicals and heavy metal ions may directly alter MHC molecules and are recognized by T cells.

- MHC molecules bind mainly peptides and not other types of antigens. Among various classes of molecules, only peptides have the structural and charge characteristics that permit binding to the clefts of MHC molecules. This is why MHC-restricted CD4+ T cells and CD8+ T cells can recognize and respond to protein antigens, the natural source of peptides. The MHC is also involved in the reactions of T cells to some nonpeptide antigens, such as small molecules and metal ions. The recognition of such antigens is discussed briefly later in the chapter.

- MHC molecules acquire their peptide cargo during their biosynthesis, assembly, and transport inside cells. Therefore, MHC molecules display peptides derived from protein antigens that are inside host cells (produced inside cells or ingested from the extracellular environment). This explains why MHC-restricted T cells recognize cell-associated microbes and not free antigens in the circulation, tissue fluids, or mucosal lumens. Class I MHC molecules acquire peptides from cytosolic proteins and class II molecules from proteins that are taken up into intracellular vesicles. The mechanisms and significance of these pathways of peptide-MHC association are discussed later.

- Only peptide-loaded MHC molecules are stably expressed on cell surfaces. The reason for this is that MHC molecules must assemble both their chains and bound peptides to achieve a stable structure, and empty molecules are degraded inside cells. This requirement for peptide binding ensures that only useful MHC molecules—that is, those displaying peptides—are expressed on cell surfaces for recognition by T cells. Once peptides bind to MHC molecules, they stay bound for a long time, up to days for some peptides. The slow off-rate ensures that after an MHC molecule has acquired a peptide, it will display the peptide long enough to allow a particular T cell that can recognize the peptide-MHC complex to find the bound peptide and initiate a response.

- In each individual, the MHC molecules can display peptides derived from the individual's own proteins, as well as peptides from foreign (i.e., microbial) proteins. This inability of MHC molecules to discriminate between self antigens and foreign antigens raises two questions. First, at any time, the quantity of self proteins in an APC is likely to be much greater than that of any microbial proteins. Why, then, are the available MHC molecules not constantly occupied by self peptides and unable to present foreign antigens?

The likely answer is that new MHC molecules are constantly being synthesized, ready to accept peptides, and they are adept at capturing any peptides that are present in cells. Also, a single T cell may need to see a peptide displayed by only as few as 0.1% to 1% of the approximately 10^5 MHC molecules on the surface of an APC, so that even rare MHC molecules displaying a peptide are enough to initiate an immune response. In addition, during viral infections, host protein synthesis is suppressed and viral proteins dominate and therefore are preferentially presented by MHC molecules. The second problem is that if MHC molecules are constantly displaying self peptides, why do we not develop immune responses to self antigens, so-called autoimmune responses? The answer is that T cells specific for self antigens are either killed or inactivated (see Chapter 9). Thus, T cells are constantly patrolling the body, looking at MHC-associated peptides, and if there is an infection, only those T cells that recognize microbial peptides will respond, while self peptide–specific T cells will either be absent or will have been previously inactivated.

MHC molecules are capable of displaying peptides but not intact protein antigens, which are too large to fit into the MHC cleft. Therefore, mechanisms must exist for converting naturally occurring proteins into peptides able to bind to MHC molecules. This conversion, called **antigen processing**, is described next.

PROCESSING AND PRESENTATION OF PROTEIN ANTIGENS

Proteins in the cytosol of any nucleated cell are processed in proteolytic complexes called proteasomes and displayed by class I MHC molecules, whereas extracellular proteins that are internalized by specialized APCs (dendritic cells, macrophages, B cells) are processed in late endosomes and lysosomes and displayed by class II molecules (Fig. 3.12). These two pathways of antigen processing involve different cellular proteins (Fig. 3.13). They are designed to sample all the proteins present in the extracellular and intracellular environments. The segregation of antigen-processing pathways also ensures that different classes of T lymphocytes recognize antigens from different compartments. Next we discuss the mechanisms of antigen processing, beginning with the class I MHC pathway.

Fig. 3.12 Pathways of intracellular processing of protein antigens. The class I MHC pathway converts proteins in the cytosol into peptides that bind to class I MHC molecules for recognition by CD8+ T cells. The class II MHC pathway converts protein antigens that are endocytosed into vesicles of antigen-presenting cells into peptides that bind to class II MHC molecules for recognition by CD4+ T cells. *CTL*, Cytotoxic T lymphocyte; *ER*, endoplasmic reticulum; *TAP*, transporter associated with antigen processing.

Processing of Cytosolic Antigens for Display by Class I MHC Molecules

The main steps in antigen presentation by class I MHC molecules include the tagging of antigens in the cytosol or nucleus for proteolysis, proteolytic generation of peptide fragments of the antigen by a specialized cytosolic enzyme complex, transport of peptides into the ER, binding of peptides to newly synthesized class I molecules, and transport of peptide-MHC complexes to the cell surface (Fig. 3.14).

Proteolysis of Cytosolic Proteins

The peptides that bind to class I MHC molecules are derived from cytosolic proteins following digestion by the ubiquitin-proteasome pathway. Antigenic proteins may be produced in the cytoplasm from viruses that are living inside infected cells, from some phagocytosed microbes that may leak from or be transported out of phagosomes into the cytosol, and from mutated or altered host genes that encode cytosolic or nuclear proteins, as in tumors. All of these proteins, as well as the cell's own misfolded cytosolic and nuclear proteins, are targeted for proteolytic digestion by the ubiquitin-proteasome pathway. These proteins are unfolded, covalently tagged with multiple copies of a peptide called ubiquitin, and threaded through a protein complex called the **proteasome** that is composed of stacked rings of proteolytic enzymes. The proteasomes degrade the unfolded proteins into peptides. In cells that have been exposed to inflammatory cytokines (as in an infection), the enzymatic composition of the proteasomes changes. As a result, these cells become very efficient at cleaving cytosolic and nuclear proteins into peptides with the size and sequence properties that enable the peptides to bind well to class I MHC molecules.

Feature	Class I MHC pathway	Class II MHC Pathway
Composition of stable peptide-MHC complex	Polymorphic α chain of MHC, β2-microglobulin, peptide	Polymorphic α and β chains of MHC, peptide
Cells that express that MHC	All nucleated cells	Dendritic cells, mononuclear phagocytes, B lymphocytes; endothelial cells, thymic epithelium
Responsive T cells	CD8+ T cells	CD4+ T cells
Source of protein antigens	Cytosolic proteins (mostly synthesized in the cell; may enter cytosol from phagosomes)	Endosomal/lysosomal proteins (mostly internalized from extracellular environment)
Enzymes responsible for peptide generation	Protease components of cytosolic proteasome	Endosomal and lysosomal proteases (e.g., cathepsins)
Site of peptide loading of MHC	Endoplasmic reticulum	Late endosomes and lysosomes
Molecules involved in transport of peptides and loading of MHC molecules	TAP	Invariant chain, DM

Fig. 3.13 Features of the pathways of antigen processing. Some of the comparative features of the two major antigen processing pathways. *MHC,* Major histocompatibility complex; *TAP,* transporter associated with antigen processing.

Binding of Peptides to Class I MHC Molecules

In order to form peptide-MHC complexes, the peptides must be transported into the endoplasmic reticulum (ER). The peptides produced by proteasomal digestion are in the cytosol, while the MHC molecules are being synthesized in the ER, and the two need to come together. This transport function is provided by a molecule, called the **transporter associated with antigen processing** (TAP), located in the ER membrane. TAP binds proteasome-generated peptides on the cytosolic side of the ER membrane, then actively pumps them into the interior of the ER. Newly synthesized class I MHC molecules, which do not contain bound peptides, associate with a bridging protein called tapasin that links them to TAP molecules in the ER membrane. Thus, as peptides enter the ER, they can easily be captured by the empty class I molecules. (As we discuss later, in the ER, the newly synthesized class II MHC molecules are not able to bind peptides because of the associated invariant chain.)

Transport of Peptide-MHC Complexes to the Cell Surface

Peptide loading stabilizes class I MHC molecules, which are exported to the cell surface. Once the class I MHC molecule binds tightly to one of the peptides generated from proteasomal digestion and delivered into the ER by TAP, this peptide-MHC complex

Fig. 3.14 Class I MHC pathway of processing of cytosolic antigens. Proteins enter the cytoplasm of cells either from endogenous synthesis by microbes, such as viruses, that reside in the cytosol (or nucleus, not shown) of infected cells or from microbes that are ingested but whose antigens are transported into the cytosol (the process of cross-presentation, described later). Cytoplasmic proteins are unfolded, ubiquitinated, and degraded in proteasomes. The peptides that are produced are transported by the transporter associated with antigen processing (TAP) into the endoplasmic reticulum (ER), where the peptides may be further trimmed. Newly synthesized class I MHC molecules are initially stabilized by chaperones and attached to TAP by a linker protein called tapasin, so the MHC molecules are strategically located to receive peptides that are transported into the ER by TAP. The peptide–class I MHC complexes are transported to the cell surface and are recognized by CD8+ T cells. *Ub*, Ubiquitin; $\beta_2 m$, β_2-microglobulin.

becomes stable and is delivered to the cell surface. If the MHC molecule does not find a peptide it can bind, the empty molecule is unstable and is eventually degraded in the ER. One protein antigen may give rise to many peptides, only a few of which (perhaps only one or two from each antigen) can bind to the MHC molecules present in the individual and have the potential to stimulate immune responses in that individual. The class I MHC-peptide complexes are recognized by CD8+ T cells.

The evolutionary struggle between microbes and their hosts is well illustrated by the numerous strategies that viruses have developed to block the class I MHC pathway of antigen presentation. These strategies include removing newly synthesized MHC molecules from the ER, inhibiting the transcription of MHC genes, and blocking peptide transport by TAP. By inhibiting

the class I MHC pathway, viruses reduce presentation of their own antigens to CD8+ T cells and are thus able to evade the adaptive immune system. These mechanisms of immune evasion are discussed in Chapter 6.

Processing of Internalized Antigens for Display by Class II MHC Molecules

The main steps in the presentation of peptides by class II MHC molecules include internalization of the antigen, proteolysis in endocytic vesicles, association of peptides with class II molecules, and transport of peptide-MHC complexes to the cell surface (Fig. 3.15).

Internalization and Proteolysis of Antigens

Antigens destined for the class II MHC pathway are usually internalized from the extracellular environment. Dendritic cells and macrophages may ingest

Fig. 3.15 Class II major histocompatibility complex (MHC) pathway of processing of internalized vesicular antigens. Protein antigens are ingested by antigen-presenting cells (APCs) into vesicles, where they are degraded into peptides. Class II MHC molecules enter the same vesicles, where the class II invariant chain peptide (CLIP) that occupies the cleft of newly synthesized class II molecules is removed. These class II molecules are then able to bind peptides derived from the endocytosed protein. The DM molecule facilitates the removal of CLIP and subsequent binding of the antigenic peptide. The peptide–class II MHC complexes are transported to the cell surface and are recognized by CD4+ T cells. *ER*, Endoplasmic reticulum; *I$_i$*, invariant chain.

extracellular microbes or microbial proteins by several mechanisms, including phagocytosis and receptor-mediated endocytosis. Microbes may bind to surface receptors specific for microbial products or to receptors that recognize antibodies or products of complement activation (opsonins) attached to the microbes. B lymphocytes efficiently internalize proteins that specifically bind to the cells' antigen receptors (see Chapter 7). Certain APCs, especially dendritic cells, may also pinocytose proteins without any specific recognition event. After internalization into APCs by any of these pathways, the microbial proteins enter acidic intracellular vesicles, called endosomes or phagosomes, which fuse with lysosomes. In these vesicles, the proteins are broken down by proteolytic enzymes, generating many peptides of varying lengths and sequences.

Binding of Peptides to Class II MHC Molecules

Peptides bind to newly synthesized class II MHC molecules in specialized vesicles. Class II MHC–expressing APCs constantly synthesize these MHC molecules in the ER. Each newly synthesized class II molecule carries with it an attached protein called the **invariant chain** (I$_i$), which contains a sequence called the class II invariant chain peptide (CLIP) that binds to the peptide-binding cleft of the class II molecule. Thus, the cleft of the newly synthesized class II molecule is occupied and prevented from accepting peptides in the ER that are destined to bind to class I MHC molecules (discussed earlier). This class II molecule with its associated I$_i$ migrates from the ER through the Golgi stacks and then, instead of traveling directly to the plasma membrane, is targeted by the cytosolic tail of the invariant chain to acidic vesicles (endosomes and lysosomes).

Fig. 3.16 Class I MHC-restricted cross-presentation of microbial antigens from infected cells by dendritic cells. Fragments of cells infected with intracellular microbes (e.g., viruses) or antigens produced in these cells are ingested by dendritic cells, and the antigens of the infectious microbes are broken down and presented in association with class I MHC molecules of the antigen-presenting cells *(APCs)*. T cells recognize the microbial antigens expressed on the APCs, and the T cells are activated. By convention, the term *cross-presentation* (or *cross-priming*) is applied to CD8+ T cells (cytotoxic T lymphocytes) recognizing class I MHC–associated antigens (as shown); the same cross-presenting APC may display class II MHC–associated antigens from the microbe for recognition by CD4+ helper T cells.

In this compartment, the invariant chain is degraded, leaving only CLIP in the peptide-binding cleft. Ingested proteins are digested into peptides in the same compartment. The vesicles also contain a class II MHC–like protein called DM, whose function is to exchange CLIP in the class II MHC molecule with other peptides that may be available in this compartment that can bind to the MHC molecule with higher affinity.

Transport of Peptide-MHC Complexes to the Cell Surface

Peptide loading stabilizes class II MHC molecules, which are exported to the cell surface. If a class II molecule binds a peptide with the right fit, the complex is stabilized and transported to the cell surface, where it can be recognized by a CD4+ T cell. Class II molecules that do not find peptides they can bind are eventually degraded by lysosomal proteases. As for the class I pathway, only a few of the peptides produced from any protein antigen can bind to MHC molecules present in the individual and stimulate immune responses in each individual.

Cross-Presentation of Internalized Antigens to CD8+ T Cells

Some dendritic cells can present ingested antigens on class I MHC molecules to CD8+ T lymphocytes. This

pathway of antigen presentation is contrary to the general rule for APCs that most internalized proteins are displayed by class II MHC molecules to CD4+ T cells. The initial response of naive CD8+ T cells, similar to CD4+ cells, requires that the antigens be presented by mature dendritic cells in lymph nodes through which the naïve T cells circulate. However, some viruses may infect only particular cell types and not dendritic cells, and these infected cells may not travel to lymph nodes or produce all the signals needed to initiate T cell activation. How, then, are naive CD8+ T lymphocytes in lymph nodes able to respond to the intracellular antigens of infected cells? Similarly, tumors arise from many different types of cells, so how can diverse tumor antigens be presented to naive CD8+ T cells in lymph nodes by dendritic cells?

A subset of classical dendritic cells has the ability to ingest infected host cells, dead tumor cells, microbes, and microbial and tumor antigens and transport the ingested antigens into the cytosol, where they are processed by the proteasome. The antigenic peptides that are generated then enter the ER and bind to class I molecules, which display the antigens for recognition by CD8+ T lymphocytes (Fig. 3.16). This process is called **cross-presentation** (or cross-priming), to indicate that one type of cell, dendritic cells, can present the antigens of other infected or dying cells or cell fragments and prime (or activate) naive CD8$^+$ T lymphocytes specific for these antigens. Once the CD8$^+$ T cells have differentiated into CTLs, they kill infected host cells or tumor cells without the need for dendritic cells or signals other than recognition of antigen (see Chapter 6). The same pathway of cross-presentation is involved in initiating CD8$^+$ T cell responses to some antigens in organ transplants (see Chapter 10).

Physiologic Significance of MHC-Associated Antigen Presentation

Many fundamental features of T cell–mediated immunity are closely linked to the peptide display function of MHC molecules:

- The restriction of T cell recognition to MHC-associated peptides ensures that T cells see and respond only to cell-associated antigens. This is because MHC molecules are cell membrane proteins and because peptide loading and subsequent expression of MHC molecules depend on intracellular biosynthetic and assembly steps. In other words, MHC molecules can be loaded with peptides only inside cells, where intracellular and ingested antigens are present. Therefore, T lymphocytes can recognize the antigens of intracellular microbes, which require T cell–mediated effector mechanisms, as well as antigens ingested from the extracellular environment, such as those against which antibody responses are generated.
- By segregating the class I and class II pathways of antigen processing, the immune system is able to respond to extracellular and intracellular microbes in different ways that are specialized to defend against these microbes (Fig. 3.17). Cytosolic antigens are processed and displayed by class I MHC molecules, which are expressed on all nucleated cells—as expected, because all nucleated cells can be infected with one or more species of viruses. Class I–associated peptides are recognized by CD8$^+$ T lymphocytes, which differentiate into CTLs. The CTLs kill the infected cells and eradicate the infection, this being the most effective mechanism for eliminating cytoplasmic microbes. CTLs also kill tumor cells which produce cytosolic proteins from mutated genes. Many bacteria, fungi, and even extracellular viruses are typically captured and ingested by macrophages and their antigens are presented by class II molecules. Because of the specificity of CD4 for class II, class II–associated peptides are recognized by CD4$^+$ T lymphocytes, which function as helper cells. These T cells help the macrophages to destroy ingested microbes, thereby activating an effector mechanism that can eliminate microbes that are internalized from the extracellular environment. B lymphocytes ingest protein antigens of microbes and also present processed peptides for recognition by CD4$^+$ helper T cells. These helper cells stimulate the production of antibodies, which serve to eliminate extracellular microbes. Neither phagocytes nor antibodies are effective against intracellular viruses and other pathogens that can survive and replicate in the cytoplasm of host cells; cells harboring these cytosolic microbes are eliminated by CD8$^+$ CTLs.

    Thus, the nature of the protective immune response to different microbes is optimized by linking several features of antigen presentation and T cell recognition: the pathways of processing of vesicular and cytosolic antigens, the cellular expression of class I and class II MHC molecules, the specificity of CD8 and CD4 coreceptors for class I and class II molecules, and the functions of CD8$^+$ cells as CTLs and of CD4$^+$ cells as helper cells. The function of linking the type of microbe to one of the the two antigen-processing pathways is important because the antigen receptors of T cells cannot distinguish between intracellular and extracellular microbes. In fact, as previously mentioned, the same virus can be extracellular early after infection and becomes intracellular once the infection is established. During its extracellular life, the virus is fought by antibodies and phagocytes, whose production or functions are stimulated by helper T cells, but once the virus has found a haven in the cytoplasm of cells, it can be eradicated only by CTL-mediated killing of the infected cells. The segregation of class I and class II antigen presentation pathways ensures the correct, specialized immune response against microbes in different locations.
- **The structural constraints on peptide binding to different MHC molecules, including length and anchor residues, account for the immunodominance of some peptides derived from complex protein antigens and for the inability of some individuals to respond to certain protein antigens.** When any protein is proteolytically degraded in APCs, many peptides may be generated, but only those peptides able to bind to the MHC molecules in that individual can be presented for recognition by T cells. These MHC-binding peptides are the

Fig. 3.17 Role of MHC-associated antigen presentation in recognition of microbial antigens by CD8+ and CD4+ effector T cells. **A,** Protein antigens of microbes that live in the cytoplasm of infected cells enter the class I MHC pathway of antigen processing. As a result, these proteins are recognized by CD8+ cytotoxic T lymphocytes, whose function is to kill infected cells. **B,** Protein antigens of microbes that are endocytosed from the extracellular environment by macrophages and B lymphocytes enter the class II MHC pathway of antigen processing. As a result, these proteins are recognized by CD4+ helper T lymphocytes, whose functions are to activate macrophages to destroy phagocytosed microbes and activate B cells to produce antibodies against extracellular microbes and toxins.

immunodominant peptides of the antigen. Even microbes with complex protein antigens express a limited number of immunodominant peptides. Many attempts have been made to identify these peptides in order to develop vaccines, but it is difficult to select a small number of peptides from any microbe that would be immunogenic in a large number of people, because of the enormous polymorphism of MHC molecules in the population. The polymorphism of the MHC also means that some individuals may not express MHC molecules capable of binding any peptide derived from a particular antigen. These individuals would be nonresponders to that antigen. One of the earliest observations that established the physiologic importance of the MHC was the discovery that some inbred animals did not respond to simple protein antigens and responsiveness (or lack of) mapped to genes called immune response (Ir) genes, later shown to be class II MHC genes.

Finally, it should be mentioned that T cells also recognize and react against small molecules and even metal ions in an MHC-restricted manner. In fact, exposure to some small molecules that are used as therapeutic drugs and to metals such as nickel and beryllium often leads to pathologic T cell reactions (so-called hypersensitivity reactions; see Chapter 11). There are several ways in which these nonpeptide antigens may be recognized by MHC-restricted CD4+ and CD8+ T cells. Some of the chemicals are thought to covalently modify self peptides or the MHC molecules themselves, creating altered molecules that are recognized as foreign. Other chemicals may bind noncovalently to MHC molecules and alter the structure of the peptide-binding cleft such that the MHC molecule can display peptides that are not normally presented and these peptide-MHC complexes are seen as being foreign.

This chapter began with two questions: how do rare antigen-specific lymphocytes find antigens, and how are the appropriate immune responses generated against extracellular and intracellular microbes? Understanding the biology of APCs and the role of MHC molecules in displaying the peptides of protein antigens has provided satisfying answers to both questions, specifically for T cell–mediated immune responses.

FUNCTIONS OF ANTIGEN-PRESENTING CELLS IN ADDITION TO ANTIGEN DISPLAY

Antigen-presenting cells not only display peptides for recognition by T cells but, in response to microbes, also express additional signals for T cell activation. The two-signal hypothesis of lymphocyte activation was introduced in Chapters 1 and 2 (see Fig. 2.19), and we will return to this concept when we discuss the responses of T and B cells in Chapters 5 and 7. Recall that antigen is the necessary signal 1, and for T cells, signal 2 is provided by APCs reacting to microbes. The expression of molecules in APCs that serve as second signals for lymphocyte activation is part of the innate immune response to different microbial products. For example, many bacteria produce a substance called lipopolysaccharide (LPS, endotoxin). When the bacteria are captured by APCs for presentation of their protein antigens, LPS acts on the same APCs, through a TLR, and stimulates the expression of costimulators and the secretion of cytokines. The costimulators and cytokines act in concert with antigen recognition by

the T cell to stimulate the proliferation of the T cells and their differentiation into effector and memory cells.

ANTIGEN RECOGNITION BY B CELLS AND OTHER LYMPHOCYTES

B lymphocytes use membrane-bound antibodies to recognize a wide variety of antigens, including proteins, polysaccharides, lipids, and small chemicals. These antigens may be expressed on microbial surfaces (e.g., capsular or envelope antigens) or may be in soluble form (e.g., secreted toxins). B cells differentiate in response to antigen and other signals into cells that secrete antibodies (see Chapter 7). The secreted antibodies enter the circulation and mucosal fluids and bind to the antigens, leading to their neutralization and elimination. The antigen receptors of B cells and the antibodies that are secreted usually recognize antigens in the native conformation, with no requirement for antigen processing or display by a specialized system. Macrophages in lymphatic sinuses and dendritic cells adjacent to follicles may capture antigens that enter lymph nodes and present the antigens, in intact (unprocessed) form, to B lymphocytes in the follicles.

The B cell–rich lymphoid follicles of the lymph nodes and spleen contain a population of cells called **follicular dendritic cells** (FDCs), whose function is to display antigens to activated B cells. FDCs are not bone-marrow derived or related to the dendritic cells that process and present antigens to T cells. FDCs express receptors that bind antigens coated with antibodies or complement by-products such as C3b and C3d, with no role for MHC molecules. The antigens displayed by FDCs are seen by specific B lymphocytes during humoral immune responses, and they function to select B cells that bind the antigens with high affinity. This process is discussed in Chapter 7.

Although this chapter has focused on peptide recognition by MHC-restricted CD4+ and CD8+ T cells, there are other, smaller populations of T cells that recognize different types of antigens. Natural killer T cells (called NK-T cells), which are distinct from the natural killer (NK) cells described in Chapter 2, are specific for lipids displayed by class I–like CD1 molecules. Mucosal associated innate T cells (MAIT cells) are specific for bacterial-derived vitamin B metabolites displayed by class I–like MR1 molecules. γδ T cells recognize a wide variety of molecules, some displayed by class I–like molecules and others apparently requiring no specific processing or display. The functions of these cells and the significance of their unusual specificities are poorly understood.

SUMMARY

- The induction of immune responses to the protein antigens of microbes depends on a specialized system for capturing and displaying these antigens for recognition by the rare naive T cells specific for any antigen. Microbes and microbial antigens that enter the body through epithelia are captured by dendritic cells located in the epithelia and transported to regional lymph nodes or captured by dendritic cells in lymph nodes and spleen. The protein antigens of the microbes are displayed by the antigen-presenting cells (APCs) to naive T lymphocytes that recirculate through the lymphoid organs.

- Molecules encoded in the major histocompatibility complex (MHC) perform the function of displaying peptides derived from protein antigens.

- MHC genes are highly polymorphic. Their major products are class I and class II MHC molecules, which contain peptide-binding clefts, where the polymorphic residues are concentrated, and invariant regions, which bind the coreceptors CD8 and CD4, respectively.

- Proteins that are produced in the cytosol of infected and tumor cells, or that enter the cytosol from phagosomes, are degraded by proteasomes, transported into the endoplasmic reticulum by TAP and bind to the clefts of newly synthesized class I MHC molecules. CD8 binds the invariant part of class I MHC molecules, so CD8+ cytotoxic T lymphocytes can be activated only by class I MHC–associated peptides derived from proteosomal degradation of cytosolic proteins.

- Proteins that are ingested by APCs from the extracellular environment are proteolytically degraded within the vesicles of the APCs, and the peptides generated bind to the clefts of newly synthesized class II MHC molecules. CD4 binds to class II MHC, because of which CD4+ helper T cells can only be activated by class II MHC–associated peptides derived mainly from proteins degraded in vesicles, which are typically ingested extracellular proteins.

- The role of MHC molecules in antigen display ensures that T cells only recognize cell-associated protein antigens and that the correct type of T cell (helper or cytotoxic) responds to the type of microbe the T cell is best able to combat.

- Microbes activate APCs to express membrane proteins (costimulators) and to secrete cytokines that provide signals that function in concert with antigens to stimulate specific T cells. The requirement for these second signals ensures that T cells respond to microbial antigens and not to harmless, nonmicrobial substances.

- B lymphocytes recognize proteins as well as nonprotein antigens, even in their native conformations. Follicular dendritic cells display antigens to germinal center B cells and select high-affinity B cells during humoral immune responses.

REVIEW QUESTIONS

1. When antigens enter through the skin, in what organs are they concentrated? What cell type(s) plays an important role in this process of antigen capture?
2. What are MHC molecules? What are human MHC molecules called? How were MHC molecules discovered, and what is their function?
3. What are the differences between the antigens that are displayed by class I and class II MHC molecules?
4. Describe the sequence of events by which class I and class II MHC molecules acquire antigens for display.
5. Which subsets of T cells recognize antigens presented by class I and class II MHC molecules? What molecules on T cells contribute to their specificity for either class I or class II MHC–associated peptide antigens?

Answers to and discussion of the Review Questions are available at Student Consult.

Antigen Recognition in the Adaptive Immune System
Structure of Lymphocyte Antigen Receptors and Development of Immune Repertoires

CHAPTER OUTLINE

Antigen receptors serve critical roles in the maturation of lymphocytes from progenitors and in all adaptive immune responses. In adaptive immunity, naive lymphocytes recognize antigens to initiate responses, and effector T cells and antibodies recognize antigens to perform their functions.

B and T lymphocytes express different receptors that recognize antigens: membrane-bound antibodies on B cells and T cell receptors (TCRs) on T lymphocytes. The principal function of cellular receptors in the immune system, as in other biologic systems, is to detect external stimuli and trigger responses of the cells on which the receptors are expressed. To recognize a large variety of different antigens, the antigen receptors of lymphocytes must be able to bind to and distinguish between many, often closely related, chemical structures. Antigen receptors are clonally distributed, meaning that each lymphocyte clone is specific for a distinct antigen and has a unique receptor, different from the receptors of all other clones. (Recall that a *clone* consists of a parent cell and its progeny.) The total number of distinct lymphocyte clones is very large, and this entire collection makes up the immune **repertoire**. Although each clone of B lymphocytes or T lymphocytes recognizes a different antigen, the antigen receptors transmit biochemical signals that are fundamentally the same in all lymphocytes and are unrelated to specificity.

These features of lymphocyte recognition and antigen receptors raise the following questions:

- How do the antigen receptors of lymphocytes recognize extremely diverse antigens and transmit activating signals to the cells?
- What are the differences in the recognition properties of antigen receptors on B cells and T cells?
- How is the vast diversity of receptor structures in the lymphocyte repertoire generated? The diversity of antigen recognition implies the existence of many structurally different antigen receptor proteins, more than can be encoded in the inherited genome (germline). Therefore, special mechanisms must exist for generating this diversity.

In this chapter, we describe the structures of the antigen receptors of B and T lymphocytes and how these receptors recognize antigens. We also discuss how the diversity of antigen receptors is generated during the process of lymphocyte development, thus giving rise to the repertoire of mature lymphocytes. The process of antigen-induced lymphocyte activation is described in later chapters.

ANTIGEN RECEPTORS OF LYMPHOCYTES

The antigen receptors of B and T lymphocytes have several features that are important for their functions in adaptive immunity (Fig. 4.1). Although these receptors have many similarities in terms of structure and mechanisms of signaling, there are fundamental differences related to the types of antigenic structures that B cells and T cells recognize.

- Membrane-bound antibodies, which serve as the antigen receptors of B lymphocytes, can recognize many types of chemical structures, while T cell antigen receptors recognize only peptides bound to major histocompatibility complex (MHC) molecules. B lymphocyte antigen receptors and the antibodies that B cells secrete can recognize the shapes, or conformations, of macromolecules, including proteins, lipids, carbohydrates, and nucleic acids, as well as simpler, smaller chemical moieties. This broad specificity of B cells for structurally different types of molecules in their native form enables the humoral immune system to recognize, respond to, and eliminate diverse microbes and toxins. In striking contrast, T cells see only peptides displayed on antigen-presenting cells (APCs) bound to MHC molecules. This specificity ensures that T cells never interact with free or soluble antigens and that they only interact with microbial or tumor antigens present inside other cells in the body.

- Antigen receptor molecules consist of regions (domains) involved in antigen recognition—therefore varying between clones of lymphocytes—and other regions required for structural integrity and effector functions—thus relatively conserved among all clones. The antigen-recognizing domains of the receptors are called variable (V) regions, and the conserved portions are the constant (C) regions. Even within each V region, most of the sequence variation is concentrated within short stretches, which are called hypervariable regions, or complementarity-determining regions (CDRs), because they form the parts of the receptor that bind antigens (i.e., they are complementary to the shapes of antigens). By concentrating sequence variation in small regions of the receptor, it is possible to maximize the variability of the antigen-binding part while retaining the basic structure of the receptors. As discussed later, special mechanisms exist in developing lymphocytes to create genes that encode different variable regions of antigen receptor proteins in individual clones.

- Antigen receptor chains are associated with invariant membrane proteins whose function is to deliver intracellular signals following antigen recognition (see Fig. 4.1). These signals, which are transmitted to the cytosol and the nucleus, may cause a lymphocyte to divide, to differentiate, to perform effector functions, or in certain circumstances to die. Thus, the two functions of lymphocyte receptors for antigen—specific antigen recognition and signal transduction—are mediated by different polypeptides. This again allows variability to be segregated in one set of molecules—the antigen receptors themselves—while leaving the conserved function of signal transduction to the other invariant proteins. The set of plasma membrane antigen receptor and signaling molecules in B lymphocytes is called the B cell receptor (BCR) complex, and in T lymphocytes it is called the T cell receptor (TCR) complex. When antigens bind to the extracellular portions of the antigen receptors of lymphocytes, intracellular portions of the associated signaling proteins are phosphorylated on conserved tyrosine residues by enzymes called protein tyrosine kinases. Phosphorylation triggers complex signaling cascades that culminate in the transcriptional

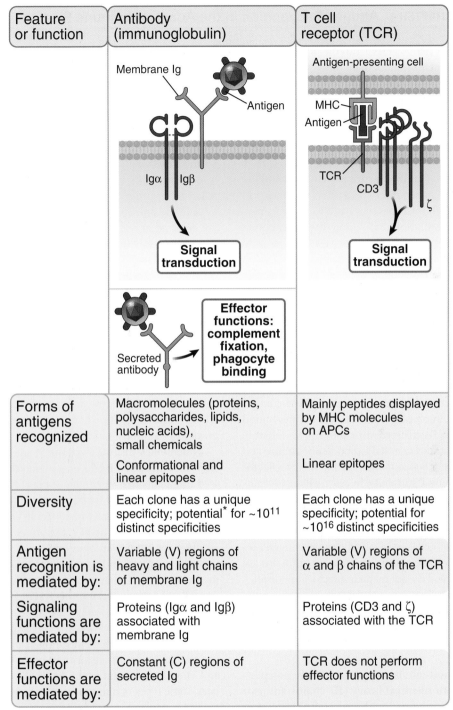

Feature or function	Antibody (immunoglobulin)	T cell receptor (TCR)
	Membrane Ig — Antigen; Igα Igβ → Signal transduction; Secreted antibody → Effector functions: complement fixation, phagocyte binding	Antigen-presenting cell; MHC — Antigen; TCR; CD3; ζ → Signal transduction
Forms of antigens recognized	Macromolecules (proteins, polysaccharides, lipids, nucleic acids), small chemicals Conformational and linear epitopes	Mainly peptides displayed by MHC molecules on APCs Linear epitopes
Diversity	Each clone has a unique specificity; potential* for ~10^{11} distinct specificities	Each clone has a unique specificity; potential for ~10^{16} distinct specificities
Antigen recognition is mediated by:	Variable (V) regions of heavy and light chains of membrane Ig	Variable (V) regions of α and β chains of the TCR
Signaling functions are mediated by:	Proteins (Igα and Igβ) associated with membrane Ig	Proteins (CD3 and ζ) associated with the TCR
Effector functions are mediated by:	Constant (C) regions of secreted Ig	TCR does not perform effector functions

Fig. 4.1 Properties of antibodies and T cell antigen receptors *(TCRs).* Antibodies (also called immuno-globulins) may be expressed as membrane receptors or secreted proteins; TCRs only function as membrane receptors. When immunoglobulin *(Ig)* or TCR molecules recognize antigens, signals are delivered to the lymphocytes by proteins associated with the antigen receptors. The antigen receptors and attached signaling proteins form the B cell receptor (BCR) and TCR complexes. Note that single antigen receptors are shown recognizing antigens, but signaling typically requires the binding of two or more receptors to adjacent antigen molecules. The important characteristics of these antigen-recognizing molecules are summarized. *The total number of possible receptors with unique binding sites is very large, but only ~10^7–10^9 clones with distinct specificities are present in adults. *APCs,* Antigen-presenting cells; *Ig,* immunoglobulin; *MHC,* major histocompatibility complex.

activation of many genes and the production of numerous proteins that mediate the responses of the lymphocytes. We return to the processes of T and B lymphocyte activation in Chapters 5 and 7, respectively.

- Antibodies exist in two forms—as membrane-bound antigen receptors on B cells and as secreted proteins—but TCRs exist only as membrane receptors on T cells. Secreted antibodies are present in the blood and mucosal secretions, where they provide protection against microbes (i.e., they are the effector molecules of humoral immunity). Antibodies are also called immunoglobulins (Igs), referring to immunity-conferring proteins with the physical characteristics of globulins. Secreted antibodies recognize microbial antigens and toxins by their variable domains, the same as the membrane-bound antigen receptors of B lymphocytes. The constant regions of some secreted antibodies have the ability to bind to other molecules that participate in the elimination of antigens: these molecules include receptors on phagocytes and proteins of the complement system. Thus, antibodies serve different functions at different stages of humoral immune responses: membrane-bound antibodies on B cells recognize antigens to initiate B cell activation, and secreted antibodies neutralize and eliminate microbes and their toxins in the effector phase of humoral immunity. In cell-mediated immunity, the effector function of microbe elimination is performed by T lymphocytes themselves and by other leukocytes responding to the T cells. The antigen receptors of T cells are involved only in antigen recognition and T cell activation, and these proteins are not secreted and do not mediate effector functions.

With this introduction, we describe next the antigen receptors of lymphocytes, first antibodies and then TCRs.

Antibodies

An antibody molecule is composed of four polypeptide chains—two identical heavy (H) chains and two identical light (L) chains—with each chain containing a variable region and a constant region (Fig. 4.2). The four chains are assembled to form a Y-shaped molecule. Each light chain is attached to one heavy chain, and the two heavy chains are attached to each other, all by disulfide bonds. A light chain is made up of one V and one C domain, and a heavy chain has one V and three or

four C domains. Each domain folds into a characteristic three-dimensional shape, called the immunoglobulin (Ig) domain (see Fig. 4.2D). An Ig domain consists of two layers of a β-pleated sheet held together by a disulfide bridge. The adjacent strands of each β-sheet are connected by short, protruding α-helical loops; in the V regions of Ig molecules, three of these loops make up the three CDRs responsible for antigen recognition. Ig domains without hypervariable loops are present in many other proteins in the immune system, as well as outside the immune system, and most of these proteins are involved in responding to stimuli from the environment and from other cells. All of these proteins are said to be members of the immunoglobulin superfamily.

The antigen-binding site of an antibody is composed of the V regions of both the heavy chain and the light chain, and the core antibody structure contains two identical antigen binding sites (see Fig. 4.2). Each variable region of the heavy chain (called V_H) or of the light chain (called V_L) contains three hypervariable regions, or CDRs. Of these three, the greatest variability is in CDR3, which is located at the junction of the V and C regions. As may be predicted from this variability, CDR3 is also the portion of the Ig molecule that contributes most to antigen binding.

Functionally distinct portions of antibody molecules were first identified based on proteolysis, which generated fragments that were composed of different parts of antibody proteins. The fragment of an antibody that contains a whole light chain (with its single V and C domains) attached to the V and first C domains of a heavy chain is required for antigen recognition and is therefore called the **Fab** (fragment, antigen-binding) region. The remaining heavy-chain C domains make up the **Fc** (fragment, crystalline) region; because this fragment is identical in all antibody molecules of a particular type, it tends to crystallize in solution. In each Ig molecule, there are two identical Fab regions that bind antigen attached to one Fc region that is responsible for most of the biologic activity and effector functions of the antibodies. (As discussed later, some types of antibodies exist as multimers of two or five Ig molecules attached to one another.) Linking the Fab and Fc regions of most antibody molecules is a flexible portion called the hinge region. The hinge allows the two antigen-binding Fab regions of each antibody molecule to move independent of each other, enabling them to simultaneously bind antigen epitopes that are separated from one another by varying distances.

A Secreted IgG

Heavy chain

Antigen-binding site

N

N

VH N

N

VL

CH1

CL

Light chain

C

C

Hinge

Fab region

Fc receptor/complement binding sites

CH2

Fc region

CH3

Tail piece C C

Disulfide bond S–S   Ig domain

B Membrane IgM

Antigen-binding site

N

N

N

VH N

N

CH1

VL

CL

CH2

CH3

CH4

Plasma membrane of B cells

C C

C Crystal structure of secreted IgG

VL

CL

VH

CH1

CH2

CH3

D

N

Complementarity determining region (CDR) loops

1

7

2

6

5

3 4

3b

C

Fig. 4.2 Structure of antibodies. Schematic diagrams of **A,** a secreted immunoglobulin G *(IgG)* molecule, and **B,** a molecule of a membrane-bound form of IgM, illustrating the domains of the heavy and light chains and the regions of the proteins that participate in antigen recognition and effector functions. N and C refer to the amino-terminal and carboxy-terminal ends of the polypeptide chains, respectively. **C,** The crystal structure of a secreted IgG molecule illustrates the domains and their spatial orientation; the heavy chains are colored *blue* and *red,* the light chains are *green,* and carbohydrates are *gray.* **D,** The ribbon diagram of the Ig V domain shows the basic β-pleated sheet structure and the projecting loops that form the three CDRs. *CDR,* Complementarity-determining region. (**C,** Courtesy Dr. Alex McPherson, University of California, Irvine, CA.)

The C-terminal end of the heavy chain may be anchored in the plasma membrane, as seen in BCRs, or it may terminate in a tail piece that lacks the membrane anchor so that the antibody is produced as a secreted protein. Light chains in Ig molecules are not directly attached to cell membranes.

There are five types of Ig heavy chains, called μ, δ, γ, ε, and α, which differ in their C regions; in humans, there are four subtypes of γ chain, called γ1, γ2, γ3, γ4, and two of the α chain, called α1 and α2. Antibodies that contain different heavy chains belong to different **classes**, or **isotypes**, and are named according to their heavy chains (IgM, IgD, IgG, IgE, and IgA). Each isotype has distinct physical and biologic properties and effector functions (Fig. 4.3). The IgG subtypes also differ from one another in functional properties, but the IgA subtypes do not. The antigen receptors of naive B lymphocytes, which are mature B cells that have not encountered antigen, are membrane-bound IgM and IgD. After stimulation by antigen and helper T lymphocytes, the antigen-specific B lymphocyte clone may expand and differentiate into progeny that secrete antibodies. Some of the progeny of IgM and IgD expressing B cells may secrete IgM, and other progeny of the same B cells may produce antibodies of other heavy-chain classes. This change in Ig isotype production is called **heavy-chain class** (or **isotype**) **switching**; its mechanism and importance are discussed in Chapter 7.

The two types of light chains, called κ and λ, differ in their C regions. Each antibody has only κ or λ light chains, but not both, and all the antibodies made by any B cell have the same type of light chain. Each type of light chain may complex with any type of heavy chain in an antibody molecule. The light-chain class (κ or λ) also remains fixed throughout the life of each B cell clone, regardless of whether or not heavy-chain class switching has occurred. The function of light chains is to form the antigen-binding surface of antibodies, along with the heavy chains; light chains do not participate in effector functions, except binding and neutralizing microbes and toxins.

Binding of Antigens to Antibodies

Antibodies are capable of binding a wide variety of antigens, including macromolecules and small chemicals. The reason for this is that the antigen-binding CDR loops of antibody molecules can either come together to form clefts capable of accommodating small molecules or form more extended surfaces capable of accommodating larger molecules (Fig. 4.4). Antibodies bind to antigens by reversible, noncovalent

interactions, including hydrogen bonds, hydrophobic interactions, and charge-based interactions. The parts of antigens that are recognized by antibodies are called **epitopes**, or determinants. Some epitopes of protein antigens may be a contiguous stretch of amino acids in the primary structure of the protein; these are called linear epitopes. Sometimes, amino acids that are not next to one another in the primary structure may be brought into proximity when the protein folds, forming a distinct shape that is recognized by an antibody; such determinants are called conformational epitopes.

The strength with which one antigen-binding site of an antibody binds to one epitope of an antigen is called the **affinity** of the interaction. Affinity often is expressed as the dissociation constant (K_d), which is the molar concentration of an antigen required to occupy half the available antibody molecules in a solution; the lower the K_d, the higher the affinity. Most antibodies produced in a primary immune response have a K_d in the range of 10^{-6} to 10^{-9} M, but with repeated stimulation (e.g., in a secondary immune response), the affinity increases to a K_d of 10^{-8} to 10^{-11} M. This increase in antigen-binding strength is called **affinity maturation** (see Chapter 7).

Each IgG, IgD, and IgE antibody molecule has two antigen-binding sites. Secreted IgA is a dimer of two linked IgA molecules and therefore has four antigen-binding sites, and secreted IgM is a pentamer, with 10 antigen-binding sites. Therefore, each antibody molecule can bind 2 to 10 epitopes of an antigen, or epitopes on two or more neighboring antigens. The total strength of binding is much greater than the affinity of a single antigen-antibody bond and is called the **avidity** of the interaction. Antibodies produced against one antigen may bind other, structurally similar antigens. Such binding to similar epitopes is called a **cross-reaction**.

In B lymphocytes, membrane-bound Ig molecules are noncovalently associated with two other proteins, called Igα and Igβ; these latter proteins combine with the membrane Ig to make up the BCR complex. When the BCR recognizes antigen, Igα and Igβ transmit signals to the interior of the B cell that initiate the process of B cell activation. These and other signals in humoral immune responses are discussed in Chapter 7.

Monoclonal Antibodies

The realization that one clone of B cells makes an antibody of only one specificity has been exploited to produce **monoclonal antibodies**, one of the most important

Isotype of antibody	Subtypes (H chain)	Plasma concentration (mg/ml)	Plasma half-life (days)	Secreted form	Functions
IgA	IgA1,2 (α1 or α2)	3.5	6	Mainly dimer, also monomer, trimer	Mucosal immunity
IgD	None (δ)	Trace	3	Monomer	Naive B cell antigen receptor
IgE	None (ε)	0.05	2	Monomer	Defense against helminthic parasites, immediate hypersensitivity
IgG	IgG1-4 (γ1, γ2, γ3 or γ4)	13.5	23	Monomer	Opsonization, complement activation, antibody-dependent cell-mediated cytotoxicity, neonatal immunity, feedback inhibition of B cells
IgM	None (μ)	1.5	5	Pentamer	Naive B cell antigen receptor (monomeric form), complement activation

Fig. 4.3 Features of the major isotypes (classes) of antibodies. This figure summarizes some important features of the major antibody isotypes of humans. Isotypes are classified on the basis of their heavy (H) chains; each isotype may contain either κ or λ light chain. The schematic diagrams illustrate the distinct shapes of the secreted forms of these antibodies. Note that IgA consists of two subclasses, called IgA1 and IgA2, and IgG consists of four subclasses, called IgG1, IgG2, IgG3, and IgG4. Most of the opsonizing and complement fixation functions of IgG are attributable to IgG1 and IgG3. The domains of the heavy chains in each isotype are labeled. The plasma concentrations and half-lives are average values in normal individuals. Ig, Immunoglobulin.

Fig. 4.4 Binding of an antigen by an antibody. This model of a protein antigen bound to an antibody molecule shows how the antigen-binding site can accommodate soluble macromolecules in their native (folded) conformation. The heavy chains of the antibody are *red*, the light chains are *yellow*, and the antigens are *blue*. (Courtesy Dr. Dan Vaughn, Cold Spring Harbor Laboratory, Cold Spring Harbor, NY.)

technical advances in immunology, with far-reaching implications for clinical medicine and research. To produce monoclonal antibodies, B cells, which have a short life span in vitro, are obtained from an animal immunized with an antigen and fused in vitro with myeloma cells (tumors of plasma cells), which can be propagated indefinitely in tissue culture (Fig. 4.5). The myeloma cell line lacks a specific enzyme, as a result of which these cells cannot grow in the presence of a certain toxic drug; fused cells, containing both myeloma and normal B cell nuclei, however, do grow in the presence of this drug because the normal B cells provide the missing enzyme. Thus, by fusing the two cell populations and culturing them with the drug, it is possible to grow out fused cells that are hybrids of the B cells and the myeloma, and are called **hybridomas**. These hybridoma cells produce antibodies, like normal B cells, but grow continuously, having acquired the immortal property of the myeloma tumor. From a population of hybridomas, one can select and expand individual cells that secrete the antibody of desired specificity; such antibodies, derived from a single B cell clone, are homogeneous monoclonal antibodies. Monoclonal antibodies against virtually any epitope on any antigen can be produced using this technology.

Most monoclonal antibodies to molecules of interest are made by fusing cells from mice immunized with that antigen with mouse myelomas. Such mouse monoclonal antibodies cannot be injected repeatedly into human subjects, because the human immune system sees the mouse

Ig as foreign and mounts an immune response against the injected antibodies. This problem has been partially overcome by genetic engineering approaches that retain the antigen-binding V regions of the mouse monoclonal antibody and replace the rest of the antibody with human Ig; such humanized antibodies are less immunogenic and more suitable for administration to people. More recently, monoclonal antibodies have been generated by using recombinant DNA technology to clone the DNA encoding human antibodies of desired specificity. Another approach is to replace the Ig genes of mice with human antibody genes and then immunize these mice with an antigen to produce specific human antibodies. Monoclonal antibodies are now in widespread use as therapeutic agents and diagnostic reagents for many diseases in humans (Fig. 4.6).

T Cell Receptors for Antigens

The TCR, which recognizes peptide antigens displayed by MHC molecules, is a membrane-bound heterodimeric protein composed of an α chain and a β chain, each chain containing one variable (V) region and one constant (C) region (Fig. 4.7). The V and C regions are homologous to immunoglobulin V and C regions. In the V region of each TCR chain, there are three hypervariable, or complementarity-determining, regions, each corresponding to a loop in the V domain. As in antibodies, CDR3 is the most variable among different TCRs.

Antigen Recognition by the T Cell Receptor

Both the α chain and the β chain of the TCR participate in specific recognition of MHC molecules and bound peptides (Fig. 4.8). One of the features of T cell antigen recognition that has emerged from x-ray crystallographic analyses of TCRs bound to MHC-peptide complexes is that each TCR interacts with as few as one to three amino acid residues of the MHC-associated peptide, and also interacts with the MHC molecule presenting the peptide.

The TCR recognizes antigen, but as with membrane Ig on B cells, it is incapable of transmitting signals to the T cell on its own. Associated with the TCR is a group of proteins, called the CD3 and ζ proteins, which together with the TCR make up the TCR complex (see Fig. 4.1). The CD3 and ζ chains are crucial for the initiation of signaling when the TCR recognizes antigen. In addition, T cell activation requires engagement of the coreceptor molecule CD4 or CD8, which recognize

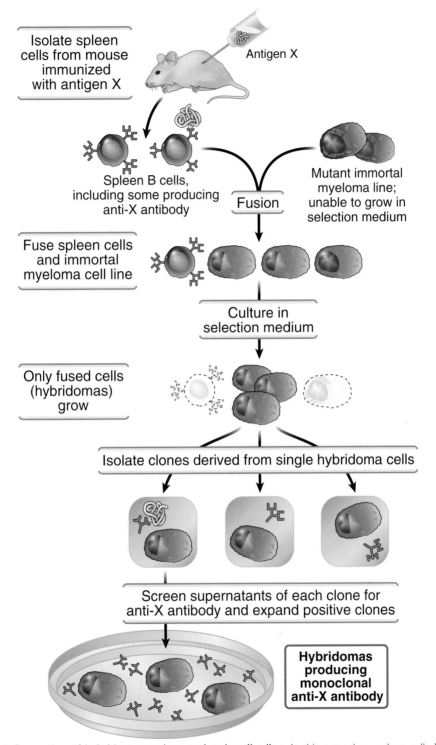

Fig. 4.5 Generation of hybridomas and monoclonal antibodies. In this procedure, spleen cells from a mouse that has been immunized with a known antigen are fused with an enzyme-deficient myeloma cell line that does not secrete its own immunoglobulins. The fused cells are then placed in a selection medium that permits the survival of only immortalized hybrids; the normal B cells provide the enzyme that the myeloma lacks, and unfused B cells cannot survive indefinitely. These hybrid cells are then grown as single-cell clones and tested for the secretion of antibody of the desired specificity. The clone producing this antibody is expanded and becomes a source of the monoclonal antibody.

Inflammatory (immunological) diseases

Target	Effect	Diseases
CD20	Depletion of B cells	Rheumatoid arthritis, multiple sclerosis, other autoimmune diseases; B cell lymphoma
IgE	Blocking IgE function	Allergy-related asthma
IL-6 receptor	Blocking inflammation	Rheumatoid arthritis
TNF	Blocking inflammation	Rheumatoid arthritis, Crohn disease, psoriasis

Cancer

Target	Effect	Diseases
CD52	Depletion of lymphocytes	Chronic lymphocytic leukemia
CTLA-4	Activation of T cells	Melanoma
EGFR	Growth inhibition of epithelial tumors	Colorectal, lung, and head and neck cancers
HER2/Neu	Inhibition of EGF signaling; depletion of tumor cells	Breast cancer
PD-1	Activation of effector T cells	Many tumors
PD-L1	Activation of effector T cells	Many tumors
VEGF	Blocking tumor angiogenesis	Breast cancer, colon cancer, age-related macular degeneration

Other diseases

Target	Effect	Diseases
Glycoprotein IIb/IIIa	Inhibition of platelet aggregation	Cardiovascular disease

Fig. 4.6 Selected monoclonal antibodies in clinical use. The figure lists some of the monoclonal antibodies that are approved for the treatment of various types of diseases.

nonpolymorphic portions of MHC molecules. The functions of these TCR-associated proteins and coreceptors are discussed in Chapter 5.

Antigen recognition by B and T lymphocyte receptors differs in important ways (Fig. 4.9). Antibodies can bind many different types of chemical structures, often with high affinities, which is why antibodies can bind to and neutralize many different microbes and toxins that may be present at low concentrations in the circulation or in the lumens of mucosal organs. TCRs only recognize peptide-MHC complexes and bind these

with relatively low affinity, which may be why the binding of T cells to APCs has to be strengthened by additional cell surface adhesion molecules (see Chapter 5). The three-dimensional structure of the TCR is similar to that of the Fab region of an Ig molecule. In contrast to membrane antibodies, in which only the heavy chain is membrane-anchored, both TCR chains are anchored in the plasma membrane. TCRs are not produced in a secreted form and do not undergo isotype switching or affinity maturation during the life of a T cell.

About 5% to 10% of T cells in the body express receptors composed of gamma (γ) and delta (δ) chains.

Fig. 4.7 Structure of the T cell antigen receptor (TCR). The schematic diagram of the αβ TCR *(left)* shows the domains of a TCR specific for a peptide-MHC complex. The antigen-binding portion of the TCR is formed by the V domains of the α and β chains. *N* and *C* refer to the amino-terminal and carboxy-terminal ends of the polypeptides. The ribbon diagram *(right)* shows the structure of the extracellular portion of a TCR as revealed by x-ray crystallography. *Ig,* Immunoglobulin; *MHC,* major histocompatibility complex. (From Bjorkman PJ: MHC restriction in three dimensions: a view of T cell receptor/ligand interactions, *Cell* 89:167–170, 1997. Copyright Cell Press; with permission.)

These receptors are structurally similar to the αβ TCR but have very different specificities. The γδ TCR may recognize a variety of protein and nonprotein antigens, usually not displayed by classical MHC molecules. T cells expressing γδ TCRs are abundant in epithelia. This observation suggests that γδ T cells recognize microbes usually encountered at epithelial surfaces, but neither the specificity nor the function of these T cells is well established. Another subpopulation of T cells, comprising less than 5% of all T cells, express αβ TCRs and surface molecules found on natural killer cells, and are therefore called natural killer T cells (NK-T cells). NK-T cells express αβ TCRs with limited diversity, and they recognize lipid antigens displayed by nonpolymorphic class I MHC–like molecules called CD1. A third subset of T cells called mucosal associated invariant T (MAIT) cells also express αβ TCRs with limited diversity, some of which are specific for bacterially derived vitamin B metabolites bound to an MHC-like protein called MR1. MAIT cells account for only about 5% of blood T cells, but up to 20%–40% of human liver T cells. The physiologic functions of NK-T cells and MAIT cells also are not well understood.

DEVELOPMENT OF B AND T LYMPHOCYTES

Now that we have discussed the structure of antigen receptors of B and T lymphocytes and how these receptors recognize antigens, the next question is how the enormous diversity of these receptors is generated. As the clonal selection hypothesis predicted, there are many clones of lymphocytes with distinct specificities, perhaps as many as 10^7–10^9, and these clones arise before an encounter with antigen. There are not enough genes in the human genome for every possible receptor to be encoded by a different gene. In fact, the immune system

Fig. 4.8 Recognition of peptide-MHC complex by a T cell antigen receptor. This ribbon diagram is drawn from the crystal structure of the extracellular portion of a peptide-MHC complex bound to a TCR that is specific for the peptide displayed by the MHC molecule. The peptide can be seen attached to the cleft at the top of the MHC molecule, and one residue of the peptide contacts the V region of a TCR. The structure of MHC molecules and their function as peptide display proteins are described in Chapter 3. *MHC,* Major histocompatibility complex; *TCR,* T cell receptor; β_2m, β_2-microglobulin. (From Bjorkman PJ: MHC restriction in three dimensions: a view of T cell receptor/ligand interactions, *Cell* 89:167–170, 1997. Copyright Cell Press; with permission.)

has developed mechanisms for generating extremely diverse antigen receptors from a limited number of inherited genes, and the generation of diverse receptors is intimately linked to the process of B and T lymphocyte maturation.

The process of lymphocyte maturation first generates a very large number of cells, each with a different antigen receptor, and then preserves the cells with useful receptors. The generation of millions of receptors is a molecular process that cannot be influenced by what the receptors recognize, because recognition can only occur after receptor generation and expression. Once these antigen receptors are expressed on developing lymphocytes, selection processes come into play that promote the survival of cells with receptors that can recognize antigens, such as microbial antigens, and eliminate cells that cannot recognize any antigens or

recognize self antigens well enough to pose danger of causing autoimmune disease. We discuss each of these events next.

Lymphocyte Development

The development of lymphocytes from bone marrow stem cells involves commitment of hematopoietic progenitors to the B or T cell lineage, the proliferation of these progenitors, the rearrangement and expression of antigen receptor genes, and selection events to preserve and expand cells that express potentially useful antigen receptors (Fig. 4.10). These steps are common to B and T lymphocytes, even though B lymphocytes mature in the bone marrow and T lymphocytes mature in the thymus. Each of the processes that occurs during lymphocyte maturation plays a special role in the generation of the lymphocyte repertoire.

- The maturation of common lymphoid progenitors in the bone marrow results in commitment to the B cell or T cell lineage. This commitment is associated with the activation of several lineage-specific transcription factors and increased accessibility of Ig and TCR genes to the gene recombination machinery, described later.
- Developing lymphocytes undergo proliferation at several stages during their maturation. Proliferation of developing lymphocytes is necessary to ensure that an adequate number of cells will be available to express antigen receptors and mature into functionally competent lymphocytes. Survival and proliferation of the earliest lymphocyte precursors are stimulated mainly by growth factors that are produced by stromal cells in the bone marrow and the thymus. In humans, IL-7 maintains and expands the number of T lymphocyte progenitors before they express antigen receptors. The growth factors required for expansion of human B cell progenitors are not defined. This proliferative expansion generates a large pool of cells in which diverse antigen receptors may be produced. Even greater proliferation of the B and T cell lineages occurs after the developing lymphocytes have completed their first antigen receptor gene rearrangement and assembled a so-called preantigen receptor (described later). This step is a quality control checkpoint in lymphocyte development that ensures preservation of cells with functional receptors.
- Lymphocytes are selected at multiple steps during their maturation to preserve useful specificities. Selection

Feature	Antigen-binding molecule	
	Immunoglobulin (Ig)	T cell receptor (TCR)
Antigen binding	Made up of three CDRs in V_H and three CDRs in V_L	Made up of three CDRs in $V\alpha$ and three CDRs in $V\beta$
Changes in constant regions	Heavy-chain class switching and change from membrane to secretory Ig	None
Affinity of antigen binding	K_d 10^{-7}-10^{-11} M; average affinity of Igs increases during immune responses to protein antigens	K_d 10^{-5}-10^{-7} M; No change during immune responses
On-rate and off-rate	Rapid on-rate, variable off-rate	Slow on-rate, slow off-rate

Fig. 4.9 Features of antigen recognition by immunoglobulins and T cell antigen receptors. The important similarities and differences of Ig and TCR molecules, the antigen receptors of B and T lymphocytes, respectively.

is based on the expression of intact antigen receptor components and what they recognize. As discussed later, many attempts to generate antigen receptors fail because of errors during the gene recombination process. Therefore, checkpoints are needed at which only cells that can express functional components of antigen receptors are selected to survive and proliferate. Prelymphocytes and immature lymphocytes that fail to express antigen receptor proteins die by apoptosis (see Fig. 4.10). The gene rearrangements in the developing lymphocytes randomly generate antigen receptors with highly diverse specificities. Some of these may be incapable of recognizing antigens in the individual—for instance, if the TCR cannot recognize MHC alleles present in the individual. In order to preserve the T cells that will be functional, immature T cells are selected to survive only if they have some affinity for MHC molecules in the thymus. This

process, called positive selection, ensures that cells that complete maturation will be capable of recognizing microbial peptides displayed by the same MHC molecules on APCs (which are the only MHC molecules these cells can normally encounter). Other antigen receptors may strongly recognize certain peptides of self proteins bound to self MHC, or strongly recognize self MHC regardless of the peptide displayed. Another selection process is needed to eliminate these potentially dangerous lymphocytes and prevent the development of autoimmune responses. The elimination of strongly self-reactive B and T lymphocytes is called negative selection.

The processes of B and T lymphocyte maturation and selection share some important features but also differ in many respects. We start with the central event that is common to both lineages: the recombination and expression of antigen receptor genes.

Fig. 4.10 Steps in maturation of lymphocytes. During their maturation, B and T lymphocytes go through cycles of proliferation and expression of antigen receptor proteins by gene recombination. Cells that fail to express intact, functional receptors die by apoptosis, because they do not receive the necessary survival signals. At the end of the process, the cells undergo positive and negative selection. The lymphocytes shown may be B or T cells.

Production of Diverse Antigen Receptors

The formation of functional genes that encode B and T lymphocyte antigen receptors is initiated by somatic recombination of gene segments that code for the variable regions of the receptors, and diversity is generated during this process.

Inherited Antigen Receptor Genes

Hematopoietic stem cells in the bone marrow and early lymphoid progenitors contain Ig and TCR genes in their inherited, or germline, configuration. In this configuration, Ig heavy-chain and light-chain loci and the TCR α chain and β chain loci each contain multiple variable region (V) gene segments, numbering about 30 to 45, and one or a few constant region (C) genes (Fig. 4.11). Between the V and C gene segments are groups of several short coding sequences called diversity (D) and joining (J) gene segments. (All antigen receptor gene loci contain V, J, and C gene segments, but only the Ig heavy chain and TCR β chain loci also contain D gene segments.) These separated gene segments cannot code for functional antigen receptor proteins, so they have to be brought together as lymphocytes mature.

Somatic Recombination and Expression of Antigen Receptor Genes

The commitment of a lymphocyte progenitor to become a B lymphocyte is associated with the recombination of randomly selected gene segments in the Ig heavy-chain locus—first one D gene segment with one J segment to form a fused DJ complex, followed by the rearrangement of a V segment to the fused DJ complex (Fig. 4.12).

Fig. 4.11 Germline organization of antigen receptor gene loci. In the germline, inherited antigen receptor gene loci contain coding segments (exons, shown as colored blocks of various sizes) that are separated by segments that are not expressed (introns, shown as *gray* sections). Each immunoglobulin (*Ig*) heavy-chain constant (*C*) region and T cell receptor (*TCR*) C region consists of multiple exons, which are not shown, that encode the domains of the C regions; the organization of the $C\mu$ exons in the Ig heavy-chain locus is shown as an example. The diagrams illustrate the antigen receptor gene loci in humans; the basic organization is the same in all species, although the precise order and number of gene segments may vary. The numbers of V, D, and J gene segments are estimates of functional gene segments (those that can code for proteins). The sizes of the segments and the distances between them are not drawn to scale. *D,* Diversity; *J,* joining; *L,* leader sequence (a small stretch of nucleotides that encodes a peptide that guides proteins through the endoplasmic reticulum and is cleaved from the mature proteins); *V,* variable.

Thus, the committed but still-developing B cell now has a recombined VDJ exon in the heavy-chain locus. This gene is transcribed, and in the primary RNA transcript, the VDJ exon is spliced to the C-region exons of the μ chain, the most 5′ C region, to form a complete μ messenger RNA (mRNA). The μ mRNA is translated to produce the μ heavy chain, which is the first Ig protein synthesized during B cell maturation.

Fig. 4.12 Recombination and expression of immunoglobulin (Ig) genes. The expression of an Ig heavy chain involves two gene recombination events (D-J joining, followed by joining of a V region to the DJ complex, with deletion of intervening gene segments). The recombined gene is transcribed, and the VDJ complex is spliced onto the C region exons of the first heavy-chain RNA (which is μ), to give rise to the μ messenger RNA (mRNA). The mRNA is translated to produce the μ heavy-chain protein. The recombination of other antigen receptor genes—that is, the Ig light chain and the T cell receptor (TCR) α and β chains—follows essentially the same sequence, except that in loci lacking D segments (Ig light chains and TCR α), a V gene recombines directly with a J gene segment.

Essentially the same sequence of DNA recombination and RNA splicing leads to production of a light chain in B cells, except that the light-chain loci lack D segments, so a V region exon recombines directly with a J segment. The rearrangement of TCR α chain and β chain genes in T lymphocytes is similar to that of Ig L and H chains, respectively.

Mechanisms of V(D)J Recombination

The somatic recombination of V and J, or of V, D, and J, gene segments is mediated by a lymphoid-specific enzyme, the VDJ recombinase, and additional enzymes, most of which are not lymphocyte specific and are involved in repair of double-stranded DNA breaks introduced by the recombinase. The VDJ recombinase is composed of the recombination-activating gene 1 and 2 (RAG-1 and RAG-2) proteins. It recognizes DNA sequences that flank all antigen receptor V, D, and J gene segments. As a result of this recognition, the recombinase brings two Ig or TCR gene segments close together and cleaves the DNA at specific sites. The DNA breaks are then repaired by ligases, producing a full-length recombined VJ or VDJ exon without the intervening DNA segments (see Fig. 4.12). The VDJ recombinase is expressed only in immature B and T lymphocytes. Although the same enzyme can mediate recombination of all Ig and TCR genes, intact Ig heavy-chain and light-chain genes are rearranged and expressed only in B cells, and TCR α and β genes are rearranged and expressed only in T cells. The lineage specificity of receptor gene rearrangement appears to be linked to the expression of lineage-specific transcription factors. In B cells, B lineage-specific transcription factors "open" the Ig gene locus at the chromatin level but not the TCR locus, whereas in developing T cells, transcriptional regulators help open the TCR locus but not the Ig locus. The "open" loci are the ones that are accessible to the recombinase.

Generation of Ig and TCR Diversity

Diversity of antigen receptors is produced by the use of different combinations of V, D, and J gene segments in different clones of lymphocytes (called combinatorial diversity) and even more by changes in nucleotide sequences introduced at the junctions of the recombining V, D, and J gene segments (called junctional diversity; Fig. 4.13). Combinatorial diversity is limited by the number of available V, D, and J gene segments, but junctional diversity is almost unlimited. Junctional diversity is produced by three mechanisms, which generate more sequences than are present in the germline genes:

- Exonucleases may remove nucleotides from V, D, and J gene segments at the sites of recombination.
- A lymphocyte-specific enzyme called terminal deoxyribonucleotidyl transferase (TdT) catalyzes the random addition of nucleotides that are not part of germline genes to the junctions between V and D segments and D and J segments, forming so-called N regions.
- During an intermediate stage in the process of V(D)J recombination, the two broken strands of the DNA at each end of the cut DNA form hairpin loops. As a first step in the repair process, the loops are asymmetrically

cut, forming overhanging DNA sequences. These overhangs have to be filled in with new nucleotides, which are called P-nucleotides, introducing even more variability at the sites of recombination.

As a result of these mechanisms, the nucleotide sequence at the site of V(D)J recombination in antibody or TCR genes in one clone of lymphocytes differs from the sequence at the V(D)J site of antibody or TCR molecules made by every other clone. These junctional sequences and the D and J segments encode the amino acids of the CDR3 loop, mentioned earlier as the most variable of the CDRs and the most important for antigen recognition. Thus, junctional diversity maximizes the variability in the antigen-recognizing portions of antibodies and TCRs. In the process of creating junctional diversity, many genes may be produced with out-of-frame sequences that cannot code for proteins and are therefore useless. This is the price the immune system pays for generating tremendous diversity. The risk of producing nonfunctional genes also is why the process of lymphocyte maturation contains checkpoints at which only cells with useful receptors are selected to survive.

The uniqueness of CDR3 sequences in every lymphocyte clone can be exploited to distinguish neoplastic and reactive proliferations of B and T lymphocytes. In tumors arising from these cells, all the cells of the tumor will have the same CDR3 (because they all arose from a single B or T cell clone), but in proliferations that are reactions to external stimuli, many CDR3 sequences will be present. The same principle can be used to define the magnitude of an immune response—measuring the number of CDR3 sequences present in a population before and during a response is an indicator of the amount of proliferative expansion of a B or T cell clone.

Maturation and Selection of B Lymphocytes

The maturation of B lymphocytes occurs mainly in the bone marrow (Fig. 4.14). Progenitors committed to the B cell lineage proliferate, giving rise to a large number of precursors of B cells, called **pro-B cells**. Subsequent maturation involves antigen receptor gene expression and selection.

Early Steps in B Cell Maturation

The Ig heavy-chain locus rearranges first, and only cells that are able to make an Ig μ heavy-chain protein are selected to survive and become pre-B cells.

	Immunoglobulin			T cell receptor	
	Heavy chain	κ	λ	α	β
Number of variable (V) gene segments	~45	35	30	45	48
Number of diversity (D) gene segments	23	0	0	0	2
Number of joining (J) gene segments	6	5	4	50	12

Mechanism

Combinatorial diversity:

Number of possible V(D)J combinations — Ig: ~3x10⁶   TCR: ~6x10⁶

Junctional diversity:

Removal of nucleotides   Addition of nucleotides (N-region or P-nucleotides)

Total potential repertoire with junctional diversity — Ig: ~10¹¹   TCR: ~10¹⁶

Fig. 4.13 Mechanisms of diversity in antigen receptors. Diversity in immunoglobulins and T cell receptors is produced by random combinations of V, D, and J gene segments, which is limited by the numbers of these segments and by removal and addition of nucleotides at the V-J or V-D-J junctions, which is almost unlimited. The numbers of gene segments refer to the average numbers of functional genes (which are known to be expressed as RNA or protein) in humans. Junctional diversity maximizes the variations in the CDR3 regions of the antigen receptor proteins, because CDR3 includes the junctions at the site of V-J and V-D-J recombination. The diversity is further enhanced by the juxtaposition of the V regions of the two types of chains in Ig or TCRs to form the complete antigen binding sites, and thus the total diversity is theoretically the product of the total diversity of each of the juxtaposed V regions. The estimated contributions of these mechanisms to the total possible numbers of distinct B and T cell antigen receptors are shown. Although the upper limit on the number of immunoglobulin *(Ig)* and TCR proteins that may be expressed is extremely large, each individual contains on the order of only 10⁷–10⁹ clones of B cells and T cells with distinct specificities and receptors; in other words, only a fraction of the potential repertoire may actually be expressed. (Modified from Davis MM, Bjorkman PJ: T-cell antigen receptor genes and T-cell recognition, *Nature* 334:395–402, 1988.)

	HSC	Pro-B	Large Pre-B	Small Pre-B	Immature B	Mature B
Ig H chain gene	Germline	D to J rearrangement	V to DJ rearrangement	Rearranged VDJ	Rearranged VDJ	Rearranged VDJ
Ig L chain gene	Germline	Germline	Germline	V to J rearrangement	Rearranged VJ	Rearranged VJ
Ig protein	None	None	pre-BCR	Intracellular μ	IgM	IgM, IgD

Fig. 4.14 Steps in the maturation and selection of B lymphocytes. The maturation of B lymphocytes proceeds through sequential steps, each of which is characterized by particular changes in immunoglobulin *(Ig)* gene expression and in the patterns of Ig protein expression. Pro-B cells begin to rearrange Ig heavy-chain genes and large pre-B cells are selected to survive and proliferate if they successfully rearrange an Ig heavy-chain gene and assemble a pre-BCR. The pre-BCR consists of a membrane-associated Ig μ protein attached to two other proteins called surrogate light chains because they take the place of the light chain in a complete Ig molecule. Small pre-B cells initiate Ig light-chain gene rearrangement, immature B cells assemble a complete membrane IgM receptor, and mature B cells coexpress IgD, with the same V regions and specificity as in the first Ig produced. *BCR,* B cell receptor; *HSC,* hematopoietic stem cell; *mRNA,* messenger RNA.

Pro-B cells cease to divide, and then any one D segment of the Ig heavy-chain locus is joined to a randomly selected J segment at the same locus. Next, a random upstream Ig V gene segment is recombined to the previously rearranged DJ unit in each pro-B cell. Given that junctional nucleotides are randomly added both when the D-J joint is made and when a V segment fuses with a DJ unit, in the majority of cells, the number of junctional nucleotides will not add up to a multiple of three. Because three nucleotides code for one amino acid, only some pro-B cells will create junctions that allow a functional Ig heavy-chain protein to be made. The cells that successfully make functional heavy-chain gene rearrangements and synthesize the Ig heavy-chain μ protein are called pre-B cells. Pre-B cells are therefore defined by the presence of the Ig μ heavy-chain protein. As cells become pre-B cells, they express the μ protein on the cell surface in association with two other invariant proteins called surrogate light chains because they resemble light chains and associate with the μ heavy chain. The complex of μ chain and surrogate light chains associates with the Igα and Igβ signaling molecules to form the pre-B cell receptor (pre-BCR) complex.

Role of the Pre-BCR Complex in B Cell Maturation

The assembled pre-BCR serves essential functions in the maturation of B cells:

- Signals from the pre-BCR complex promote the survival and proliferation of B lineage cells that have made a productive rearrangement at the Ig H chain locus. This is the first checkpoint in B cell development, and it selects and expands the pre-B cells that express a functional μ heavy chain (which is an essential component of the pre-BCR and BCR). Pre-B cells that make out-of-frame (nonproductive) rearrangements at the heavy-chain locus fail to make the μ protein, cannot express a pre-BCR or receive pre-BCR signals, and die by programmed cell death (apoptosis). The pre-BCR signaling pathway includes a downstream tyrosine kinase called Btk, which is encoded on the X chromosome. Mutations in Btk in boys results in the failure of pre-B cells to survive and the subsequent absence of B cells. This disease is called **X-linked agammaglobulinemia**.

- The pre-BCR complex signals to shut off recombination of Ig heavy-chain genes on the second chromosome, so each B cell can express an Ig heavy chain from only one of the two inherited parental alleles.

This process is called allelic exclusion, and it helps ensure that each cell can only express a receptor of a single specificity.

- Signals from the pre-BCR complex shut off expression of the surrogate light-chain genes and open up the Ig κ light-chain locus making it available for recombination. The cells transiently stop dividing, and can express the μ protein only in the cytoplasm (and not on the cell surface) because they have no surrogate light-chain proteins or regular light-chain proteins. At this stage, these cells are called small pre-B cells.

- In small pre-B cells, V to J rearrangement of the κ light-chain gene is initiated, leading to production of the κ protein and the assembly of cell surface IgM. The cells at this next stage of differentiation are called immature B cells. The λ light chain is produced only if the rearranged κ chain locus fails to express a functional protein or if the κ chain generates a potentially harmful self-reactive receptor and has to be eliminated, by a process called receptor editing, described later.

In immature B cells, the BCR complex delivers signals that promote survival, thus preserving cells that express complete antigen receptors; this is the second checkpoint during B cell maturation. Signals from the antigen receptor also shut off production of the recombinase enzyme and further recombination at light-chain loci. As a result, each B cell produces either one κ or one λ light chain from one of the inherited parental alleles. The presence of two sets of light-chain genes in the genome simply increases the chance of completing successful gene recombination and receptor expression.

Completion of B Cell Maturation

Further maturation occurs after the immature B cells leave the bone marrow and enter the spleen. The final maturation step involves coexpression of IgD with IgM; this occurs because in any given B cell, the recombined heavy-chain VDJ unit may be spliced either to Cμ or Cδ exons in the primary RNA transcript, giving rise to μ or δ mRNA, respectively. We know that the ability of B cells to respond to antigens develops together with the coexpression of IgM and IgD, but why both classes of receptor are needed is not known. The IgM⁺IgD⁺ cell is the mature B cell, able to respond to antigen in peripheral lymphoid tissues.

Selection of Mature B Cells

Developing B cells are positively selected based mainly on expression of complete antigen receptors and not on the recognition specificity of these cells. (This is fundamentally different in maturing T cells, as discussed later.) The B cell repertoire is further shaped by negative selection. In this process, if an immature B cell binds an antigen in the bone marrow with high affinity, it may re-express the VDJ recombinase enzyme, undergo additional light-chain V-J recombination, generate a different light chain, and thus change the specificity of the antigen receptor, a process called **receptor editing** (see Chapter 9). Some B cells that encounter antigens in the bone marrow may die by apoptosis, also known as deletion. The antigens that developing B cells may recognize in the bone marrow are mostly self antigens that are abundantly expressed throughout the body (i.e., are ubiquitous), such as blood proteins, and membrane molecules common to all cells. Negative selection therefore eliminates potentially dangerous cells that can recognize and react against ubiquitous self antigens.

The process of Ig gene recombination is random and cannot be inherently biased toward recognition of microbes. However, the receptors produced are able to recognize the antigens of many, varied microbes that the immune system must defend against. The repertoire of B lymphocytes is selected positively for expression of functional receptors and selected negatively against strong recognition of self antigens. What is left after these selection processes is a large collection of mature B cells, which by chance include cells that are able to recognize almost any microbial antigen that may be encountered.

Subsets of Mature B Cells

Most mature B cells are called follicular B cells because they are found within lymph node and spleen follicles. Marginal-zone B cells, which are found at the margins of splenic follicles, develop from bone-marrow–derived hematopoietic stem cells, as do follicular B cells. B-1 lymphocytes, a distinct population found at mucosal sites and the peritoneal cavity, develop earlier from fetal-liver–derived hematopoietic stem cells. The role of these B cell subsets in humoral immunity is described in Chapter 7.

Maturation and Selection of T Lymphocytes

T cell progenitors migrate from the bone marrow to the thymus, where the entire process of maturation occurs (Fig. 4.15). The process of T lymphocyte maturation has some unique features, primarily related to the specificity of different subsets of T cells for peptides displayed by different classes of MHC molecules.

Fig. 4.15 Steps in the maturation and selection of major histocompatibility complex (MHC)–restricted T lymphocytes. The maturation of T lymphocytes in the thymus proceeds through sequential steps often defined by the expression of the CD4 and CD8 coreceptors. The T cell receptor *(TCR)* β chain is first expressed at the double-negative pre-T cell stage, and the complete T cell receptor is expressed in double-positive cells. The pre-TCR consists of the TCR β chain associated with a protein called pre-Tα. Maturation culminates in the development of CD4+ and CD8+ single-positive T cells. As with B cells, failure to express antigen receptors at any stage leads to death of the cells by apoptosis. Only class II MHC is shown for negative selection, but the same process eliminates self-reactive class I MHC–restricted CD8+ T cells.

Early Steps in T Cell Maturation

The least developed progenitors in the thymus are called **pro-T cells or double-negative T cells** because they do not express CD4 or CD8. These cells expand in number mainly under the influence of IL-7 produced in the thymus. TCR β gene recombination, mediated by the VDJ recombinase, occurs in some of these double-negative cells. (The γδ T cells undergo similar recombination involving TCR γ and δ loci, but they belong to a distinct lineage and are not discussed further.) If VDJ recombination is successful in one of the two inherited loci and a TCR β chain protein is synthesized, it is expressed on

the cell surface in association with an invariant protein called pre-Tα, to form the pre-TCR complex of **pre-T cells**. If the recombination in one of the two inherited loci is not successful, recombination will take place on the other locus. If that too fails and a complete TCR β chain is not produced in a pro-T cell, the cell dies.

The pre-TCR complex delivers intracellular signals once it is assembled, similar to the signals from the pre-BCR complex in developing B cells. These signals promote survival, proliferation, and TCR α gene recombination and inhibit VDJ recombination in the second β chain locus (allelic exclusion). Failure to express the α chain and the complete TCR again results in death of the cell. The surviving cells express the complete αβ TCR and both the CD4 and CD8 coreceptors; these cells are called **double-positive T cells**.

Selection of Mature T Cells

Different clones of double-positive T cells express different αβ TCRs. If the TCR of a T cell recognizes an MHC molecule in the thymus, which must be a self MHC molecule displaying a self peptide, and if the interaction is of low or moderate affinity, this T cell is selected to survive. T cells that do not recognize an MHC molecule in the thymus die by apoptosis; these T cells would not be useful because they would be incapable of seeing MHC-displayed cell-associated antigens in that individual. This preservation of self MHC–restricted (i.e., useful) T cells is the process of **positive selection**. During this process, T cells whose TCRs recognize class I MHC–peptide complexes preserve the expression of CD8, the coreceptor that binds to class I MHC, and lose expression of CD4, the coreceptor specific for class II MHC molecules. Conversely, if a T cell recognizes class II MHC–peptide complexes, this cell maintains expression of CD4 and loses expression of CD8. Thus, what emerges are **single-positive T cells** (or single-positive thymocytes), which are either CD8+ class I MHC restricted or CD4+ class II MHC restricted. During positive selection, the T cells also become committed to different functional fates: the CD8+ T cells will differentiate into CTLs on activation, and the CD4+ cells will differentiate into cytokine-producing helper T cells.

Immature, double-positive T cells whose receptors strongly recognize MHC-peptide complexes in the thymus undergo apoptosis. This is the process of **negative selection**, and it serves to eliminate T lymphocytes that could react in a harmful way against self proteins that are expressed in the thymus. If a T cell that recognizes a self peptide with high avidity were allowed to mature, recognition of the same self antigen in the periphery could lead to harmful immune responses against self tissues, so such a T cell must be eliminated. Some immature T cells that recognize self antigens in the thymus do not die but develop into regulatory T cells (see Chapter 9). Most of the proteins present in the thymus are self proteins, because foreign (microbial and tumor) antigens are typically captured and taken to secondary lymphoid organs. Some of these self proteins are present throughout the body, and others are proteins that are restricted to particular tissues but are expressed in thymic epithelial cells by special mechanisms, as discussed in Chapter 9 in the context of self-tolerance.

It may seem surprising that both positive selection and negative selection are mediated by recognition of the same set of self MHC–self peptide complexes in the thymus. The two factors that determine the choice between positive and negative selection are the affinity of the TCR and the concentration of the self antigen in the thymus. If a TCR strongly recognizes an abundant self antigen in the thymus, that T cell will be negatively selected, which makes sense because strong recognition of an abundant self antigen has the potential for causing autoimmunity. However, if a TCR recognizes a self peptide–self MHC complex weakly, that T cell will be positively selected because there is a reasonable chance the T cell will recognize a foreign peptide presented by self MHC strongly. This is the process that gives rise to the repertoire of functional T cells.

▮ SUMMARY

- In the adaptive immune system, the molecules responsible for specific recognition of antigens are antibodies and T cell antigen receptors.
- Antibodies (also called immunoglobulins) may be produced as membrane receptors of B lymphocytes and as proteins secreted by antigen-stimulated B cells that have differentiated into antibody-secreting plasma cells. Secreted antibodies are the effector molecules of humoral immunity, capable of neutralizing microbes and microbial toxins and eliminating them by activating various effector mechanisms.
- T cell receptors (TCRs) are membrane receptors and are not secreted.

- The core structure of antibodies consists of two identical heavy chains and two identical light chains, forming a disulfide-linked complex. Each chain consists of a variable (V) region, which is the portion that recognizes antigen, and a constant (C) region, which provides structural stability and, in heavy chains, performs the effector functions of antibodies. The V region of one heavy chain and of one light chain together form the antigen-binding site, and thus the core structure has two identical antigen-binding sites.
- T cell receptors consist of an α chain and a β chain. Each chain contains one V region and one C region, and both chains participate in the recognition of

antigens, which for most T cells are peptides displayed by MHC molecules.

- The V regions of immunoglobulin (Ig) and TCR molecules contain hypervariable segments, also called complementarity-determining regions (CDRs), which are the regions of contact with antigens.

- The genes that encode antigen receptors consist of multiple segments separated in the germline and brought together during maturation of lymphocytes. In B cells, the Ig gene segments undergo recombination as the cells mature in the bone marrow, and in T cells, the TCR gene segments undergo recombination during maturation in the thymus.

- Receptors of different specificities are generated in part by different combinations of V, D, and J gene segments. The process of recombination introduces variability in the nucleotide sequences at the sites of recombination by adding or removing nucleotides from the junctions. The result of this introduced variability is the development of a diverse repertoire of lymphocytes, in which clones of cells with different antigen specificities express receptors that differ in sequence and recognition, and most of the differences are concentrated at the regions of gene recombination.

- During their maturation, lymphocytes are selected to survive at several checkpoints; only cells with complete functional antigen receptors are preserved and expanded. In addition, T lymphocytes are positively selected to recognize peptide antigens displayed by self MHC molecules and to ensure that the recognition of the appropriate type of MHC molecule matches the coreceptor preserved.

- Immature lymphocytes that strongly recognize self antigens are negatively selected and prevented from completing their maturation, thus eliminating cells with the potential of reacting in harmful ways against self tissues.

REVIEW QUESTIONS

1. What are the functionally distinct domains (regions) of antibody and TCR molecules? What features of the amino acid sequences in these regions are important for their functions?

2. What are the differences in the types of antigens recognized by antibodies and TCRs?

3. What mechanisms contribute to the diversity of antibody and TCR molecules? Which of these mechanisms contributes the most to the diversity?

4. What are some of the checkpoints during lymphocyte maturation that ensure survival of the useful cells?

5. What is the phenomenon of negative selection, and what is its importance?

Answers to and discussion of the Review Questions are available at Student Consult.

5

T Cell–Mediated Immunity
Activation of T Lymphocytes

CHAPTER OUTLINE

T lymphocytes perform multiple functions in defending against infections by various kinds of microbes. A major role for T lymphocytes is in **cell-mediated immunity**, which provides defense against infections by microbes that live and reproduce inside host cells. In all viral and some bacterial, fungal, and protozoan infections, microbes may find a haven inside cells, from where they must be eliminated by cell-mediated immune responses (Fig. 5.1).

- Many microbes are ingested by phagocytes as part of the early defense mechanisms of innate immunity and are killed by microbicidal mechanisms that are largely limited to phagocytic vesicles (to protect the cells themselves from damage by these mechanisms). However, some of these microbes have evolved to resist the microbicidal activities of phagocytes and are able to survive, and even replicate, in the vesicles of phagocytes. In such infections, T cells stimulate the ability of macrophages to kill the ingested microbes.

- Some extracellular microbes, such as bacteria and fungi, are readily destroyed if they are phagocytosed, especially by neutrophils. Other extracellular pathogens, such as helminthic parasites, are destroyed by special types of leukocytes (eosinophils). In these infections, T cells provide defense by recruiting the leukocytes that destroy the microbes.

- Some microbes, notably viruses, are able to infect and replicate inside a wide variety of cells, and parts of the life cycles of the viruses take place in the cytosol and nucleus. These infected cells often do not possess intrinsic mechanisms for destroying the microbes, especially outside vesicles. Even some phagocytosed microbes within macrophages can escape into the cytosol and evade the microbicidal mechanisms of the vesicular compartment. T cells kill the infected cells, thus eliminating the reservoir of infection.

Other populations of T cells help B cells to produce antibodies as part of humoral immune responses (see Chapter 7). Although our emphasis in this chapter is on defense against infections, the principal physiologic function of the immune system, some T cells, especially

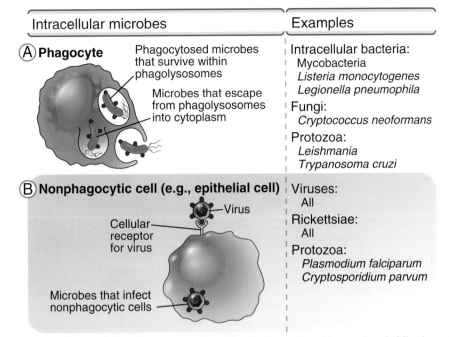

Fig. 5.1 Types of intracellular microbes combated by T cell–mediated immunity. **A**, Microbes may be ingested by phagocytes and may survive within vesicles (phagolysosomes) or escape into the cytosol, where they are not susceptible to the microbicidal mechanisms of the phagocytes. **B**, Viruses may infect many cell types, including nonphagocytic cells, and replicate in the nucleus and cytosol of the infected cells. Rickettsiae and some protozoa are obligate intracellular parasites that reside in nonphagocytic cells.

CD8+ T cells, also destroy cancerous cells. This role of T cells is discussed in Chapter 10.

Most of the functions of T lymphocytes—activation of phagocytes, killing of infected and tumor cells, and help for B cells—require that the T lymphocytes interact with other cells, which may be phagocytes, infected host cells, or B lymphocytes. Furthermore, the initiation of T cell responses requires that naive T cells recognize antigens displayed by dendritic cells, which capture antigens and concentrate them in lymphoid organs. Thus, T lymphocytes work by communicating with other cells. Recall that the specificity of T cells for peptides displayed by major histocompatibility complex (MHC) molecules ensures that the T cells can see and respond only to antigens associated with other host cells (see Chapters 3 and 4). This chapter discusses the way in which T lymphocytes are activated by recognition of cell-associated antigens and other stimuli. We address the following questions:

- What signals are needed to activate T lymphocytes, and what cellular receptors are used to sense and respond to these signals?

- How are the few naive T cells specific for any microbe converted into the large number of effector T cells that have specialized functions and the ability to eliminate diverse microbes?
- What molecules are produced by T lymphocytes that mediate their communications with other cells, such as macrophages, B lymphocytes, and other leukocytes?

After describing here how T cells recognize and respond to the antigens of cell-associated microbes, in Chapter 6, we discuss how these T cells function to eliminate the microbes.

PHASES OF T CELL RESPONSES

Naive T lymphocytes recognize antigens in the peripheral (secondary) lymphoid organs, which initiates proliferation of the T cells and their differentiation into effector and memory cells, and the effector cells perform their functions when they are activated by the same antigens in any infected tissue (Fig. 5.2). Naive T cells express antigen receptors and coreceptors that function in recognizing cells harboring microbes, but naive

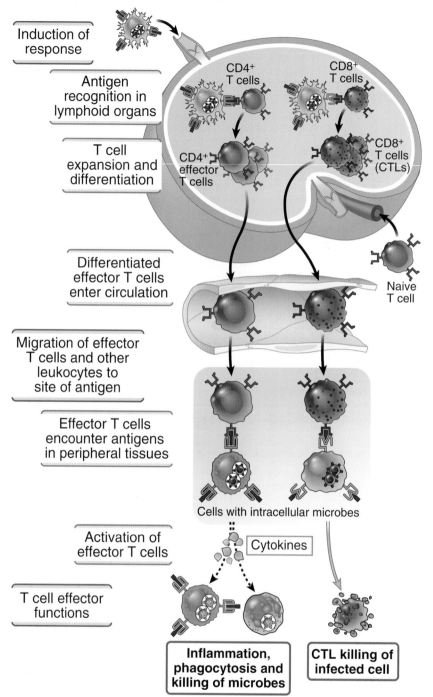

Induction of response

Antigen recognition in lymphoid organs

CD4+ T cells

CD8+ T cells

T cell expansion and differentiation

CD4+ effector T cells

CD8+ T cells (CTLs)

Naive T cell

Differentiated effector T cells enter circulation

Migration of effector T cells and other leukocytes to site of antigen

Effector T cells encounter antigens in peripheral tissues

Cells with intracellular microbes

Activation of effector T cells

Cytokines

T cell effector functions

Inflammation, phagocytosis and killing of microbes

CTL killing of infected cell

Fig. 5.2 Induction and effector phases of cell-mediated immunity. Induction of response: Naive CD4+ T cells and CD8+ T cells recognize peptides that are derived from protein antigens and presented by dendritic cells (DCs) in peripheral lymphoid organs. The T lymphocytes are stimulated to proliferate and differentiate into effector cells, many of which enter the circulation. Some of the activated CD4+ T cells remain in the lymph node, migrate into follicles, and help B cells to produce antibodies (shown in Fig. 5.13). Migration of effector T cells and other leukocytes to site of antigen: effector T cells and other leukocytes migrate through blood vessels in peripheral tissues by binding to endothelial cells that have been activated by cytokines produced in response to infection in these tissues. T cell effector functions: CD4+ T cells recruit and activate phagocytes to destroy microbes, and CD8+ cytotoxic T lymphocytes *(CTLs)* kill infected cells.

cells are incapable of performing the effector functions required for eliminating the microbes. Differentiated effector cells are capable of performing these functions, which they do at any site of infection. In this chapter, we focus on the initial responses of naive T cells to antigens. The development of effector T lymphocytes and their functions in cell-mediated immunity are described in Chapter 6 and the roles of helper T cells in antibody responses in Chapter 7.

The responses of naive T lymphocytes to cell-associated microbial antigens consist of a series of sequential steps that result in an increase in the number of antigen-specific T cells and the conversion of naive T cells to effector and memory cells (Fig. 5.3).

- One of the earliest responses is the secretion of **cytokines** required for growth and differentiation and increased expression of receptors for various cytokines. The cytokine interleukin-2 (IL-2), which is produced by antigen-activated T cells, stimulates proliferation of these cells, resulting in a rapid increase in the number of antigen-specific lymphocytes, a process called **clonal expansion.**
- The activated lymphocytes **differentiate,** resulting in the conversion of naive T cells into a population of **effector T cells,** which function to eliminate microbes.

- Many of the effector T cells leave the lymphoid organs, enter the circulation, and migrate to any site of infection, where they can eradicate the infection. Some activated T cells may remain in the lymph node, where they provide signals to B cells that promote antibody responses against the microbes.
- Some of the progeny of the T cells that have proliferated in response to antigen develop into **memory T cells,** which are long-lived, circulate or reside in tissues for years, and are ready to respond rapidly to subsequent exposure to the same microbe.
- As effector T cells eliminate the infectious agent, the stimuli that triggered T cell expansion and differentiation also are eliminated. As a result, most of the cells in the greatly expanded clones of antigen-specific effector lymphocytes die, returning the system to a resting state, with only memory cells remaining from the immune response.

This sequence of events is common to both CD4+ and CD8+ T lymphocytes, although there are important differences in the properties and effector functions of CD4+ and CD8+ cells, as discussed in Chapter 6.

Naive and effector T cells have different patterns of circulation and migration through tissues, which are critical for their different roles in immune responses.

Fig. 5.3 Steps in the activation of T lymphocytes. Naive T cells recognize major histocompatibility complex (MHC)-associated peptide antigens displayed on antigen-presenting cells and other signals (not shown). The T cells respond by producing interleukin-2 (IL-2) and expressing receptors for IL-2, leading to an autocrine pathway of cell proliferation. The result is expansion of the clone of T cells that are specific for the antigen. Some of the progeny differentiate into effector cells, which serve various functions in cell-mediated immunity, and memory cells, which survive for long periods. Other changes associated with activation, such as the expression of various surface molecules, are not shown. *APC,* Antigen-presenting cell; *CTL,* cytotoxic T lymphocyte; *IL-2R,* interleukin-2 receptor.

As discussed in previous chapters, naive T lymphocytes constantly recirculate through peripheral lymphoid organs searching for foreign protein antigens. The antigens of microbes are transported from the portals of entry of the microbes to the same regions of peripheral lymphoid organs through which naive T cells recirculate. In these organs, the antigens are processed and displayed by MHC molecules on dendritic cells, the antigen-presenting cells (APCs) that are the most efficient stimulators of naive T cells (see Chapter 3). When a T cell recognizes antigen, it is transiently arrested on the dendritic cell and it initiates an activation program. Activation results in proliferation and differentiation, and then the cells may leave the lymphoid organ and migrate preferentially to the inflamed tissue, the original source of the antigen. The control of this directed migration is discussed later in this chapter.

With this overview, we proceed to a description of the stimuli required for T cell activation and regulation. We then describe the biochemical signals that are generated by antigen recognition and the biologic responses of the lymphocytes.

ANTIGEN RECOGNITION AND COSTIMULATION

The initiation of T cell responses requires multiple receptors on the T cells recognizing their specific ligands on APCs (Fig. 5.4).
- The T cell receptor (TCR) recognizes MHC-associated peptide antigens.
- CD4 or CD8 coreceptors on the T cells bind to MHC molecules on the APC and work with the TCR complex to deliver activating signals.
- Adhesion molecules strengthen the binding of T cells to APCs.
- Molecules called costimulators, which are expressed on APCs after encounter with microbes, bind to costimulatory receptors on the naive T cells, thus promoting responses to infectious pathogens.
- Cytokines amplify the T cell response and direct it along various differentiation pathways.

The roles of these molecules in T cell responses to antigens are described next. Cytokines are discussed mainly in Chapter 6.

Recognition of Peptide-MHC Complexes

The TCR for antigen and the CD4 or CD8 coreceptor together recognize complexes of peptide antigens and MHC molecules on APCs, and this recognition provides the initiating, or first, signal for T cell activation (Fig. 5.5). The TCRs expressed on all CD4+ and CD8+ T cells consist of an α chain and a β chain, both of which participate in antigen recognition (see Fig. 4.7). (A small subset of T cells expresses TCRs composed of γ and δ chains, which do not recognize MHC-associated peptide antigens.) The TCR of a T cell specific for a foreign (e.g., microbial) peptide recognizes the displayed peptide and simultaneously recognizes residues of the MHC molecule located around the peptide-binding cleft. Every mature MHC-restricted T cell expresses either CD4 or CD8, both of which are called coreceptors because they bind to the same MHC molecules that the TCR binds and are required for initiation of signaling from the TCR complex. At the time when the TCR is recognizing the peptide-MHC complex, CD4 or CD8 binds the class II or class I MHC molecule, respectively, at a site separate from the peptide-binding cleft. As discussed in Chapter 3, when

Fig. 5.4 Receptors and ligands involved in T cell activation and inhibition. **A**, Major surface molecules of CD4+ T cells involved in the activation of these cells and their corresponding ligands on antigen-presenting cells. CD8+ T cells use most of the same molecules, except that the TCR recognizes peptide-class I MHC complexes, and the coreceptor is CD8, which recognizes class I MHC. CD3 is composed of three polypeptide chains, δ, ε, and γ, arranged in two pairs (δε and γε); we show CD3 as three chains. Immunoreceptor tyrosine-based activation motifs *(ITAMs)* are the regions of cytosolic tails of signaling proteins that are phosphorylated on tyrosine residues and become docking sites for other tyrosine kinases (see Fig. 5.10). Immunoreceptor tyrosine-based inhibitory motifs are the regions of signaling proteins that are sites for tyrosine phosphatases that counteract actions of ITAMs. **B**, Important properties of major surface molecules of T cells involved in functional responses. Cytokines and cytokine receptors are not listed here. The functions of most of these molecules are described in this chapter; the role of CTLA-4 and PD-1 in shutting off T cell responses is described in Chapter 9. LFA-1 is an integrin involved in leukocyte binding to endothelium and other cells. *APC*, Antigen-presenting cell; *ICAM-1*, intercellular adhesion molecule 1; *LFA-1*, leukocyte function–associated antigen 1; *MHC*, major histocompatibility complex; *PD-1*, programmed death-1; *TCR*, T cell receptor.

protein antigens are ingested by APCs from the extracellular milieu into vesicles, these antigens are processed into
peptides that are displayed by class II MHC molecules. In
contrast, protein antigens present in the cytosol are processed by proteasomes into peptides displayed by class I
MHC molecules. Thus, because of the specificity of the
coreceptors for different classes of MHC molecules, CD4+
and CD8+ T cells recognize peptides generated through
different protein processing pathways. The TCR and its
coreceptor need to be engaged simultaneously to initiate
the T cell response, and multiple TCRs likely need to be
triggered for T cell activation to occur. Once these conditions are achieved, the T cell begins its activation program.

**The biochemical signals that lead to T cell activa-
tion are triggered by a set of proteins linked to the
TCR that are part of the TCR complex and by the
CD4 or CD8 coreceptor** (see Fig. 5.5). In lymphocytes, antigen recognition and subsequent signaling are
performed by different sets of molecules. The TCR αβ

**Fig. 5.5 Antigen recognition and signal transduction during
T cell activation.** Different T cell molecules recognize antigen
and deliver biochemical signals to the interior of the cell as a
result of antigen recognition. The CD3 and ζ proteins are noncovalently attached to the T cell receptor *(TCR)* α and β chains
by interactions between charged amino acids in the transmembrane domains of these proteins (not shown). The figure illustrates a CD4+ T cell; the same interactions are involved in the
activation of CD8+ T cells, except that the coreceptor is CD8
and the TCR recognizes a peptide–class I MHC complex. *APC,*
Antigen-presenting cell; *ITAM,* immunoreceptor tyrosine-based
activation motifs; *MHC,* major histocompatibility complex.

heterodimer recognizes antigens, but it is not able to
transmit biochemical signals to the interior of the cell.
The TCR is noncovalently associated with a complex of
transmembrane signaling proteins including three CD3
proteins and a protein called the ζ chain. The TCR, CD3,
and ζ chain make up the TCR complex. Although the
α and β TCRs must vary among T cell clones in order
to recognize diverse antigens, the signaling functions of
TCRs are the same in all clones, and therefore the CD3
and ζ proteins are invariant among different T cells. The
mechanisms of signal transduction by these proteins of
the TCR complex are discussed later in the chapter.

T cells can also be activated by molecules that bind to
the TCRs of many or all clones of T cells, regardless of
the peptide-MHC specificity of the TCR. For instance,
some microbial toxins may bind to the TCRs of many
T cell clones and also bind to MHC class II molecules on
APCs without occupying the peptide-binding cleft. By
activating a large number of T cells, these toxins induce
excessive cytokine release and cause systemic inflammatory disease. They are called superantigens because, like
conventional antigens, they bind to MHC molecules and
to TCRs, but to many more than typical antigens do.

Role of Adhesion Molecules in T Cell Responses

**Adhesion molecules on T cells recognize their ligands
on APCs and stabilize the binding of the T cells to the
APCs.** Most TCRs bind the peptide-MHC complexes
for which they are specific with low affinity. To induce a
response, the binding of T cells to APCs must be stabilized
for a sufficiently long period to achieve the necessary signaling threshold. This stabilization function is performed
by adhesion molecules on the T cells that bind to ligands
expressed on APCs. The most important of these adhesion molecules belong to the family of heterodimeric
(two-chain) proteins called integrins. The major T cell
integrin involved in binding to APCs is leukocyte function–associated antigen 1 (LFA-1), whose ligand on APCs
is called intercellular adhesion molecule 1 (ICAM-1).

On resting naive T cells, which are cells that have not
previously recognized and been activated by antigen,
the LFA-1 integrin is in a low-affinity state. Antigen recognition by a T cell increases the affinity of that cell's
LFA-1. Therefore, once a T cell sees antigen, it increases
the strength of its binding to the APC presenting that
antigen, providing a positive feedback loop. Integrin-mediated adhesion is critical for the ability of T cells

to bind to APCs displaying microbial antigens. Integrins also play an important role in directing the migration of effector T cells and other leukocytes from the circulation to sites of infection. This process is described in Chapter 2 and later in this chapter.

Role of Costimulation in T Cell Activation

The full activation of T cells depends on the recognition of costimulators on APCs in addition to antigen (Fig. 5.6). We have previously referred to costimulators as second signals for T cell activation. The name costimulator derives from the fact that these molecules provide stimuli to T cells that function together with stimulation by antigen.

The best-defined costimulators for T cells are two homologous proteins called B7-1 (CD80) and B7-2 (CD86), both of which are expressed on APCs and whose expression is increased when the APCs encounter microbes. These B7 proteins are recognized by a receptor called CD28, which is expressed on most T cells. Different members of the B7 and CD28 families serve to stimulate or inhibit immune responses (Fig. 5.7). The binding of CD28 on T cells to B7 on the APCs generates signals in the T cells that work together with signals generated by TCR recognition of antigen presented by MHC proteins on the same APCs. CD28-mediated signaling is essential for the responses of naive T cells; in the absence of CD28:B7 interactions, antigen recognition by the TCR is insufficient for initiating T cell responses. The requirement for costimulation ensures that naive T lymphocytes are activated maximally by microbial antigens and not by harmless foreign substances or by self antigens, because, as stated previously, microbes stimulate the expression of B7 costimulators on APCs.

A protein called ICOS (inducible costimulator), which is homologous to CD28 and also expressed on

Fig. 5.6 Role of costimulation in T cell activation. Resting antigen-presenting cells *(APCs)*, which have not been exposed to microbes or adjuvants, may present peptide antigens, but they do not express costimulators and are unable to activate naive T cells. T cells that recognize antigen without costimulation may die or become unresponsive (tolerant) to subsequent exposure to antigen. Microbes, as well as cytokines produced during innate immune responses to microbes, induce the expression of costimulators, such as B7 molecules, on the APCs. The B7 costimulators are recognized by the CD28 receptor on naive T cells, providing signal 2. In conjunction with antigen recognition (signal 1), this recognition initiates T cell responses. Activated APCs also produce cytokines that stimulate the differentiation of naive T cells into effector cells (not shown). *IL,* Interleukin.

T cells, plays an important role in the development and function of follicular helper T cells during germinal center responses (see Chapter 7).

Another set of molecules that participate in T cell responses are CD40 ligand (CD40L, or CD154) on activated T cells and CD40 on APCs. These molecules do not directly enhance T cell activation. Instead, CD40L expressed on an antigen-stimulated T cell binds to CD40 on APCs and activates the APCs to express more B7 costimulators and to secrete cytokines (e.g., IL-12) that enhance T cell differentiation. Thus, the CD40L-CD40 interaction promotes T cell activation by making APCs better at stimulating T cells. CD40L on effector CD4+ T cells also enhances activation of B cells and macrophages, as discussed later.

The role of costimulation in T cell activation explains an observation mentioned in earlier chapters. Protein antigens, such as those used in vaccines, fail to elicit T cell–dependent immune responses unless these antigens are administered with substances that activate APCs, especially dendritic cells. Such substances are called **adjuvants,** and they function mainly by inducing the expression of costimulators on APCs and by stimulating the APCs to secrete cytokines that activate T cells. Most adjuvants used in experimental immunology are products of microbes (e.g., killed mycobacteria, which is often used in experimental studies) or substances that mimic microbes, and they bind to pattern recognition receptors of the innate immune system, such as Toll-like receptors and NOD-like receptors (see Chapter 2). Adjuvants used in human vaccines are mainly aluminum

Name	B7-1 (CD80)	B7-2 (CD86)	ICOS-L (CD275)	PD-L1 (B7-H1, CD274)	PD-L2 (B7-DC, CD273)

| Ligands on APCs and other cells | | | | |

| Receptors on T cells | | | |

Name	CD28	CTLA-4	ICOS	PD-1
Major function	**Activation** (naive T cells)	**Inhibition** (mediates suppressive function of regulatory T cells)	**Activation** (follicular helper T cells in antibody responses)	**Inhibition**

Fig. 5.7 Proteins of the B7 and CD28 families. Ligands on *APCs* that are homologous to B7 bind to receptors on T cells that are homologous to CD28. Different ligand-receptor pairs serve distinct roles in immune responses. CD28 and *ICOS* are stimulatory receptors on T cells, and CTLA-4 and PD-1 are inhibitory receptors. Their functions are discussed in the text.

salts that induce local inflammation, which secondarily leads to dendritic cell costimulator expression. Thus, adjuvants trick the immune system into responding to purified protein antigens in a vaccine as if these proteins were parts of infectious microbes.

The increasing understanding of costimulators has led to new strategies for inhibiting harmful immune responses. Agents that block B7:CD28 interactions are used in the treatment of disorders in which T cell activation causes organ dysfunction, such as certain autoimmune diseases and graft rejection, and antibodies that block CD40:CD40L interactions are being tested in these diseases.

Inhibitory Receptors of T Cells

Inhibitory receptors are critical for limiting and terminating immune responses. These inhibitory receptors have been called **coinhibitors** to contrast them with the costimulators discussed earlier. Two important inhibitory receptors—CTLA-4 and PD-1—are structurally related to CD28 (see Fig. 5.7). CTLA-4, like CD28, recognizes B7-1 and B7-2 on APCs, and PD-1 recognizes two different but structurally related ligands, PD-L1 and PD-L2, on many cell types. Both CTLA-4 and PD-1 are induced in activated T cells, and function to terminate responses of these cells. CTLA-4 also plays an important role in the suppressive function of regulatory T cells (see Chapter 9). CTLA-4 and PD-1 prevent responses to self antigens and are also involved in inhibiting T cell responses to some tumors and chronic viral infections. These discoveries are the basis for the use of antibodies that block CTLA-4 or PD-1 to enhance immune responses to tumors in cancer patients (see Chapter 10). Because the normal function of these inhibitory receptors is to prevent immune responses against self antigens, genetic deletion or blockade of these molecules in mice and humans results in autoimmune disease. The function of these inhibitory receptors is discussed in more detail in Chapter 9, in the context of maintaining unresponsiveness to self antigens.

Stimuli for Activation of CD8+ T Cells

The activation of CD8+ T cells is stimulated by recognition of class I MHC–associated peptides and requires costimulation and helper T cells. CD8+ T cells function in much the same manner to kill infected cells and tumor cells, and their responses to microbial antigens and tumor antigens are essentially similar. However, the responses of CD8+ T cells differ in several ways from responses of CD4+ T lymphocytes:

- The initiation of CD8+ T cell activation often requires cytosolic antigen from one cell (e.g., virus-infected or tumor cells) to be cross-presented by dendritic cells (see Fig. 3.16).
- The differentiation of naive CD8+ T cells into fully active cytotoxic T lymphocytes (CTLs) and memory cells may require the concomitant activation of CD4+ helper T cells (Fig. 5.8). When virus-infected or tumor cells are ingested by dendritic cells, the APCs may present viral or tumor antigens from the cytosol in complex with class I MHC molecules and from vesicles in complex with class II MHC molecules. Thus, both CD8+ T cells and CD4+ T cells

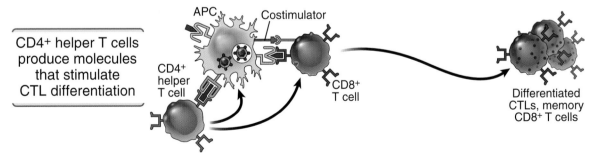

Fig. 5.8 Activation of CD8+ T cells. Antigen-presenting cells *(APCs)*, principally dendritic cells, may ingest and present microbial antigens to CD8+ T cells (cross-presentation) and to CD4+ helper T cells. Sometimes, the APC may be infected and can directly present antigens (not shown). The helper T cells then produce cytokines that stimulate the expansion and differentiation of the CD8+ T cells. Helper cells also may activate APCs to make them potent stimulators of CD8+ T cells. *CTLs,* Cytotoxic T lymphocytes.

Labels in figure:
CD4+ helper T cells produce molecules that stimulate CTL differentiation
APC
Costimulator
CD4+ helper T cell
CD8+ T cell
Differentiated CTLs, memory CD8+ T cells

specific for viral or tumor antigens are activated near one another. The CD4+ T cells may produce cytokines or membrane molecules that help to activate the CD8+ T cells. This requirement for helper T cells in CD8+ T cell responses is the likely explanation for the increased susceptibility to viral infections and cancers in patients infected with the human immunodeficiency virus (HIV), which kills CD4+ but not CD8+ T cells.

Now that we have described the stimuli required to activate naive T lymphocytes, we next consider the biochemical pathways triggered by antigen recognition and other stimuli.

BIOCHEMICAL PATHWAYS OF T CELL ACTIVATION

Following the recognition of antigens and costimulators, T cells express proteins that are involved in their proliferation, differentiation, and effector functions (Fig. 5.9). Naive T cells that have not encountered antigen have a low level of protein synthesis. Within minutes of antigen recognition, new gene transcription and protein synthesis are seen in the activated T cells. These newly expressed proteins mediate many of the subsequent responses of the T cells. The expression of these proteins is a consequence of signal transduction pathways emanating from the TCR complex and costimulatory receptors.

Antigen recognition activates several biochemical mechanisms that lead to T cell responses, including the activation of enzymes such as kinases, recruitment of adaptor proteins, and production or activation of functional transcription factors (Fig. 5.10). These biochemical pathways are initiated when TCR complexes and the appropriate coreceptor are brought together by binding to MHC-peptide complexes on the surface of APCs. In addition, there is an orderly movement of proteins in both the APC and T cell membranes at the region of cell-to-cell contact, such that the TCR complex, CD4/CD8 coreceptors, and CD28 coalesce to the center and the integrins move to form a peripheral ring. This redistribution of signaling and adhesion molecules is required for optimal induction of activating signals in the T cell. The region of contact between the APC and T cell, including the redistributed membrane proteins, is called the **immune synapse**. Although

the synapse was first described as the site of delivery of activating signals from membrane receptors to the cell's interior, it may serve other functions. Some effector molecules and cytokines may be secreted through this region, ensuring that they do not diffuse away but are targeted to the cell in contact with the T cell. Enzymes that degrade or inhibit signaling molecules are also recruited to the synapse, so it may be involved in terminating lymphocyte activation as well.

The cytoplasmic tails of the CD4 and CD8 coreceptors have a constitutively attached protein tyrosine kinase called Lck. As discussed in Chapter 4, several transmembrane signaling proteins are associated with the TCR, including the CD3 and ζ chains. CD3 and ζ contain motifs, each with two tyrosine residues, called **immunoreceptor tyrosine-based activation motifs** (ITAMs), which are critical for signaling. Lck, which is brought near the TCR complex by the CD4 or CD8 molecules, phosphorylates tyrosine residues contained within the ITAMs of the CD3 and ζ proteins, and this is the event that launches signal transduction in the T cells. The importance of the coreceptors is that by binding to MHC molecules, they bring the kinase close to its critical substrates in the TCR complex. The phosphorylated ITAMs of the ζ chain become docking sites for a tyrosine kinase called ZAP-70 (zeta-associated protein of 70 kD), which also is phosphorylated by Lck and thereby made enzymatically active. The active ZAP-70 then phosphorylates various adaptor proteins and enzymes, which assemble near the TCR complex and mediate additional signaling events.

The major signaling pathways linked to TCR complex activation are the calcium-NFAT pathway, the Ras– and Rac–MAP kinase pathways, the PKCθ–NF-κB pathway, and the PI-3 kinase pathway:

- **Nuclear factor of activated T cells (NFAT)** is a transcription factor present in an inactive phosphorylated form in the cytosol of resting T cells. NFAT activation and its nuclear translocation depend on the concentration of calcium (Ca^{2+}) ions in the cytosol. This signaling pathway is initiated by phosphorylation and activation of an enzyme called phospholipase Cγ (PLCγ) by a kinase, Itk, that becomes attached to one of the adaptor proteins in the signaling complex. Activated PLCγ catalyzes the hydrolysis of a plasma membrane phospholipid called phosphatidylinositol 4,5-bisphosphate

(PIP2). One by-product of PLCγ-mediated PIP2 breakdown, called inositol 1,4,5-triphosphate (IP3), binds to IP3 receptors on the endoplasmic reticulum (ER) membrane and the mitochondria and initiates release of Ca^{2+} into the cytosol. In response to the loss of calcium from intracellular stores, a plasma membrane calcium channel is opened, leading to the influx of extracellular Ca^{2+} into the cell, which further increases the cytosolic Ca^{2+} concentration and sustains this for hours. The elevated cytosolic Ca^{2+} leads to activation of a phosphatase called calcineurin. This enzyme removes phosphates from cytoplasmic NFAT, enabling the transcription factor to migrate into the nucleus, where it binds to and activates the promoters of several genes, including the genes encoding the T cell growth factor IL-2

Fig. 5.9 Proteins produced by antigen-stimulated T cells. Antigen recognition by T cells results in the synthesis and expression of a variety of proteins, examples of which are shown. The kinetics of production of these proteins **(A)** are approximations and may vary in different T cells and with different types of stimuli. The possible effects of costimulation on the patterns or kinetics of gene expression are not shown. The functions of some of the surface proteins expressed on activated T cells are shown in **(B)**. CD69 is a marker of T cell activation involved in cell migration; the interleukin-2 receptor (IL-2R) receives signals from the cytokine IL-2 that promotes T cell survival and proliferation; CD40 ligand is an effector molecule of T cells; CTLA-4 is an inhibitor of immune responses. c-Fos (shown in **A**) is a transcription factor. *TCR*, T cell receptor.

Fig. 5.10 Signal transduction pathways in T lymphocytes. Antigen recognition by T cells induces early signaling events, which include tyrosine phosphorylation of molecules of the T cell receptor *(TCR)* complex and the recruitment of adaptor proteins to the site of T cell antigen recognition. These early events lead to the activation of several biochemical intermediates, which in turn activate transcription factors that stimulate transcription of genes whose products mediate the responses of the T cells. The possible effects of costimulation on these signaling pathways are not shown. These signaling pathways are illustrated as independent of one another, for simplicity, but may be interconnected in more complex networks. *AP-1,* Activating protein 1; *APC,* antigen-presenting cell; *GTP/GDP,* guanosine triphosphate/diphosphate; *ITAM,* immunoreceptor tyrosine-based activation motif; *mTOR,* mammalian target of rapamycin; *NFAT,* nuclear factor of activated T cells; *PKC,* protein kinase C; *PLCγ1,* γ1 isoform of phosphatidylinositol-specific phospholipase C; *PI-3,* phosphatidylinositol-3; *ZAP-70,* zeta-associated protein of 70 kD.

and components of the IL-2 receptor. Calcineurin inhibitors (cyclosporine and tacrolimus) are drugs that block the phosphatase activity of calcineurin, and thus suppress the NFAT-dependent production of cytokines by T cells. These drugs are widely used as immunosuppressants to prevent graft rejection

and other T cell–mediated inflammatory conditions (see Chapter 10).

• The **Ras/Rac–MAP kinase pathways** include the guanosine triphosphate (GTP)-binding Ras and Rac proteins, several adaptor proteins, and a cascade of enzymes that eventually activate one of a family of mitogen-activated protein (MAP) kinases. These pathways are initiated by ZAP-70–dependent phosphorylation and accumulation of adaptor proteins at the plasma membrane, leading to the recruitment of Ras or Rac, and their activation by exchange of bound guanosine diphosphate (GDP) with GTP. Ras•GTP and Rac•GTP, the active forms of these proteins, initiate different enzyme cascades, leading to the activation of distinct MAP kinases. The terminal MAP kinases in these pathways, called extracellular signal–regulated kinase (ERK) and c-Jun amino-terminal (N-terminal) kinase (JNK), respectively, induce the expression of a protein called c-Fos and the phosphorylation of another protein called c-Jun. c-Fos and phosphorylated c-Jun combine to form the transcription factor **activating protein 1 (AP-1),** which enhances the transcription of several T cell genes.

- Another major pathway involved in TCR signaling consists of activation of the θ isoform of the serine-threonine kinase called protein kinase C (PKCθ), which leads to activation of the transcription factor **NF-κB.** PKC is activated by diacylglycerol, which, like IP3, is generated by PLC-mediated hydrolysis of membrane inositol lipids. PKCθ acts through adaptor proteins recruited to the TCR complex to activate NF-κB.
- TCR signal transduction also involves a lipid kinase called **PI-3 kinase,** which phosphorylates the membrane phospholipid PIP2 to generate phosphatidyl inositol (3,4,5)-trisphosphate (PIP3). PIP3 is required for the activation of a number of targets, including a serine-threonine kinase called Akt, or protein kinase B, which has many roles, including stimulating expression of antiapoptotic proteins and thus promoting survival of antigen-stimulated T cells. The PI-3 kinase/Akt pathway is triggered not only by the TCR but also by CD28 and IL-2 receptors. Akt activates mTOR (mammalian target of rapamycin), a serine-threonine kinase that is involved in stimulating protein translation and promoting cell survival and growth. Rapamycin, a drug that binds to and inactivates mTOR, is used to treat graft rejection.

The various transcription factors that are induced or activated in T cells, including NFAT, AP-1, and NF-κB, stimulate transcription and subsequent production of cytokines, cytokine receptors, cell cycle inducers, and effector molecules such as CD40L (see Fig. 5.9). All of these signals are initiated by antigen recognition, because binding of the TCR and coreceptors to peptide-MHC complexes is necessary to bring together critical enzymes and substrates in T cells.

As stated earlier, recognition of costimulators, such as B7 molecules, by their receptor CD28 is essential for full T cell responses. The biochemical signals transduced by CD28 on binding to B7 costimulators are less well defined than are TCR-triggered signals. CD28 engagement likely amplifies some TCR signaling pathways that are triggered by antigen recognition (signal 1) and may induce other signals that complement TCR signals.

Lymphocyte activation is associated with a profound change in cellular metabolism. In naive (resting) T cells, low levels of glucose are taken up and used to generate energy in the form of adenosine triphosphate (ATP) by mitochondrial oxidative phosphorylation. Upon activation, glucose uptake increases markedly, and the cells switch to aerobic glycolysis. This process generates less ATP but facilitates the synthesis of more amino acids, lipids, and other molecules that provide building blocks for organelles and for producing new cells. As a result, it is possible for activated T cells to more efficiently manufacture the cellular constituents that are needed for their rapid increase in size and for producing daughter cells.

Having described the stimuli and biochemical pathways in T cell activation, we now discuss how T cells respond to antigens and differentiate into effector cells capable of combating microbes.

FUNCTIONAL RESPONSES OF T LYMPHOCYTES TO ANTIGEN AND COSTIMULATION

The recognition of antigen and costimulators by T cells initiates an orchestrated set of responses that culminate in the expansion of the antigen-specific clones of lymphocytes and the differentiation of the naive T cells into effector cells and memory cells (see Fig. 5.3). Many of the responses of T cells are mediated by cytokines that are secreted by the T cells and act on the T cells themselves and on many other cells involved in immune defenses. Each component of the biologic responses of T cells is discussed next.

Secretion of Cytokines and Expression of Cytokine Receptors

In response to antigen and costimulators, T lymphocytes, especially CD4+ T cells, rapidly secrete the cytokine IL-2. We have already discussed cytokines in innate immune responses, which are produced mainly by dendritic cells and macrophages (see Chapter 2). In adaptive immunity, cytokines are secreted by T cells, mainly CD4+ cells. Because most of these cytokines are

Fig. 5.11 Role of interleukin-2 and IL-2 receptors in T cell proliferation. Naive T cells express the low-affinity IL-2 receptor *(IL-2R)* complex, made up of the β and γc chains (γc designates common γ chain, so called because it is a component of receptors for several cytokines). On activation by antigen recognition and costimulation, the cells produce IL-2 and express the α chain of the IL-2R (CD25), which associates with the β and γc chains to form the high-affinity IL-2 receptor. Binding of IL-2 to its receptor initiates proliferation of the T cells that recognized the antigen. *APC,* Antigen-presenting cell.

produced by effector T cells and serve diverse roles in host defense, we describe them in Chapter 6 when we discuss the effector mechanisms of cell-mediated immunity.

IL-2 is produced within 1 to 2 hours after activation of CD4+ T cells. Activation also transiently increases the expression of the high-affinity IL-2 receptor, thus rapidly enhancing the ability of the T cells to bind and respond to IL-2 (Fig. 5.11). The receptor for IL-2 is a three-chain molecule. Naive T cells express two signaling chains, β and γ, which constitute the low-affinity receptor for IL-2, but these cells do not express the α chain (CD25) that enables the receptor to bind IL-2 with high affinity. Within hours after activation by antigens and costimulators, the T cells produce the α chain of the receptor, and now the complete IL-2 receptor is able to bind IL-2 strongly. Thus, IL-2 produced by antigen-stimulated T

cells preferentially binds to and acts on the same T cells, an example of autocrine cytokine action.

The principal functions of IL-2 are to stimulate the survival and proliferation of T cells, resulting in an increase in the number of the antigen-specific T cells; because of these actions, IL-2 was originally called T cell growth factor. The high-affinity IL-2 receptor is constitutively expressed in regulatory T cells, so these cells are very sensitive to IL-2. In fact, IL-2 is essential for the maintenance of regulatory T cells and thus for controlling immune responses, as we discuss in Chapter 9. Activated CD8+ T cells and natural killer (NK) cells express the low-affinity βγ receptor and respond to higher concentrations of IL-2.

Clonal Expansion

T lymphocytes activated by antigen and costimulation begin to proliferate within 1 or 2 days, resulting

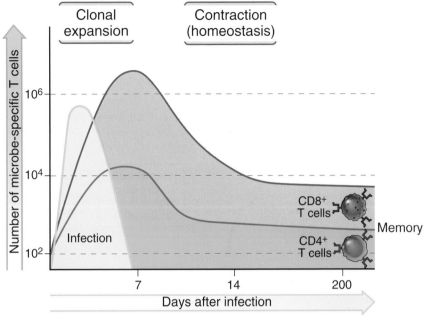

Fig. 5.12 Expansion and decline of T cell responses. The numbers of CD4+ and CD8+ T cells specific for various antigens in inbred mice and the clonal expansion and contraction during immune responses are illustrated. The numbers are approximations based on studies of model microbial and other antigens in inbred mice; in humans, the numbers of lymphocytes are approximately 1000-fold greater.

in expansion of antigen-specific clones (Fig. 5.12). This expansion quickly provides a large pool of antigen-specific lymphocytes from which effector cells can be generated to combat infection.

The magnitude of clonal expansion is remarkable, especially for CD8+ T cells. Before infection, the frequency of CD8+ T cells specific for any one microbial protein antigen is approximately 1 in 10^5 or 1 in 10^6 lymphocytes in the body. At the peak of some viral infections, possibly within a week after the infection, as many as 10% to 20% of all the lymphocytes in the lymphoid organs may be specific for that virus. This means that the numbers of cells in antigen-specific clones have increased by more than 10,000-fold, with an estimated doubling time of approximately 6 hours. This enormous expansion of T cells specific for a microbe is not accompanied by a detectable increase in bystander cells that do not recognize that microbe.

The expansion of CD4+ T cells appears to be 100-fold to 1000-fold less than that of CD8+ cells. This difference may reflect differences in the functions of the two types of T cells. CD8+ CTLs are effector cells that kill infected and tumor cells by direct contact, and many CTLs may be needed to kill large numbers of infected or tumor cells. By contrast, each CD4+ effector cell secretes cytokines that activate many other effector cells, so a relatively small number of cytokine producers may be sufficient.

Differentiation of Naive T Cells into Effector Cells

Some of the progeny of antigen-stimulated, proliferating T cells differentiate into effector cells whose function is to eradicate infections and some cancers. This process of differentiation is the result of changes in gene expression, such as the activation of genes encoding cytokines (in CD4+ T cells) or cytotoxic proteins (in CD8+ CTLs). It begins in concert with clonal expansion, and differentiated effector cells appear within 3 or 4 days after exposure to microbes. Effector cells of the CD4+ lineage acquire the capacity to produce different sets of cytokines. The subsets of T cells that are distinguished by their cytokine profiles are named Th1, Th2, and Th17 (Fig. 5.13). Many of these cells leave the peripheral lymphoid organs and migrate to sites of infection, where their cytokines recruit other leukocytes that destroy the infectious agents. The development and functions

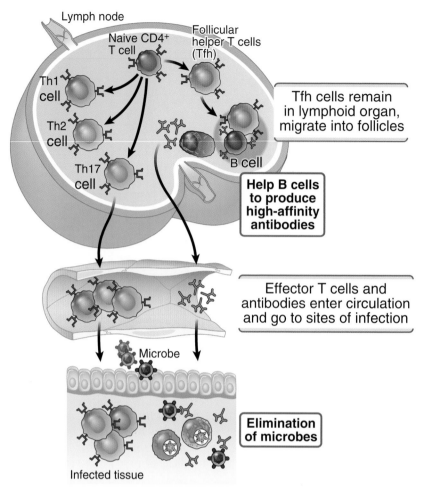

Fig. 5.13 Development of effector CD4⁺ T cells. When naive CD4⁺ T cells are activated in secondary lymphoid organs, they proliferate and differentiate into effector cells. Some of the effectors (the Th1, Th2, and Th17 populations) mostly exit the lymphoid organ and function to eradicate microbes in peripheral tissues. Other differentiated cells, called follicular helper *T (Tfh)* cells, remain in the lymphoid organ and help B cells to produce potent antibodies.

of these effector cells are described in Chapter 6, when we discuss cell-mediated immunity. Other differentiated CD4⁺ T cells remain in the lymphoid organs and migrate into lymphoid follicles, where they further differentiate into T follicular helper cells and help B lymphocytes to produce antibodies (see Chapter 7). As we discuss in Chapters 6 and 7, CD4⁺ helper T cells activate phagocytes and B lymphocytes through the actions of the plasma membrane protein CD40L and secreted cytokines. In addition, the interaction of CD40L on T cells with CD40 on dendritic cells increases the expression of costimulators on these

APCs and the production of T cell–stimulating cytokines, thus providing a positive feedback (amplification) mechanism for APC-induced T cell activation. Effector cells of the CD8⁺ lineage acquire the ability to kill infected and tumor cells; their development and function are also described in Chapter 6.

Development of Memory T Lymphocytes
A fraction of antigen-activated T lymphocytes differentiates into long-lived memory cells. These cells are a pool of lymphocytes that are induced by microbes and are ready to respond rapidly if the microbe returns. We

do not know what factors determine whether the progeny of antigen-stimulated lymphocytes will differentiate into effector cells or memory cells. Memory cells have several important characteristics.

- Memory cells survive even after the infection is eradicated and antigen is no longer present. Certain cytokines, including IL-7 and IL-15, which are produced by stromal cells in tissues, may serve to keep memory cells alive and cycling slowly.
- Memory T cells may be rapidly induced to produce cytokines or kill infected cells on encountering the antigen that they recognize. These cells do not perform any effector functions until they encounter antigen, but once activated, they respond much more vigorously and rapidly than do naive lymphocytes.
- Memory T cells can be found in lymphoid organs, in various peripheral tissues, especially mucosa and skin, and in the circulation. They can be distinguished from naive and effector cells by several criteria (see Chapter 1). A subset of memory T cells, called central memory cells, populate lymphoid organs and are responsible for rapid clonal expansion after reexposure to antigen. Another subset, called effector memory cells, localize in mucosal and other peripheral tissues and mediate rapid effector functions on reintroduction of antigen to these sites. A third subset, called tissue-resident memory cells, reside in the skin and mucosal tissues and may be incapable of entering the circulation. They mediate rapid secondary responses to antigens encountered in tissues.

Memory T cells can likely be activated in lymphoid and nonlymphoid tissues, and their activation, unlike that of naive T cells, does not require high levels of costimulation or antigen presentation by dendritic cells. In fact, various APCs, including B cells, may be capable of activating memory T cells.

MIGRATION OF T LYMPHOCYTES IN CELL-MEDIATED IMMUNE REACTIONS

As we discussed at the beginning of this chapter, T cell responses are initiated primarily in secondary lymphoid organs, and the effector phase occurs mainly in peripheral tissue sites of infection (see Fig. 5.2). **Thus, T cells at different stages of their lives have to migrate in different ways:**

- Naive T cells must migrate between blood and secondary (peripheral) lymphoid organs throughout the body, until they encounter dendritic cells within the lymphoid organ that display the antigens the T cells recognize (see Chapter 3).
- After the naive T cells are activated and differentiate into effector cells, these cells must migrate back to the sites of infection, where they function to kill microbes.

The migration of naive and effector T cells is controlled by three families of proteins—selectins, integrins, and chemokines—that regulate the migration of all leukocytes, as described in Chapter 2 (see Fig. 2.16). The routes of migration of naive and effector T cells differ significantly because of selective expression of different adhesion molecules and chemokine receptors on naive T cells versus effector T cells, together with the selective expression of endothelial adhesion molecules and chemokines in lymphoid tissues and sites of inflammation (Fig. 5.14).

Naive T cells express the adhesion molecule L-selectin (CD62L) and the chemokine receptor CCR7, which mediate the selective migration of the naive cells into lymph nodes through specialized blood vessels called high endothelial venules (HEVs) (see Fig. 5.14). HEVs are located in the T cell zones of lymphoid tissues and are lined by specialized endothelial cells, which express carbohydrate ligands that bind to L-selectin. HEVs also display chemokines that are made only in lymphoid tissues and are specifically recognized by CCR7. The migration of naive T cells proceeds in a multistep sequence like that of migration of all leukocytes through blood vessels (see Chapter 2):

- Naive T cells in the blood engage in L-selectin–mediated rolling interactions with the HEV, allowing chemokines to bind to CCR7 on the T cells.
- CCR7 transduces intracellular signals that activate the integrin LFA-1 on the naive T cell, increasing the binding affinity of the integrin.
- The increased affinity of the integrin for its ligand, ICAM-1, on the HEV results in firm adhesion and arrest of the rolling T cells.
- The T cells then exit the vessel through the endothelial junctions and are retained in the T cell zone of the lymph node because of the chemokines produced there.

Thus, many naive T cells that are carried by the blood into an HEV migrate to the T cell zone of the lymph node stroma. This happens constantly in all lymph nodes and mucosal lymphoid tissues in the body. Effector T cells

T cell homing receptor	Ligand on endothelial cell	Function of receptor: ligand pair
Naive T cells L-selectin	L-selectin ligand	Adhesion of naive T cells to high endothelial venule (HEV) in lymph node
LFA-1 (β₂-integrin)	ICAM-1	Stable arrest on HEV
CCR7	CCL19 or CCL21	Activation of integrins and chemotaxis
Activated (effector and memory) T cells E- and P-selectin ligand	E- or P-selectin	Initial weak adhesion of effector and memory T cells to cytokine-activated endothelium at peripheral site of infection
LFA-1 (β₂-integrin) or VLA-4 (β₁ integrin)	ICAM-1 or VCAM-1	Stable arrest on cytokine-activated endothelium at peripheral site of infection
CXCR3, others	CXCL10, others	Activation of integrins and chemotaxis

do not express CCR7 or L-selectin, and thus they are not drawn into lymph nodes.

The phospholipid sphingosine 1-phosphate (S1P) plays a key role in the egress of T cells from lymph nodes. The levels of S1P are higher in the blood and lymph than inside lymph nodes. S1P binds to and induces internalization of its receptor, which keeps the expression of the receptor on circulating naive T cells low. When a naive T cell enters the node, it is exposed to lower concentrations of S1P, and expression of the receptor begins to increase. If the T cell does not recognize any antigen, the cell leaves the node through efferent lymphatic vessels, following the gradient of S1P into the lymph. If the T cell does encounter specific antigen and is activated, the surface expression of the S1P receptor is suppressed for several days by CD69, which is transiently expressed following T cell activation. As a result, recently activated T cells stay in the lymph node long enough to undergo clonal expansion and differentiation. When this process is completed, S1P receptor is reexpressed on the cell surface; at the same time, the cells lose expression of L-selectin and CCR7, which previously attracted the naive T cells to the lymph nodes. Therefore, activated T cells are drawn out of the nodes into the draining lymph, which then transports the cells to the circulation. The net result of these changes is that differentiated effector T cells leave the lymph nodes and enter the circulation. The importance of the S1P pathway has been highlighted by the development of a drug (fingolimod) that binds to the S1P receptor and blocks the exit of T cells from lymph nodes. This drug is approved for the treatment of the inflammatory disease multiple sclerosis.

Effector T cells migrate to sites of infection because they express adhesion molecules and chemokine receptors that bind to ligands expressed or displayed on vascular endothelium at sites of infection. The process of differentiation of naive T lymphocytes into effector cells is accompanied by changes in the types of adhesion molecules and chemokine receptors expressed on these cells (see Fig. 5.14). The migration of activated T cells into peripheral tissues is controlled by the same kinds of interactions involved in the migration of other leukocytes into tissues (see Chapter 2):

- Activated T cells express high levels of the glycoprotein ligands for E- and P-selectins and the integrins LFA-1 and VLA-4 (very late antigen 4). Innate immune cytokines produced in response to the infection, such as TNF and IL-1, act on the endothelial cells to increase expression of E- and P-selectins, as well as ligands for integrins, especially ICAM-1 and vascular cell adhesion molecule 1 (VCAM-1), the ligand for the VLA-4 integrin.
- Effector T cells that are passing through the blood vessels at the infection site bind first to the endothelial selectins, leading to rolling interactions.
- Effector T cells also express receptors for chemokines that are produced by macrophages and endothelial cells at these inflammatory sites and are displayed on the surface of the endothelium. The rolling T cells bind these chemokines, leading to increased affinity of the integrins for their ligands and firm adhesion of the T cells to the endothelium.
- After the effector T lymphocytes are arrested on the endothelium, they engage other adhesion molecules at the junctions between endothelial cells, crawling through these junctions into the tissue. Chemokines that were produced by macrophages and other cells in the tissues stimulate the motility of the transmigrating T cells.

The net result of these molecular interactions between the T cells and endothelial cells is that the T cells migrate out of the blood vessels to the area of infection. Naive T cells do not express ligands for E- or P-selectin and do not express receptors for chemokines produced at inflammatory sites. Therefore, naive T cells do not migrate into sites of infection or tissue injury.

Fig. 5.14 Migration of naive and effector T lymphocytes. A, Naive T lymphocytes home to lymph nodes as a result of L-selectin, integrin, and chemokine receptor CCR7 binding to their ligands on high endothelial venules *(HEVs)*. Chemokines expressed in lymph nodes bind to CCR7 on naive T cells, enhancing integrin-dependent adhesion and migration through the HEV. The phospholipid, sphingosine 1-phosphate *(S1P)*, plays a role in the exit of T cells from lymph nodes, by binding to its receptor, called S1PR1 (type 1 sphingosine 1-phosphate receptor). Activated T lymphocytes, including the majority of effector cells, home to sites of infection in peripheral tissues, and this migration is mediated by E-selectin and P-selectin, integrins, and chemokines secreted at inflammatory sites. Follicular helper T *(Tfh)* cells (not shown) are effector cells that remain in lymphoid organs, because they express a chemokine receptor (CXCR5) that draws them into lymphoid follicles, where they can interact with resident B lymphocytes. **B,** This table summarizes the functions of the principal T cell homing receptors and chemokine receptors and their ligands. *ICAM-1*, Intercellular adhesion molecule 1; *LFA-1*, leukocyte function–associated antigen 1; *VCAM-1*, vascular cell adhesion molecule 1; *VLA-4*, very late antigen 4.

The homing of effector T cells to an infected tissue is independent of antigen recognition, but lymphocytes that recognize antigens are preferentially retained and activated at the site. The homing of effector T cells to sites of infection mainly depends on adhesion molecules and chemokines. Therefore, any effector T cell present in the blood, regardless of antigen specificity, can enter the site of any infection. This nonselective migration presumably maximizes the chances of effector lymphocytes entering tissues where they may encounter the microbes they recognize. The effector T cells that leave the circulation and that specifically recognize microbial antigen presented by local tissue APCs become reactivated and contribute to the killing of the microbe in the APC. One consequence of this reactivation is an increase in the expression of VLA integrins on the T cells. Some of these integrins specifically bind to molecules present in the extracellular matrix, such as hyaluronic acid and fibronectin. Therefore, the antigen-stimulated lymphocytes adhere firmly to the tissue matrix proteins near the antigen, which may serve to keep the cells at the inflammatory sites. This selective retention contributes to accumulation of more and more T cells specific for microbial antigens in the region of the infection.

As a result of this sequence of T cell migration events, the effector phase of T cell–mediated immune responses may occur at any site of infection. Whereas the activation of naive T cells requires antigen presentation and costimulation by dendritic cells, differentiated effector cells are less dependent on costimulation. Therefore, the proliferation and differentiation of naive T cells are confined to lymphoid organs, where dendritic cells (which express abundant costimulators) display antigens, but the functions of effector T cells may be reactivated by any host cell displaying microbial peptides bound to MHC molecules, not just dendritic cells.

Elucidation of the molecular interactions involved in leukocyte migration has spurred many attempts to develop agents to block the process of cell migration into tissues. Antibodies against integrins are effective in the inflammatory diseases multiple sclerosis and inflammatory bowel disease. The clinical utility of these drugs is limited by the increased risk of new infection or reactivation of latent infections, because the immune surveillance function of the T cells is impaired when their migration into tissues is blocked. A small-molecule inhibitor of the S1P pathway is used for treating multiple sclerosis, as mentioned previously. Small molecules that bind to and block chemokine receptors have also been developed, and some have shown efficacy in inflammatory bowel disease.

DECLINE OF THE IMMUNE RESPONSE

Because of the remarkable expansion of antigen-specific lymphocytes at the peak of an immune response, it is predictable that once the response is over, the system must return to its steady state, called homeostasis, so that it is prepared to respond to the next infectious pathogen (see Fig. 5.12). During the response, the survival and proliferation of T cells are maintained by antigen, costimulatory signals from CD28, and cytokines such as IL-2. Once an infection is cleared and the stimuli for lymphocyte activation disappear, many of the cells that had proliferated in response to antigen are deprived of these survival signals. As a result, these cells die by apoptosis (programmed cell death). The response subsides within 1 or 2 weeks after the infection is eradicated, and the only sign that a T cell–mediated immune response had occurred is the pool of surviving memory lymphocytes.

To summarize, numerous mechanisms have evolved to overcome the challenges that T cells face in the generation of a useful cell-mediated immune response:

- Naive T cells need to find the antigen. This problem is solved by APCs that capture the antigen and concentrate it in specialized lymphoid organs in the regions through which naive T cells recirculate.
- The correct type of T lymphocytes (i.e., CD4$^+$ helper T cells or CD8$^+$ CTLs) must respond to antigens from the endosomal and cytosolic compartments. This selectivity is determined by the specificity of the CD4 and CD8 coreceptors for class II and class I MHC molecules and by the segregation of extracellular (vesicular) and intracellular (cytosolic) protein antigens for display by class II and class I MHC molecules, respectively.
- T cells should respond to microbial antigens but not to harmless proteins. This preference for microbes is maintained because T cell activation requires costimulators that are induced on APCs by microbes.
- Antigen recognition by a small number of T cells must lead to a response that is large enough to be effective. This is accomplished by robust clonal expansion after stimulation and by several amplification mechanisms induced by microbes and activated T cells themselves that enhance the response.
- The response must be optimized to combat different types of microbes. This is accomplished largely by the development of specialized subsets of effector T cells.

SUMMARY

- T lymphocytes are the mediators of the cell-mediated arm of the adaptive immune system, which combats microbes that are ingested by phagocytes and live within these cells or microbes that infect host cells. T lymphocytes also mediate defense against some extracellular microbes, help B lymphocytes to produce antibodies, and destroy cancer cells.

- The responses of T lymphocytes consist of sequential phases: recognition of cell-associated microbes by naive T cells, expansion of the antigen-specific clones by proliferation, and differentiation of some of the progeny into effector cells and memory cells.

- T cells use their antigen receptors to recognize peptide antigens displayed by MHC molecules on antigen-presenting cells (APCs), which accounts for the specificity of the ensuing response, and also recognize polymorphic residues of the MHC molecules, accounting for the MHC restriction of T cell responses.

- Antigen recognition by the T cell receptor (TCR) triggers signals that are delivered to the interior of the cells by molecules associated with the TCR (CD3 and ζ chains) and by the coreceptors CD4 and CD8, which recognize class II and class I MHC molecules, respectively.

- The binding of T cells to APCs is enhanced by adhesion molecules, notably the integrins, whose affinity for their ligands is increased by antigen recognition by the TCR.

- APCs exposed to microbes or to cytokines produced as part of the innate immune reactions to microbes express costimulators that bind to receptors on T cells and deliver necessary second signals for T cell activation.

- The biochemical signals triggered in T cells by antigen recognition and costimulation result in the activation of various transcription factors that stimulate the expression of genes encoding cytokines, cytokine receptors, and other molecules involved in T cell responses.

- The signaling pathways involve protein tyrosine kinases which phosphorylate proteins that become docking sites for additional kinases and other signaling molecules. The signaling pathways include the calcineurin/NFAT, RAS-MAP kinase, and PI-3 kinase/MTOR pathways.

- In response to antigen recognition and costimulation, T cells secrete cytokines that induce proliferation of the antigen-stimulated T cells and mediate the effector functions of T cells.

- T cells proliferate following activation by antigen and costimulators, resulting in expansion of the antigen-specific clones. The survival and proliferation of activated T cells are driven by the growth factor IL-2.

- Some of the T cells differentiate into effector cells that are responsible for eradicating infections. CD4$^+$ effector cells produce surface molecules, notably CD40L, and secrete various cytokines that activate other leukocytes to destroy microbes. CD8$^+$ effector cells are able to kill infected and tumor cells.

- Other activated T cells differentiate into memory cells, which survive even after the antigen is eliminated and are capable of rapid responses to subsequent encounter with the antigen.

- Naive T cells migrate to peripheral lymphoid organs, mainly lymph nodes draining sites of microbe entry, whereas many of the effector T cells generated in lymphoid organs are able to migrate to any site of infection.

- The pathways of migration of naive and effector T cells are controlled by adhesion molecules and chemokines. The migration of T cells is independent of antigen, but cells that recognize microbial antigens in tissues are retained at these sites.

REVIEW QUESTIONS

1. What are the components of the TCR complex? Which of these components are responsible for antigen recognition and which for signal transduction?
2. What are some of the molecules in addition to the TCR that T cells use to initiate their responses to antigens, and what are the functions of these molecules?
3. What is costimulation? What is the physiologic significance of costimulation? What are some of the ligand-receptor pairs involved in costimulation?
4. Summarize the links among antigen recognition, the major biochemical signaling pathways in T cells, and the production of transcription factors.

5. What is the principal growth factor for T cells? Why do antigen-specific T cells expand more than other (bystander) T cells on exposure to an antigen?

6. What are the mechanisms by which CD4+ effector T cells activate other leukocytes?

7. What are the major properties of memory T lymphocytes?

8. Why do naive T cells migrate preferentially to lymphoid organs and differentiated effector T cells (which have been activated by antigen) migrate preferentially to tissues that are sites of infection?

Answers to and discussion of the Review Questions are available at Student Consult.

Effector Mechanisms of T Cell–Mediated Immunity
Functions of T Cells in Host Defense

Host defense in which T lymphocytes serve as effector cells is called cell-mediated immunity. T cells are essential for eliminating microbes that survive and replicate inside cells and for eradicating infections by some extracellular microbes, often by recruiting other leukocytes to clear the infectious pathogens. T cells also destroy tumors that produce proteins that are recognized as foreign antigens (see Chapter 10). In this chapter, we focus on the role of T cell responses in defense against pathogenic microbes. Cell-mediated immune responses begin with the activation of naive T cells to proliferate and to differentiate into effector cells. The majority of these effector T cells then migrate to sites of infection, where they function to eliminate the microbes. Some CD4+ effector cells stay in lymphoid organs and help B lymphocytes to produce high-affinity antibodies (humoral immunity, see Chapter 7). In Chapter 3 we described the function of major histocompatibility complex (MHC) molecules in displaying the antigens of intracellular microbes for recognition by T lymphocytes, and in Chapter 5 we discussed the early events in the activation of naive T

lymphocytes. In this chapter, we address the following questions:
• What types of effector T cells are involved in the elimination of microbes?
• How do effector T cells develop from naive T cells, and how do effector cells eradicate infections by diverse microbes?
• What are the roles of macrophages and other leukocytes in the destruction of infectious pathogens?

TYPES OF T CELL–MEDIATED IMMUNE REACTIONS

Two main types of cell-mediated immune reactions eliminate different types of microbes: CD4+ helper T cells express molecules that recruit and activate other leukocytes to phagocytose (ingest) and destroy microbes, and CD8+ cytotoxic T lymphocytes (CTLs) kill infected cells containing microbial proteins in the cytosol, thus eliminating cellular reservoirs of infection (Fig. 6.1). Microbial infections may occur anywhere in the body, and some infectious pathogens

Fig. 6.1 Cell-mediated Immunity. A, Effector T cells of the CD4+ Th1 and Th17 subsets recognize microbial antigens and secrete cytokines that recruit leukocytes (inflammation) and activate phagocytes to kill the microbes. Effector cells of the Th2 subset (not shown) recruit eosinophils, which destroy helminthic parasites. **B,** CD8+ cytotoxic T lymphocytes (CTLs) kill infected cells with microbial antigens in the cytosol. CD8+ T cells also produce cytokines that induce inflammation and activate macrophages (not shown).

are able to infect and live within host cells. Pathogenic microbes that infect and survive inside host cells include (1) many bacteria, fungi, and protozoa that are ingested by phagocytes but resist the killing mechanisms of these phagocytes and thus survive in vesicles or in the cytosol, and (2) viruses that infect phagocytic and nonphagocytic cells and replicate in these cells (see Chapter 5, Fig. 5.1). CD4+ and CD8+ T cells recognize microbes in different cellular compartments and differ in the nature of the reactions they elicit. In general, CD4+ T cells recognize antigens of microbes that may be intracellular or extracellular (based on where the microbes survive and replicate) but whose antigens are internalized into endocytic vesicles. These T cells secrete cytokines that recruit and activate phagocytes and other leukocytes that kill the microbes. In contrast, CD8+ T cells recognize microbial antigens that are present in the cytosol of infected cells and destroy these cells.

Cell-mediated immunity against pathogens was discovered as a form of immunity to an intracellular bacterial infection that could be transferred from immune animals to naive animals by cells (now known to be T lymphocytes) but not by serum antibodies (Fig. 6.2). It

was known from early studies that lymphocytes were responsible for the specificity of cell-mediated immunity against different microbes, but the elimination of the microbes was a function of activated macrophages. As already mentioned, CD4+ T cells are mainly responsible for this classical type of cell-mediated immunity, whereas CD8+ T cells can eradicate infections without a requirement for phagocytes.

T cell–mediated immune reactions consist of multiple steps (see Chapter 5, Fig. 5.2). Naive T cells are stimulated by microbial antigens in peripheral (secondary) lymphoid organs, giving rise to effector T cells whose function is to eradicate the infections. The differentiated effector T cells then migrate to the site of infection. Phagocytes at these sites that have ingested the microbes or microbial proteins into intracellular vesicles display peptide fragments of the protein antigens bound to cell surface class II MHC molecules for recognition by CD4+ effector T cells. Peptide antigens derived from microbial proteins in the cytosol of infected cells are displayed by class I MHC molecules for recognition by CD8+ effector T cells. Antigen recognition activates the effector T cells to perform their

Fig. 6.2 Cell-mediated immunity to an intracellular bacterium, *Listeria monocytogenes*. In these experiments, a sample of lymphocytes or serum (a source of antibodies) was taken from a mouse that had previously been exposed to a sublethal dose of *Listeria* organisms (immune mouse) and transferred to a normal (naive) mouse, and the recipient of the adoptive transfer was challenged with the bacteria. The number of bacteria were measured in the spleen of the recipient mouse to determine if the transfer had conferred immunity. Protection against bacterial challenge (seen by reduced recovery of live bacteria) was induced by the transfer of immune lymphoid cells, now known to be T cells (**A**), but not by the transfer of serum (**B**). The bacteria were killed in vitro by activated macrophages but not by T cells (**C**). Therefore protection depends on antigen-specific T lymphocytes, but bacterial killing is the function of activated macrophages.

task of eliminating the infectious pathogens. Thus, in cell-mediated immunity, T cells recognize protein antigens at two stages. First, naive T cells recognize antigens in lymphoid tissues and respond by proliferating and by differentiating into effector cells (see Chapter 5). Second, effector T cells recognize the same antigens anywhere in the body and respond by eliminating these microbes.

This chapter describes how CD4+ and CD8+ effector T cells develop in response to microbes and eliminate these microbes. Because CD4+ helper T lymphocytes and CD8+ CTLs use distinct mechanisms to combat infections, we discuss the development and functions of the effector cells of these lymphocyte classes individually. We conclude by describing how the two classes of lymphocytes may cooperate to eliminate intracellular microbes.

DEVELOPMENT AND FUNCTIONS OF CD4+ EFFECTOR T LYMPHOCYTES

In Chapter 5 we introduced the concept that effector cells of the CD4+ lineage could be distinguished on the basis of the cytokines they produce. These subsets of CD4+ T cells differ in their functions and serve distinct roles in cell-mediated immunity.

Subsets of CD4+ Helper T Cells Distinguished by Cytokine Profiles

Analysis of cytokine production by helper T (Th) cells has revealed that functionally distinct subsets of CD4+ T cells exist that produce different cytokines and that eliminate different types of pathogens. The existence of these subsets illustrates how the immune system mounts specialized responses that are optimized to combat diverse microbes. For example, intracellular microbes such as mycobacteria are ingested by phagocytes but resist intracellular killing. The adaptive immune response to such microbes results in the activation of the phagocytes, enabling them to kill the ingested microbes. In contrast, the immune response to helminths is dominated by the production of immunoglobulin E (IgE) antibodies and the activation of eosinophils, which destroy the helminths. The immune response to extracellular bacteria and fungi requires cytokines that help to drive neutrophilic inflammation, because neutrophils in large numbers are needed to eliminate these pathogens. All these types of immune responses depend on CD4+ helper T cells, but for many years it was not clear how the CD4+ helper cells are able to stimulate such distinct immune effector mechanisms. We now know that these responses are mediated by subpopulations of CD4+ effector T cells that produce different cytokines.

CD4+ helper T cells may differentiate into three subsets of effector cells that produce distinct sets of cytokines that function to defend against different types of microbial infections in tissues, and a fourth subset that activates B cells in secondary lymphoid organs (Fig. 6.3). The subsets that were defined first are called Th1 cells and Th2 cells (for type 1 helper T cells and type 2 helper T cells, respectively); the third population, which was identified later, is called Th17 cells because its signature cytokine is interleukin (IL)-17. The T cells that help B lymphocytes, called follicular helper T (Tfh) cells, are described in Chapter 7 and will not be considered further in this chapter. The discovery of these subpopulations has been an important milestone in understanding immune responses and provides models for studying the process of cell differentiation. However, it should be noted that some activated CD4+ T cells may produce mixtures of cytokines and therefore cannot be readily classified into these subsets, and there may be plasticity in these populations so that one subset may convert into another under some conditions. Despite these caveats, considering the functions of CD4+ effector cells in the context of the major subsets is helpful for understanding the mechanisms of cell-mediated immunity.

The cytokines produced in adaptive immune responses include those made by the Th subsets, as well as cytokines produced by CD4+ regulatory T cells and CD8+ T cells. These cytokines of adaptive immunity share some general properties, but they each have different biologic activities and play unique roles in the effector phase or regulation of these responses (Fig. 6.4). The functions of the CD4+ T cell subsets reflect the actions of the cytokines they produce. Similar sets of cytokines may be produced early in immune responses by innate lymphoid cells, such as ILC1, ILC2, and ILC3 (see Chapter 2), and later by Th1, Th2, and Th17 cells, respectively. These combined innate and adaptive responses with similar cytokine profiles and functional outcomes are sometimes grouped under "type 1 immunity," "type 2 immunity," and "type 3 immunity."

Effector T cells	Defining cytokines	Principal target cells	Major immune reactions	Host defense	Role in disease
Th1	IFN-γ	Macrophages	Macrophage activation	Intracellular pathogens	Autoimmunity; chronic inflammation
Th2	IL-4 IL-5 IL-13	Eosinophils	Eosinophil and mast cell activation; alternative macrophage activation	Helminths	Allergy
Th17	IL-17 IL-22	Neutrophils	Neutrophil recruitment and activation	Extracellular bacteria and fungi	Autoimmunity; inflammation
Tfh	IL-21 (and IFN-γ or IL-4)	B cells	Antibody production	Extracellular pathogens	Autoimmunity (autoantibodies)

Fig. 6.3 Characteristics of subsets of CD4+ helper T lymphocytes. A naive CD4+ T cell may differentiate into subsets that produce different cytokines that recruit and activate different cell types (referred to as *target cells*) and combat different types of infections in host defense. These subsets also are involved in various kinds of inflammatory diseases. The table summarizes the major differences among *Th1, Th2, Th17,* and *Tfh* subsets of helper T cells. *IFN,* Interferon; *IL,* interleukin.

Each subset of CD4+ T cells develops in response to the types of microbes that subset is best at eradicating. Different microbes elicit the production of different cytokines from dendritic cells and other cells, and these cytokines drive the differentiation of antigen-activated T cells to one or another subset. We next discuss the functions and development of each of the major subsets of CD4+ effector T cells.

Th1 Cells

The Th1 subset is induced by microbes that are ingested by and activate phagocytes, primarily macrophages, and Th1 cells stimulate phagocyte-mediated killing of ingested microbes (Fig. 6.5). The signature cytokine of Th1 cells is interferon-γ (IFN-γ), the most potent macrophage-activating cytokine known. (Despite its similar name, IFN-γ is a much less potent antiviral cytokine than the type I IFNs [see Chapter 2]).

Th1 cells, acting through CD40 ligand and IFN-γ, increase the ability of macrophages to kill phagocytosed microbes (Fig. 6.6). Macrophages ingest and

attempt to destroy microbes as part of the innate immune response (see Chapter 2). The efficiency of this process is greatly enhanced by the interaction of Th1 cells with the macrophages. When microbes are ingested into phagosomes of the macrophages, microbial peptides are presented on class II MHC molecules and are recognized by CD4+ T cells. If these T cells belong to the Th1 subset, they are induced to express CD40 ligand (CD40L, or CD154) and to secrete IFN-γ. Binding of CD40L to CD40 on macrophages functions together with IFN-γ binding to its receptor on the same macrophages to trigger biochemical signaling pathways that lead to the generation of reactive oxygen species (ROS) and nitric oxide (NO) and activation of lysosomal proteases. All these molecules are potent destroyers of microbes. The net result of CD40-mediated and IFN-γ–mediated activation is that macrophages become strongly microbicidal and can destroy most ingested microbes. This pathway of macrophage activation by CD40L and IFN-γ is called **classical macrophage activation**, in contrast to Th2-mediated alternative macrophage activation, discussed later. Classically

A **General properties of T cell cytokines**

Property	Significance
Produced transiently in response to antigen	Provides cytokine only when needed
Usually acts on same cell that produces the cytokine (autocrine) or nearby cells (paracrine)	Systemic effects of cytokines usually reflect severe infections or autoimmunity
Pleiotropism: each cytokine has multiple biological actions	Provides diversity of actions but may limit clinical utility of cytokines because of unwanted effects
Redundancy: multiple cytokines may share the same or similar biological activities	Blocking any one cytokine may not achieve a desired effect

B **Biologic actions of selected T cell cytokines**

Cytokine	Principal action	Cellular source(s)
IL-2	T cell proliferation; regulatory T cell survival	Activated T cells
Interferon-γ (IFN-γ)	Activation of macrophages (classical pathway)	CD4+ Th1 and CD8+ T cells, natural killer (NK) cells
IL-4	B cell switching to IgE; alternative macrophage activation	CD4+ Th2 T cells, mast cells
IL-5	Activation of eosinophils	CD4+ Th2 T cells, mast cells, innate lymphoid cells
IL-13	B cell switching to IgE; alternative macrophage activation	CD4+ Th2 T cells, mast cells, innate lymphoid cells
IL-17	Stimulation of acute inflammation	CD4+ Th17 T cells, other cells
IL-21	B cell activation; Tfh differentiation	CD4+ Tfh T cells
IL-22	Maintenance of epithelial barrier function	CD4+ Th17 T cells, NK cells, innate lymphoid cells

Fig. 6.4 Properties of the major cytokines produced by CD4+ helper T lymphocytes. **A,** General properties of cytokines produced during adaptive immune responses. **B,** Functions of cytokines involved in T cell–mediated immunity. Note that IL-2, which is produced by T cells early after activation and is the first identified T cell cytokine, was discussed in Chapter 5 in the context of T cell activation. Transforming growth factor β (TGF-β) functions mainly as an inhibitor of immune responses; its role is discussed in Chapter 9. The cytokines of innate immunity are shown in Fig. 2.14; several of these are also made by T cells and thus function in adaptive immunity as well. More information about these cytokines and their receptors is provided in Appendix III. *IgE,* Immunoglobulin E; *IL,* interleukin.

Fig. 6.5 Functions of Th1 cells. Th1 cells produce the cytokine interferon-γ *(IFN-γ)*, which activates macrophages to kill phagocytosed microbes (classical pathway of macrophage activation). In mice, IFN-γ stimulates the production of IgG antibodies, but this has not been established in humans. *APC*, Antigen-presenting cell.

activated macrophages, often called M1 macrophages, also secrete cytokines that stimulate inflammation and express increased levels of MHC molecules and costimulators, which amplify the T cell response. CD8+ T cells secrete IFN-γ as well, and may contribute to macrophage activation and killing of ingested microbes.

The critical role of Th1 cells in defense against intracellular microbes is demonstrated by the fact that individuals with inherited defects in the development or function of this subset are susceptible to infections with such microbes, especially prevalent nontuberculous mycobacterial species that do not infect immunocompetent individuals.

Essentially the same reaction, consisting of leukocyte recruitment and activation, may be elicited by injecting a microbial (or other) protein into the skin of an individual who has been immunized with the protein or previously infected with the microbe. This reaction is called **delayed-type hypersensitivity** (DTH), and it is described in Chapter 11 when we discuss injurious immune reactions.

Development of Th1 Cells

The differentiation of naive CD4+ T cells to Th1 effector cells is driven by a combination of antigen-induced T cell receptor (TCR) signaling and the cytokines IL-12 and IFN-γ (Fig. 6.7A). In response to many bacteria (especially intracellular bacteria) and viruses, dendritic cells and macrophages produce IL-12, and natural killer (NK) cells produce IFN-γ. Therefore, when naive T cells recognize the antigens of these microbes, the T cells are also exposed to IL-12 and IFN-γ. Type I IFNs, produced in response to viral infections, also promote Th1 differentiation. IL-12 and IFN-γ activate the transcription factors Stat4 and Stat1, respectively, and antigen-induced signals in combination with the cytokines induce expression of a transcription factor called T-bet that is essential for Th1 development and function. These transcription factors work together to stimulate the expression of IFN-γ and other proteins involved in the migration of Th1 cells to sites of infection. Note that IFN-γ not only activates macrophages to kill ingested microbes but also promotes more Th1 development and inhibits the development of Th2 and Th17 cells. Thus, IFN-γ increasingly polarizes the response to the Th1 subset.

Th2 Cells

Th2 cells are induced by parasitic worm infections and promote IgE-, mast cell- and eosinophil-mediated destruction of these parasites (Fig. 6.8). The signature cytokines of Th2 cells—IL-4, IL-5, and IL-13—function cooperatively in eradicating worm infections. Helminths are too large to be phagocytosed, so mechanisms other than macrophage activation are needed for their destruction. When Th2 and related Tfh cells encounter the antigens of helminths, the T cells secrete their cytokines. IL-4 produced by Tfh cells stimulates the production of IgE antibodies, which coat the helminths and thus help in their clearance. Eosinophils use their Fc receptors to bind to the IgE and are activated by IL-5 produced by the Th2 cells,

Fig. 6.6 Activation of macrophages by Th1 lymphocytes. Effector T lymphocytes of the Th1 subset recognize the antigens of ingested microbes on macrophages. In response to this recognition, the T lymphocytes express CD40L, which engages CD40 on the macrophages, and the T cells secrete interferon-γ *(IFN-γ)*, which binds to IFN-γ receptors on the macrophages. This combination of signals activates the macrophages to produce microbicidal substances that kill the ingested microbes. Activated macrophages also secrete tumor necrosis factor *(TNF)*, interleukin-1 *(IL-1)*, and chemokines, which induce inflammation, and IL-12, which promotes Th1 responses. These macrophages also express more major histocompatibility complex *(MHC)* molecules and costimulators, which further enhance T cell responses. A, Illustration shows a CD4+ T cell recognizing class II MHC–associated peptides and activating the macrophage. B, The figure summarizes macrophage responses and their roles in cell-mediated immunity.

as well as by signals from these IgE-specific Fc receptors. Activated eosinophils release their granule contents, which are toxic to the parasites. IL-13 stimulates mucus secretion and intestinal peristalsis, increasing the expulsion of parasites from the intestines. IgE also binds to mast cells and is responsible for their activation, leading to the secretion of chemical mediators that stimulate inflammation and proteases that destroy toxins.

Th2 cytokines inhibit classical macrophage activation and stimulate the alternative pathway of macrophage activation (Fig. 6.9). IL-4 and IL-13 shut down the activation of inflammatory macrophages, thus terminating these potentially damaging reactions. These cytokines also can activate macrophages to secrete growth factors that act on fibroblasts to increase collagen synthesis and induce fibrosis. This type of macrophage response is called **alternative macrophage**

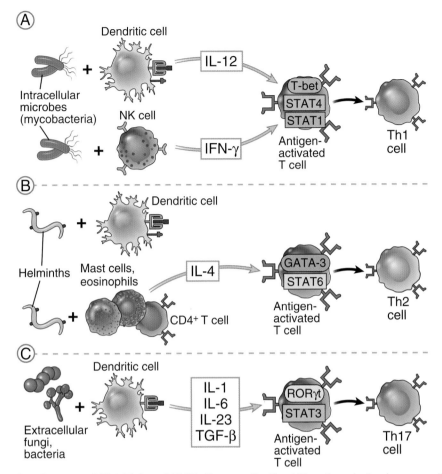

Fig. 6.7 Development of Th1, Th2, and Th17 effector cells. Dendritic cells and other immune cells that respond to different types of microbes secrete cytokines that induce the development of antigen-activated CD4+ T cells into Th1 **(A)**, Th2 **(B)**, and Th17 **(C)** subsets. The transcription factors that are involved in T cell differentiation are indicated in boxes in the antigen-activated T cells. *IFN*, Interferon-γ; *IL*, interleukin; *TGF-β*, transforming growth factor β; *NK*, natural killer.

activation, to distinguish it from classical activation, which enhances microbicidal functions. Alternative macrophage activation mediated by Th2 cytokines may play a role in tissue repair following injury and may contribute to fibrosis in a variety of disease states.

Th2 cells are involved in allergic reactions to environmental antigens. The antigens that elicit such reactions are called allergens. They induce Th2 responses in genetically susceptible individuals, and repeat exposure to the allergens triggers mast cell and eosinophil activation. Allergies are the most common type of immune disorder; we will return to these diseases in Chapter 11 when we discuss hypersensitivity reactions. Antagonists of IL-5 are approved for the treatment of asthma, and an antibody against the IL-4 receptor is approved for the allergic disease atopic dermatitis.

The relative activation of Th1 and Th2 cells in response to an infectious microbe may determine the outcome of the infection (Fig. 6.10). For example, the protozoan parasite *Leishmania major* lives inside the phagocytic vesicles of macrophages, and its elimination requires the activation of the macrophages by *L. major*–specific Th1 cells. Most inbred strains of mice make an effective Th1 response to the parasite and are thus able to eradicate the infection. However, in some inbred mouse

Fig. 6.8 Functions of Th2 cells. Th2 cells produce the cytokines interleukin-4 *(IL-4)*, IL-5, and IL-13. IL-4 (and IL-13) act on B cells to stimulate production mainly of IgE antibodies, which bind to mast cells. Help for antibody production may be provided by Tfh cells that produce Th2 cytokines and reside in lymphoid organs and not by classical Th2 cells. IL-5 activates eosinophils, a response that is important in the destruction of helminths. *APC,* Antigen-presenting cell; *Ig,* immunoglobulin; *IL,* interleukin.

strains, the response to *L. major* is dominated by Th2 cells, and these mice succumb to the infection. *Mycobacterium leprae,* the bacterium that causes leprosy, is a pathogen for humans that also lives inside macrophages and may be eliminated by cell-mediated immune mechanisms. Some people infected with *M. leprae* are unable to eradicate the infection, which, if left untreated, will progress to a destructive form of the disease, called lepromatous leprosy. By contrast, in other patients, the bacteria induce strong cell-mediated immune responses with activated T cells and macrophages around the infection site and few surviving microbes; this form of less injurious infection is called tuberculoid leprosy.

The tuberculoid form is associated with the activation of *M. leprae*–specific Th1 cells, whereas the destructive lepromatous form is associated with a defect in Th1 cell activation and sometimes a strong Th2 response. The same principle—that the T cell cytokine response to an infectious pathogen is an important determinant of the outcome of the infection—may be true for other infectious diseases.

Development of Th2 Cells

Differentiation of naive CD4+ T cells to Th2 cells is stimulated by IL-4, which may be produced by mast cells, other tissue cells, and T cells themselves at sites

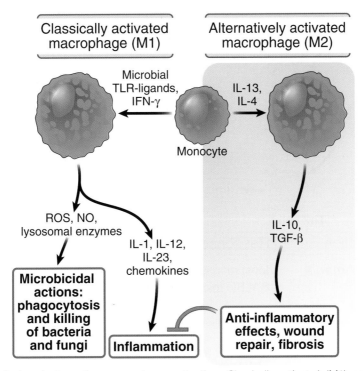

Fig. 6.9 Classical and alternative macrophage activation. Classically activated *(M1)* macrophages are induced by microbial products binding to TLRs and cytokines, particularly interferon-γ *(IFN-γ)*, and are microbicidal and proinflammatory. Alternatively activated *(M2)* macrophages are induced by interleukin-4 *(IL-4)* and IL-13 (produced by certain subsets of T lymphocytes and other leukocytes) and are important in tissue repair and fibrosis. The M1 and M2 populations may represent extreme phenotypes, and there may be other macrophage populations that express different sets of proteins. Also, in most immune responses, various mixtures of these macrophages are likely induced. *NO,* Nitric oxide; *ROS,* reactive oxygen species; *TGF-β,* transforming growth factor β; *TLR,* Toll-like receptor.

of helminth infection (see Fig. 6.7B). IL-4 activates the transcription factor Stat6 and antigen-induced signals in combination with IL-4 induce expression of a transcription factor GATA-3, which is required for Th2 differentiation. Analogous to Th1 cells, these transcription factors stimulate the expression of Th2 cytokines and proteins involved in cell migration and thus promote Th2 responses. IL-4 produced by Th2 cells enhances further Th2 differentiation, thus amplifying the Th2 response.

Th17 Cells

Th17 cells develop in response to extracellular bacterial and fungal infections and induce inflammatory reactions that destroy these organisms (Fig. 6.11). The major cytokines produced by Th17 cells are IL-17 and IL-22. This T cell subset was discovered during studies of

inflammatory diseases, many years after Th1 and Th2 subsets were described, and its role in host defense was established later.

The major function of Th17 cells is to stimulate the recruitment of neutrophils and, to less extent, monocytes, thus inducing the inflammation that accompanies many T cell–mediated adaptive immune responses. Recall that inflammation also is one of the principal reactions of innate immunity (see Chapter 2). Typically, when T cells stimulate inflammation, the reaction is stronger and more prolonged than when it is elicited by innate immune responses only. IL-17 secreted by Th17 cells stimulates the production of chemokines from other cells, and these chemokines are responsible for leukocyte recruitment. Th17 cells also stimulate the production of antimicrobial substances, called defensins, that

Infection	Response	Outcome
Leishmania major	Most mouse strains: Th1 ⇒	Recovery
	BALB/c mice: Th2 ⇒	Disseminated infection
Mycobacterium leprae	Some patients: Th1 ⇒	Tuberculoid leprosy
	Some patients: Defective Th1 or dominant Th2 ⇒	Lepromatous leprosy (high bacterial count)

Fig. 6.10 Balance between Th1 and Th2 cell activation determines outcome of intracellular infections. Naive CD4+ T lymphocytes may differentiate into Th1 cells, which activate phagocytes to kill ingested microbes, and Th2 cells, which inhibit classical macrophage activation. The balance between these two subsets may influence the outcome of infections, as illustrated by *Leishmania* infection in mice and leprosy in humans. *IFN,* Interferon; *IL,* interleukin; *TNF,* tumor necrosis factor.

function like locally produced endogenous antibiotics. IL-22 produced by Th17 cells induces epithelial cell defensin production, helps to maintain the integrity of epithelial barriers and may promote repair of damaged epithelia.

These reactions of Th17 cells are critical for defense against fungal and bacterial infections, especially in epithelial barrier tissues. These microbes can survive outside cells but are rapidly destroyed once they are phagocytosed, especially by neutrophils. Rare individuals who have inherited defects in Th17 responses are prone to developing chronic mucocutaneous candidiasis and bacterial abscesses in the skin. Th17 cells are also implicated in numerous inflammatory diseases, and antagonists of IL-17 and of the Th17-inducing cytokine IL-23 are very effective treatments for psoriasis, an inflammatory skin disease. An antagonist that neutralizes IL-12 and IL-23 (by binding to a protein shared by these two-chain cytokines), and thus inhibits the

development of both Th1 and Th17 cells, is used for the treatment of inflammatory bowel disease and psoriasis.

Development of Th17 Cells

The development of Th17 cells from naive CD4+ cells is driven by cytokines secreted by dendritic cells (and macrophages) in response to fungi and extracellular bacteria (see Fig. 6.7C). Recognition of fungal glycans and bacterial peptidoglycans and lipopeptides by innate immune receptors on dendritic cells stimulates the secretion of several innate proinflammatory cytokines, including IL-1, IL-6, and IL-23. IL-6 and IL-23 activate the transcription factor Stat3. Signals induced by these innate inflammatory cytokines and another cytokine called transforming growth factor β (TGF-β), in combination with TCR signals, induce the expression of the transcription factor RORγT. These transcription factors are required for Th17 differentiation. Interestingly, TGF-β is a powerful inhibitor of immune responses, but

Fig. 6.11 Functions of Th17 cells. Th17 cells produce the cytokine interleukin-17 *(IL-17)*, which induces production of chemokines and other cytokines from various cells, and these recruit neutrophils (and monocytes, not shown) into the site of inflammation. Some of the cytokines made by Th17 cells, notably IL-22, function to maintain epithelial barrier function in the intestinal tract and other tissues. *APC,* Antigen-presenting cell; *CSFs,* colony-stimulating factors; *TNF,* tumor necrosis factor.

when present together with IL-6 or IL-1, it promotes the development of Th17 cells.

DIFFERENTIATION AND FUNCTIONS OF CD8⁺ CYTOTOXIC T LYMPHOCYTES

Phagocytes are best at killing microbes that are confined to vesicles, and microbes that directly enter the cytosol (e.g., viruses) or escape from phagosomes into the cytosol (e.g., some ingested bacteria) are relatively resistant to the microbicidal mechanisms of phagocytes. Eradication of such cytosolic pathogens requires

another effector mechanism of T cell–mediated immunity: CD8⁺ CTLs. CTLs also serve a vital role in defense against cancers (see Chapter 10).

CD8⁺ T lymphocytes activated by antigen and other signals differentiate into CTLs that are able to kill infected cells expressing the antigen. Naive CD8⁺ T cells can recognize antigens but are not capable of killing antigen-expressing cells. The differentiation of naive CD8⁺ T cells into fully active CTLs is accompanied by the synthesis of molecules involved in cell killing, giving these effector T cells the functional capacity that is the basis for their designation as cytotoxic. CD8⁺ T lymphocytes recognize class I MHC–associated peptides on infected cells and tumor cells. The sources of class I–associated peptides are protein antigens synthesized in the cytosol and protein antigens of phagocytosed microbes that escape from phagocytic vesicles into the cytosol (see Chapter 3). In addition, some dendritic cells may capture the antigens of infected cells and tumors, transfer these antigens into the cytosol, and thus present the ingested antigens on class I MHC molecules, by the process known as cross-presentation (see Fig. 3.16, Chapter 3). The differentiation of naive CD8⁺ T cells into functional CTLs and memory cells requires not only antigen recognition but also costimulation and, in some situations, help from CD4⁺ T cells (see Fig. 5.7, Chapter 5).

CD8⁺ CTLs recognize class I MHC–peptide complexes on the surface of infected cells and kill these cells, thus eliminating the reservoir of infection. The T cells recognize MHC-associated peptides by their TCR and the CD8 coreceptor. These infected cells also are called targets of CTLs, because they are destroyed by the CTLs. The TCR and CD8, as well as other signaling proteins, cluster in the CTL membrane at the site of contact with the target cell and are surrounded by the leukocyte function–associated antigen 1 (LFA-1) integrin. These molecules bind their ligands on the target cell, forming an immune synapse (see Chapter 5).

Antigen recognition by CTLs results in the activation of signal transduction pathways that lead to the exocytosis of the contents of the CTL's granules into the synapse between the CTL and the target cell (Fig. 6.12). Because all nucleated cells express class I MHC, and differentiated CTLs do not require costimulation or T cell help for activation, the CTLs can be activated by and are able to kill any infected cell in any tissue. CTLs kill target cells mainly as a result of delivery of granule proteins into the target cells. Two types of granule proteins critical for

Fig. 6.12 Mechanisms of killing of infected cells by CD8⁺ cytotoxic T lymphocytes *(CTLs)*. CTLs recognize class I major histocompatibility complex (MHC)–associated peptides of cytoplasmic microbes in infected cells and form tight adhesions (conjugates) with these cells. Adhesion molecules such as integrins stabilize the binding of the CTLs to infected cells (not shown). The CTLs are activated to release (exocytose) their granule contents (perforin and granzymes) toward the infected cell, referred to as the target cell. Granzymes are delivered to the cytosol of the target cell by a perforin-dependent mechanism. Granzymes then induce apoptosis. *ICAM-1,* Intercellular adhesion molecule 1; *LFA-1,* leukocyte function–associated antigen 1.

killing are granzymes (granule enzymes) and perforin. **Perforin** disrupts the integrity of the target cell plasma membrane and endosomal membranes, thereby facilitating the delivery of granzymes into the cytosol. **Granzymes** (granule enzymes) cleave and thereby activate enzymes called caspases (cysteine proteases that cleave proteins after aspartic acid residues) that are present in the cytosol of target cells and whose major function is to induce apoptosis.

Activated CTLs also express a membrane protein called Fas ligand, which binds to a death-inducing receptor, called Fas (CD95), on target cells. Engagement of Fas activates caspases and induces target cell apoptosis; this pathway does not require granule exocytosis and probably plays only a minor role in killing by CD8⁺ CTLs.

The net result of these effector mechanisms of CTLs is that the infected cells are killed. Cells that have undergone apoptosis are rapidly phagocytosed and eliminated. CTLs themselves are not injured during the process of killing other cells, so each CTL can kill a target cell, detach, and go on to kill additional targets.

In addition to their cytotoxic activity, CD8⁺ effector cells secrete IFN-γ. This cytokine is responsible for

activation of macrophages in infections and in disease states where excessive activation of CD8⁺ T cells may be a feature. It may also play a role in defense against some tumors.

Although we have described the effector functions of CD4⁺ T cells and CD8⁺ T cells separately, these types of T lymphocytes may function cooperatively to destroy intracellular microbes (Fig. 6.13). If microbes are phagocytosed and remain sequestered in macrophage vesicles, CD4⁺ T cells may be adequate to eradicate these infections by secreting IFN-γ and activating the microbicidal mechanisms of the macrophages. However, if the microbes are able to escape from vesicles into the cytoplasm, they become insusceptible to the killing mechanisms of activated macrophages, and their elimination requires destruction of the infected cells by CD8⁺ CTLs.

RESISTANCE OF PATHOGENIC MICROBES TO CELL-MEDIATED IMMUNITY

Different microbes have developed diverse mechanisms to resist T lymphocyte–mediated host defense (Fig. 6.14). Many intracellular bacteria,

Fig. 6.13 Cooperation between CD4+ and CD8+ T cells in eradication of intracellular infections. In a macrophage infected by an intracellular bacterium, some of the bacteria are sequestered in vesicles (phagosomes), and others may escape into the cytosol. CD4+ T cells recognize antigens derived from the vesicular microbes and activate the macrophage to kill the microbes in the vesicles. CD8+ T cells recognize antigens derived from the cytosolic bacteria and are needed to kill the infected cell, thus eliminating the reservoir of infection. *CTL*, Cytotoxic T lymphocyte; *IFN*, interferon.

such as *Mycobacterium tuberculosis, Legionella pneumophila,* and *Listeria monocytogenes,* inhibit the fusion of phagosomes with lysosomes or create pores in phagosome membranes, allowing these organisms to escape into the cytosol. Thus, these microbes are able to resist the microbicidal mechanisms of phagocytes and survive and even replicate inside phagocytes. Many viruses inhibit class I MHC–associated antigen presentation by inhibiting production or expression of class I molecules, by blocking transport of antigenic peptides from the cytosol into the endoplasmic reticulum (ER) and by removing newly synthesized class I molecules from the ER. All these viral mechanisms reduce the loading of class I MHC molecules by viral peptides. The result of this defective loading is reduced surface expression of class I MHC molecules, because empty class I molecules are unstable and are not expressed on the cell surface. It is interesting that NK cells are activated by class I–deficient cells (see Chapter 2). Thus, host defenses have evolved to combat immune evasion mechanisms of microbes: CTLs recognize class I MHC–associated viral peptides, viruses inhibit class I MHC expression, and NK cells recognize the absence of class I MHC molecules on infected or stressed cells.

Other viruses produce inhibitory cytokines or soluble (decoy) cytokine receptors that bind and neutralize cytokines such as IFN-γ, reducing the amount of cytokines available to trigger cell-mediated immune reactions. Some viruses evade elimination and establish chronic infections by stimulating expression of inhibitory receptors, including PD-1 (programmed [cell] death protein 1; see Chapter 9) on CD8+ T cells, thus inhibiting the effector functions of CTLs. This phenomenon, in which the T cells mount an initial response against the virus but the response is prematurely terminated, has been called **T cell exhaustion** (Fig. 6.15). It typically occurs as a reaction to chronic antigenic stimulation, as in chronic viral infections or tumors, and is a mechanism by which the repeatedly stimulated T cell terminates its own

Microbe	Mechanism	
Mycobacteria	Inhibition of phagolysosome fusion	
Herpes simplex virus (HSV)	Inhibition of antigen presentation: HSV peptide interferes with TAP transporter	
Cytomegalovirus (CMV)	Inhibition of antigen presentation: inhibition of proteasomal activity; removal of class I MHC molecules from endoplasmic reticulum (ER)	
Epstein-Barr virus (EBV)	Inhibition of antigen presentation: inhibition of proteasomal activity	
Epstein-Barr virus (EBV)	Production of IL-10, inhibition of macrophage and dendritic cell activation	
Pox virus	Inhibition of effector cell activation: production of soluble cytokine receptors	

Fig. 6.14 Evasion of cell-mediated immunity *(CMI)* by microbes. Select examples of different mechanisms by which bacteria and viruses resist the effector mechanisms of CMI. *CTL*, Cytotoxic T lymphocyte; *ER*, endoplasmic reticulum; *IFN*, interferon; *IL*, interleukin; *TAP*, transporter associated with antigen processing.

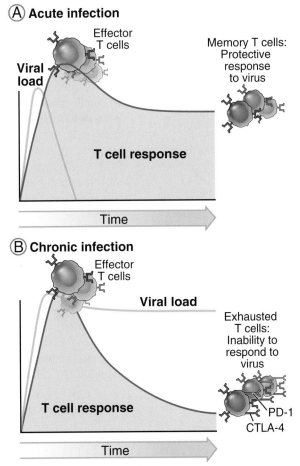

Fig. 6.15 T cell activation and exhaustion. A, In an acute viral infection, virus-specific CD8⁺ T cells proliferate, differentiate into effector CTLs and memory cells, and clear the virus. **B,** In some chronic viral infections,
CD8⁺ T cells mount an initial response but begin to express inhibitory receptors (such as PD-1 and CTLA-4)
and are inactivated, leading to persistence of the virus. This process is called *exhaustion* because the T cells
do make a response, but this is short lived.

response. Still other viruses directly infect and kill
immune cells, the best example being human immunodeficiency virus (HIV), which is able to survive in
infected persons by killing CD4⁺ T cells.

The outcome of infections is influenced by the
strength of host defenses and the ability of pathogens
to resist these defenses. The same principle is evident
when the effector mechanisms of humoral immunity
are considered. One approach for tilting the balance
between the host and microbes in favor of protective immunity is to vaccinate individuals to enhance

adaptive immune responses. The principles underlying
vaccination strategies are described at the end of Chapter 8, after the discussion of humoral immunity.

As we will discuss in Chapter 10, tumors, like infectious pathogens, have developed several mechanisms for
evading or resisting CD8⁺ T cell–mediated immunity.
These mechanisms include inhibiting expression of class
I MHC molecules and inducing T cell exhaustion. Blocking some of these evasion mechanisms provides effective strategies for unleashing antitumor immunity (see
Chapter 10).

SUMMARY

- Cell-mediated immunity is the arm of adaptive immunity that eradicates infections by cell-associated microbes. This form of host defense uses two types of T cells: CD4$^+$ helper T cells recruit and activate phagocytes to kill ingested and some extracellular microbes, and CD8$^+$ CTLs eliminate the reservoirs of infection by killing cells harboring microbes in the cytosol.

- CD4$^+$ T cells can differentiate into subsets of effector cells that make different cytokines and perform distinct functions.

- Effector cells of the Th1 subset recognize the antigens of microbes that have been ingested by macrophages. These T cells secrete IFN-γ and express CD40 ligand, which function cooperatively to activate macrophages.

- Classically activated macrophages produce substances, including ROS, NO, and lysosomal enzymes, that kill ingested microbes. Macrophages also produce cytokines that induce inflammation.

- Th2 cells stimulate eosinophilic inflammation and trigger the alternative pathway of macrophage activation, and Tfh cells induced in parallel trigger IgE production. IgE and eosinophils are important in host defense against helminthic parasites.

- The balance between activation of Th1 and Th2 cells determines the outcomes of many infections, with Th1 cells promoting and Th2 cells suppressing defense against intracellular microbes.

- Th17 cells enhance neutrophil and monocyte recruitment and acute inflammation, which is essential for defense against certain extracellular bacteria and fungi.

- CD8$^+$ T cells differentiate into CTLs that kill infected cells, mainly by inducing apoptosis of the infected cells. CD4$^+$ and CD8$^+$ T cells often function cooperatively to eradicate intracellular infections. CD8$^+$ CTLs also kill cancer cells and are the key mediators of antitumor immunity.

- Many pathogenic microbes have evolved mechanisms to resist cell-mediated immunity. These mechanisms include inhibiting phagolysosome fusion, escaping from the vesicles of phagocytes, inhibiting the assembly of class I MHC–peptide complexes, producing inhibitory cytokines or decoy cytokine receptors, and inactivating T cells, thus prematurely terminating T cell responses.

REVIEW QUESTIONS

1. What are the types of T lymphocyte–mediated immune reactions that eliminate microbes that are sequestered in the vesicles of phagocytes and microbes that live in the cytoplasm of infected host cells?

2. What are the major subsets of CD4$^+$ effector T cells, how do they differ, and what are their roles in defense against different types of infectious pathogens?

3. What are the mechanisms by which T cells activate macrophages, and what are the responses of macrophages that result in the killing of ingested microbes?

4. How do CD8$^+$ CTLs kill cells infected with viruses?

5. What are some of the mechanisms by which intracellular microbes resist the effector mechanisms of cell-mediated immunity?

Answers to and discussion of the Review Questions are available at Student Consult.

Humoral Immune Responses
Activation of B Lymphocytes and Production of Antibodies

Humoral immunity is mediated by antibodies and is the arm of the adaptive immune response that functions to neutralize and eliminate extracellular microbes and microbial toxins. Humoral immunity is the principal defense mechanism against microbes with capsules rich in polysaccharides and lipids, because antibodies can be produced against polysaccharides and lipids but T cells cannot respond to nonprotein antigens. Antibodies are produced by B lymphocytes and their progeny. Naive B lymphocytes recognize antigens but do not secrete antibodies, and activation of these cells stimulates their differentiation into antibody-secreting plasma cells.

This chapter describes the process and mechanisms of B cell activation and antibody production, focusing on the following questions:

- How are antigen receptor–expressing naive B lymphocytes activated and converted to antibody secreting cells?

- How is the process of B cell activation regulated so that the most useful types of antibodies are produced in response to different types of microbes?

Chapter 8 describes how the antibodies that are produced during humoral immune responses function to defend individuals against microbes and toxins.

PHASES AND TYPES OF HUMORAL IMMUNE RESPONSES

The activation of B lymphocytes results in their proliferation, leading to expansion of antigen-specific clones, and their differentiation into plasma cells, which secrete antibodies (Fig. 7.1). Naive B lymphocytes express two classes of membrane-bound antibodies, immunoglobulins M and D (IgM and IgD), that function as receptors for antigens. These naive B cells are activated by antigen binding to membrane

Fig. 7.1 Phases of humoral immune responses. Naive B lymphocytes recognize antigens, and under the influence of helper T cells and other stimuli (not shown), the B cells are activated to proliferate, giving rise to clonal expansion, and to differentiate into antibody-secreting plasma cells. Some of the activated B cells undergo heavy-chain isotype switching and affinity maturation, and some become long-lived memory cells.

immunoglobulin (Ig) and by other signals discussed later in the chapter. The antibodies secreted in response to an antigen have the same specificity as the surface receptors on naive B cells that recognize that antigen in order to initiate the response. One activated B cell may generate a few thousand plasma cells, each of which can produce copious amounts of antibody, in the range of several thousand molecules per hour. In this way, humoral immunity can keep pace with rapidly proliferating microbes. During their differentiation, some B cells may begin to produce antibodies of different heavy-chain isotypes (or classes) that mediate different effector functions and are specialized to combat different types of microbes. This process is called heavy-chain isotype (or class) switching. During the course of a B cell response to an infection, the affinity of antibodies specific for microbial proteins increases over time. This process is called affinity maturation, and it leads to the production of antibodies with improved capacity to bind to and neutralize microbes and their toxins.

Antibody responses to different antigens are classified as T-dependent or T-independent, based on the requirement for T cell help (Fig. 7.2). B lymphocytes recognize and are activated by a wide variety of chemically distinct antigens, including proteins, polysaccharides, lipids, nucleic acids, and small chemicals. Helper T lymphocytes play an important role in B cell activation by protein antigens. (The designation *helper* came from the discovery that some T cells stimulate, or help, B lymphocytes to produce antibodies.) T cells help B cells respond to only protein antigens because T cells can only recognize peptides derived from proteins presented as peptide–major histocompatibility complex (MHC) complexes. In the absence of T cell help, most protein antigens elicit weak or no antibody responses. Therefore, protein antigens and the antibody responses to these antigens are called T-dependent. Polysaccharides, nucleic acids, lipids, and other multivalent antigens (which contain the same structural unit repeated multiple times in tandem) can stimulate antibody production without the involvement of helper T cells. Therefore, these multivalent nonprotein antigens and the antibody responses to them are called T-independent. The antibodies produced in response to proteins exhibit more isotype switching and affinity maturation

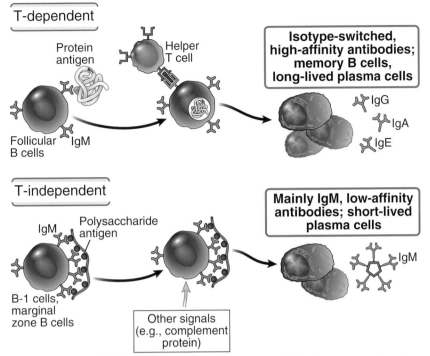

Fig. 7.2 T-dependent and T-independent antibody responses. Antibody responses to protein antigens require T cell help, and the antibodies produced typically show isotype switching and are of high affinity. Nonprotein (e.g., polysaccharide) antigens are able to activate B cells without T cell help. Most T-dependent responses are made by follicular B cells, whereas marginal zone B cells and B-1 cells play greater roles in T-independent responses. *Ig,* Immunoglobulin.

than antibodies against T-independent antigens because helper T cells stimulate these processes. Furthermore, T-dependent antigens stimulate the generation of long-lived plasma cells and memory B cells. Thus, the most specialized and long-lived antibody responses involve protein antigens and are generated under the influence of helper T cells, whereas T-independent responses are relatively simple and transient, and involve only the direct activation of B cells by antigens.

Different subsets of B cells respond preferentially to T-dependent and T-independent antigens (see Fig. 7.2). The majority of B cells are called **follicular B cells** because they reside in and circulate through the follicles of lymphoid organs (see Chapter 1). These follicular B cells make the bulk of T-dependent, class-switched, and high-affinity antibody responses to protein antigens and give rise to long-lived plasma cells. **Marginal-zone B cells,** which are located in the peripheral region of the splenic white pulp and also in the outer rim of follicles in lymph nodes, respond largely to blood-borne polysaccharide and

lipid antigens; **B-1 cells** respond to multivalent antigens in the mucosal tissues and peritoneum. Marginal-zone B cells and B-1 cells express antigen receptors of limited diversity and make predominantly T-independent IgM responses. IgM antibodies may be produced spontaneously by B-1 cells, without overt immunization. These antibodies, called **natural antibodies**, may help to clear some cells that die by apoptosis during normal cell turnover and may also provide protection against some bacterial pathogens.

Antibody responses generated during the first exposure to an antigen, called primary responses, differ quantitatively and qualitatively from responses to subsequent exposures, called secondary responses (Fig. 7.3). The amounts of antibody produced in the primary immune response are smaller than the amounts produced in secondary responses. In secondary responses to protein antigens, there is increased heavy-chain isotype switching and affinity maturation, because repeated stimulation by a protein antigen leads to an increase in the number and activity of helper T lymphocytes.

Fig. 7.3 Features of primary and secondary antibody responses. Primary and secondary antibody responses differ in several respects, illustrated schematically in (A) and summarized in (B). In a primary response, naive B cells in peripheral lymphoid tissues are activated to proliferate and differentiate into anti-body-secreting plasma cells and memory cells. Some plasma cells may migrate to and survive in the bone marrow for long periods. In a secondary response, memory B cells are activated to produce larger amounts of antibodies, often with more heavy-chain class switching and affinity maturation. These features of secondary responses are seen mainly in responses to protein antigens, because these changes in B cells are stimulated by helper T cells, and only proteins activate T cells (not shown). The kinetics of the responses may vary with different antigens and types of immunization. *Ig*, Immunoglobulin.

Table (B):

	Primary response	Secondary response
Lag after immunization	Usually 5–10 days	Usually 1–3 days
Peak response	Smaller	Larger
Antibody isotype	Usually IgM>IgG	Relative increase in IgG and, under certain situations, in IgA or IgE (heavy-chain isotype switching)
Antibody affinity	Lower average affinity, more variable	Higher average affinity (affinity maturation)

With this introduction, we now discuss B cell activation and antibody production, beginning with the responses of B cells to the initial encounter with antigen.

STIMULATION OF B LYMPHOCYTES BY ANTIGEN

Humoral immune responses are initiated when antigen-specific B lymphocytes in the spleen, lymph nodes, and mucosal lymphoid tissues recognize antigens. Some of the antigens in tissues or in the blood are transported to and concentrated in the B cell–rich follicles and marginal zones of these peripheral lymphoid organs. In lymph nodes, macrophages lining the subcapsular sinus may capture antigens and take them to the adjacent follicles, where the bound antigens are displayed to B cells. B lymphocytes specific for an antigen use their membrane-bound Ig as receptors that recognize the antigen directly, without any need for processing of the antigen. B cells are capable of recognizing the native antigen, so the antibodies that are subsequently secreted (which have the same specificity as the B cell antigen receptors) are able to bind to the native microbe or microbial product.

The recognition of antigen triggers signaling pathways that initiate B cell activation. As with T lymphocytes, B cell activation also requires signals in addition to antigen recognition, and many of these second signals are produced during innate immune reactions to microbes. In the following sections, we describe the mechanisms of B cell activation by antigen and other stimuli, followed by a discussion of the functional consequences of antigen recognition.

Antigen-Induced Signaling in B Cells

Antigen-induced clustering of membrane Ig receptors triggers biochemical signals that activate B cells (Fig. 7.4). The process of B lymphocyte activation is, in principle, similar to the activation of T cells (see Chapter 5, Fig. 5.9). In B cells, antigen receptor–mediated signal transduction requires the bringing together (cross-linking) of two or more membrane Ig molecules. Antigen receptor cross-linking occurs when two or more antigen molecules in an aggregate, or repeating epitopes of one antigen molecule, bind to adjacent membrane Ig molecules of a B cell. Polysaccharides, lipids, and other nonprotein antigens often contain multiple identical epitopes in each molecule and are therefore able to bind to numerous Ig receptors on a B cell at the same time.

Even protein antigens may be expressed in an array on the surface of microbes and are thus able to cross-link antigen receptors of a B cell.

Signals initiated by antigen receptor cross-linking are transduced by receptor-associated proteins. Membrane IgM and IgD, the antigen receptors of naive B lymphocytes, have highly variable extracellular antigen-binding regions (see Chapter 4). However, these membrane receptors have short cytoplasmic tails, so although they recognize antigens, they do not themselves transduce signals. The receptors are noncovalently associated with two proteins, called Igα and Igβ, to form the **B cell receptor (BCR) complex**, analogous to the T cell receptor (TCR) complex of T lymphocytes. The cytoplasmic domains of Igα and Igβ each contain a conserved immunoreceptor tyrosine-based activation motif (ITAM), similar to those found in signaling subunits of many other activating receptors in the immune system (e.g., CD3 and ζ proteins of the TCR complex; see Chapter 5). When two or more antigen receptors of a B cell are brought together by antigen-induced cross-linking, the tyrosines in the ITAMs of Igα and Igβ are phosphorylated by tyrosine kinases associated with the BCR complex. These phosphotyrosines recruit the Syk tyrosine kinase (equivalent to ZAP-70 in T cells), which is activated and in turn phosphorylates tyrosine residues on adaptor proteins. These phosphorylated proteins then recruit and activate a number of downstream molecules, mainly enzymes that initiate signaling cascades that activate transcription factors.

The net result of receptor-induced signaling in B cells is the activation of transcription factors that switch on the expression of genes whose protein products are involved in B cell proliferation and differentiation. Some of the important proteins are described below.

Role of Innate Immune Signals in B Cell Activation

B lymphocytes express a receptor for a complement system protein that provides second signals for the activation of these cells (Fig. 7.5A). The complement system, introduced in Chapter 2, is a collection of plasma proteins that are activated by microbes and by antibodies attached to microbes and function as effector mechanisms of host defense (see Chapter 8). When the complement system is activated by a microbe as part of the innate immune response, the microbe becomes coated with proteolytic fragments of the most abundant complement

Fig. 7.4 Antigen receptor–mediated signal transduction in B lymphocytes. Cross-linking of antigen receptors on B cells by antigen triggers biochemical signals that are transduced by the immunoglobulin (*Ig*)-associated proteins Igα and Igβ. These signals induce early tyrosine phosphorylation events, activation of various biochemical intermediates and enzymes, and activation of transcription factors. Similar signaling events are seen in T cells after antigen recognition. Note that maximal signaling requires cross-linking of at least two Ig receptors by antigens. *AP-1,* Activating protein 1; *GDP,* guanosine diphosphate; *GTP,* guanosine triphosphate; *ITAM,* immunoreceptor tyrosine-based activation motif; *NFAT,* nuclear factor of activated T cells; *NF-κB,* nuclear factor κB; *PKC,* protein kinase C; *PLC,* phospholipase C.

protein, C3. One of these fragments is called C3d. B lymphocytes express a receptor for C3d called complement receptor type 2 (CR2, or CD21). B cells that are specific for a microbe's antigens recognize the antigens by their BCRs and simultaneously recognize the bound C3d via the CR2 receptor. Engagement of CR2 greatly enhances antigen-dependent activation responses of B cells by enhancing tyrosine phosphorylation of ITAMs. This role

of complement in humoral immune responses illustrates the fundamental tenet of the two-signal hypothesis that was introduced in Chapter 2, that microbes or innate immune responses to microbes provide signals in addition to antigen that are necessary for lymphocyte activation. In humoral immunity, complement activation represents one way in which innate immunity facilitates B lymphocyte activation.

Fig. 7.5 Role of innate immune signals in B cell activation. Signals generated during innate immune responses to microbes and some antigens cooperate with recognition of antigen by antigen receptors to initiate B cell responses. **A,** Activation of complement by microbes leads to the binding of a complement breakdown product, C3d, to the microbes. The B cell simultaneously recognizes a microbial antigen (by the immunoglobulin receptor) and bound C3d by *CR2* (type 2 complement receptor). CR2 is attached to a complex of proteins (CD19, CD81) that are involved in delivering activating signals to the B cell. **B,** Molecules derived from microbes (so-called pathogen-associated molecular patterns [PAMPs]; see Chapter 2) may activate Toll-like receptors *(TLRs)* of B cells at the same time as microbial antigens are being recognized by the antigen receptor. *BCR,* B cell receptor.

Microbial products also directly activate B cells by engaging innate pattern recognition receptors (see Fig. 7.5B). B lymphocytes, similar to dendritic cells and other leukocytes, express numerous Toll-like receptors (TLRs; see Chapter 2). Pathogen-associated molecular patterns bind to TLRs on the B cells, which triggers activating signals that work in concert with signals from the antigen receptor. This combination of signals stimulates B cell proliferation, differentiation, and Ig secretion, thus promoting antibody responses against microbes.

Functional Consequences of B Cell Activation by Antigen

B cell activation by multivalent antigen (and other signals) may initiate the proliferation and differentiation of the cells and prepares them to interact with helper T lymphocytes if the antigen is a protein (Fig. 7.6). The activated B lymphocytes may begin to synthesize more IgM and to produce some of this IgM in a secreted form. Thus, antigen stimulation induces the early phase of the humoral immune response. This response is greatest when the antigen is multivalent, cross-links many antigen receptors, and activates complement and innate immune receptors strongly; all these features are typically seen with polysaccharides and other T-independent microbial antigens, as discussed later, but not most soluble proteins. Therefore, by themselves, protein antigens typically do not stimulate high levels of B cell proliferation and differentiation. However, protein antigens induce changes in B cells that enhance their ability to interact with helper T lymphocytes.

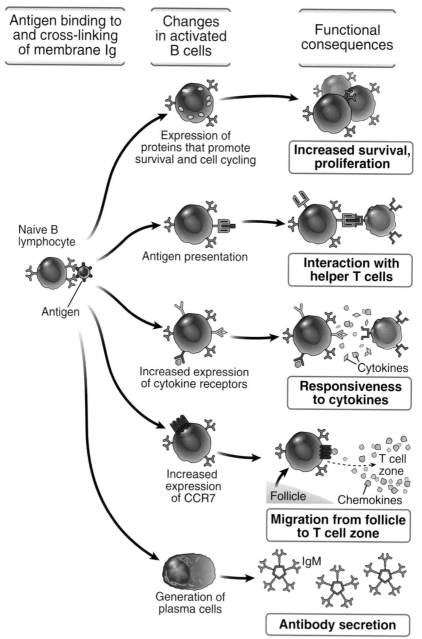

Fig. 7.6 Functional consequences of antigen receptor-mediated B cell activation. The activation of B cells by antigen in lymphoid organs initiates the process of B cell proliferation and immunoglobulin M (IgM) secretion and prepares the B cell for interaction with helper T cells.

Activated B cells endocytose protein antigen that binds specifically to the BCR, resulting in degradation of the antigen and display of peptides bound to class II MHC molecules, which can be recognized by helper T cells. Activated B cells migrate out of the follicles and toward the anatomic compartment where helper T cells are concentrated. Thus, the B cells are poised to interact with and respond to helper T cells, which were derived from naive T cells previously activated by the same antigen presented by dendritic cells.

The next section describes the interactions of helper T cells with B lymphocytes in antibody responses to T-dependent protein antigens. Responses to T-independent antigens are discussed at the end of the chapter.

FUNCTIONS OF HELPER T LYMPHOCYTES IN HUMORAL IMMUNE RESPONSES

For a protein antigen to stimulate an antibody response, B lymphocytes and helper T lymphocytes specific for that antigen must come together in lymphoid organs and interact in a way that stimulates B cell proliferation and differentiation. We know this process works efficiently because protein antigens elicit antibody responses within 3 to 7 days after antigen exposure. The efficiency of antigen-induced T-B cell interaction raises many questions. How do B cells and T cells specific for epitopes of the same antigen find one another, considering that naive B and T lymphocytes specific for any one antigen are rare, probably less than 1 in 100,000 of all the lymphocytes in the body? How do helper T cells specific for an antigen interact with B cells specific for an epitope of the same antigen and not with irrelevant B cells? What signals are delivered by helper T cells that stimulate not only the secretion of antibody but also the special features of the antibody response to proteins—namely, heavy-chain isotype switching and affinity maturation? As discussed next, the answers to these questions are now well understood.

The process of T-B cell interaction and T cell–dependent antibody responses is initiated by recognition of different epitopes of the same protein antigen by the two cell types and occurs in a series of sequential steps (Fig. 7.7):

- Naive CD4$^+$ T cells are activated in the T cell zone of a secondary lymphoid organ by antigen (in the form of processed peptides bound to class II MHC molecules) presented by dendritic cells, and differentiate into functional (cytokine-producing) helper T cells.
- Naive B cells are activated in the follicles of the same lymphoid organ by an exposed epitope on the same protein (in its native conformation) that is transported to the follicle.
- The antigen-activated helper T cells and B cells migrate toward one another and interact at the edges of the follicles, where the initial antibody response develops.

- Some of the cells migrate back into follicles to form germinal centers, where the more specialized antibody responses are induced.

Next we describe each of these steps in detail.

Activation and Migration of Helper T Cells and B cells

Helper T cells that have been activated by dendritic cells migrate toward the B cell zone and interact with antigen-stimulated B lymphocytes in parafollicular areas of the peripheral lymphoid organs (see Fig. 7.7A).

- The initial activation of T cells requires antigen recognition and costimulation, as described in Chapter 5. The antigens that stimulate CD4$^+$ helper T cells are proteins derived from microbes that are internalized, processed in late endosomes and lysosomes, and displayed as peptides bound to class II MHC molecules of antigen-presenting cells (APCs) in the T cell–rich zones of peripheral lymphoid tissues. T cell activation is induced best by microbial protein antigens and, in the case of vaccines, by protein antigens that are administered with adjuvants, which stimulate the expression of costimulators on APCs. The CD4$^+$ T cells differentiate into effector cells capable of producing various cytokines and CD40 ligand, and some of these T lymphocytes migrate toward the edges of lymphoid follicles.
- B lymphocytes are activated by antigen in the follicles, as described above, and the activated B cells begin to move out of the follicles toward the T cells.

The directed migration of activated B and T cells toward one another depends on changes in the expression of certain chemokine receptors on the activated lymphocytes. Activated T cells reduce expression of the chemokine receptor CCR7, which recognizes chemokines produced in T cell zones, and increase expression of the chemokine receptor CXCR5, which binds a chemokine produced in B cell follicles. Activated B cells undergo precisely the opposite changes, decreasing CXCR5 and increasing CCR7 expression. As a result, antigen-stimulated B and T cells migrate toward one another and meet at the edges of lymphoid follicles or in interfollicular areas. The next step in their interaction occurs here. Because antigen recognition is required for these changes, the cells that move towards one another are the ones that have been stimulated by antigen. This regulated migration is one mechanism for ensuring that rare

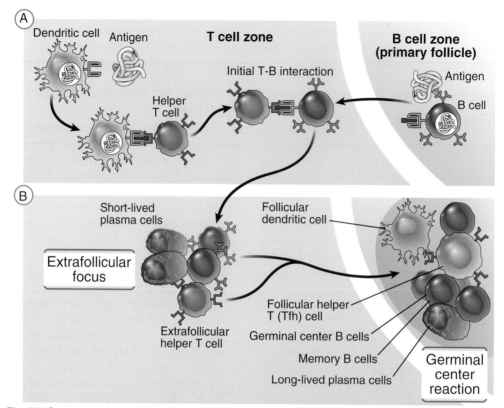

Fig. 7.7 Sequence of events in helper T cell–dependent antibody responses. A, T and B lymphocytes independently recognize the antigen in different regions of peripheral lymphoid organs and are activated. The activated cells migrate toward one another and interact at the edges of lymphoid follicles. **B,** Antibody-secreting plasma cells are initially produced in the extrafollicular focus where the antigen-activated T and B cells interact. Some of the activated B and T cells migrate back into the follicle to form the germinal center, where the antibody response develops fully.

antigen-specific lymphocytes can locate one another and interact productively during immune responses to the antigen.

Presentation of Antigens by B Lymphocytes to Helper T Cells

The B lymphocytes that bind protein antigens by their membrane Ig antigen receptors endocytose these antigens, process them in endosomal vesicles, and display class II MHC–associated peptides for recognition by CD4+ helper T cells (Fig. 7.8). The membrane Ig of B cells is a high-affinity receptor that enables a B cell to specifically bind a particular antigen, even when the extracellular concentration of the antigen is very low. In addition, antigen bound by membrane Ig is endocytosed efficiently and is delivered to late endosomal vesicles and lysosomes, where proteins are processed into peptides that bind to class II MHC molecules (see Chapter 3). Therefore, B lymphocytes are efficient APCs for the antigens they specifically recognize.

Any one B cell may bind a conformational epitope of a native protein antigen, internalize and process the protein, and display multiple peptides from that protein for T cell recognition. Therefore, B cells recognize one epitope of a protein antigen first, and helper T cells recognize different epitopes of the same protein later. Because B cells efficiently internalize and process the antigen for which they have specific receptors, and helper T cells recognize peptides derived from the same antigen, the ensuing interaction remains antigen specific. B cells are capable of activating previously differentiated effector T cells but are inefficient at initiating the responses of naive T cells.

Fig. 7.8 Antigen presentation by B lymphocytes to helper T cells. B cells specific for a protein antigen bind and internalize that antigen, process it, and present peptides attached to class II major histocompatibility complex *(MHC)* molecules to helper T cells. The B cells and helper T cells are specific for the same antigen, but the B cells recognize native (conformational) epitopes, and the helper T cells recognize peptide fragments of the antigen bound to class II MHC molecules.

The idea that a B cell recognizes one epitope of an intact antigen and displays different epitopes (peptides) for recognition by helper T cells was first demonstrated by studies using hapten-carrier conjugates. A hapten is a small chemical that is recognized by B cells but stimulates strong antibody responses only if it is attached to a carrier protein. In this situation, the B cell binds the hapten portion, ingests the conjugate, and displays peptides derived from the carrier to helper T cells. The antibody response is, of course, specific for the epitope that the B cell recognized (the hapten in this example), and the peptides derived from the carrier protein simply bring helper T cells into the reaction. This concept has been exploited to develop effective vaccines against microbial polysaccharides (Fig. 7.9). Some bacteria have polysaccharide-rich capsules, and the polysaccharides themselves stimulate T-independent antibody responses, which are weak in infants and young children. If the polysaccharide is coupled to a carrier protein, however, effective T-dependent responses are induced against the polysaccharide because helper T cells specific for the carrier are engaged in the response. In this situation, the B cell recognizes the polysaccharide (equivalent to the hapten) and the T cell recognizes peptides from the attached protein (the carrier); the antibody response is specific for the polysaccharide, but it is much stronger than conventional T-independent responses because helper T cells are "forced" to participate. Such **conjugate vaccines** have been very useful for inducing protective immunity against bacteria such as *Haemophilus influenzae*, especially in infants, and current vaccines against pneumococcus are also conjugate vaccines.

Mechanisms of Helper T Cell–Mediated Activation of B Lymphocytes

Activated helper T lymphocytes that recognize antigen presented by B cells use CD40 ligand (CD40L) and secreted cytokines to activate the antigen-specific B cells (Fig. 7.10). The process of helper T cell–mediated B lymphocyte activation is analogous to the process of T cell–mediated macrophage activation in cell-mediated immunity (see Chapter 6, Fig. 6.6). CD40L expressed on activated helper T cells binds to CD40 on B lymphocytes. Engagement of CD40 generates signals in the B cells that stimulate proliferation and the synthesis and secretion of antibodies. At the same time, cytokines produced by the helper T cells bind to cytokine receptors on B lymphocytes and stimulate more B cell proliferation and Ig production. The requirement for the CD40L-CD40 interaction ensures that only T and B lymphocytes in physical contact engage in productive interactions. As described previously, the antigen-specific lymphocytes are the cells that physically interact, thus ensuring that the antigen-specific B cells are the cells that receive T cell help and are activated. The CD40L-CD40 interaction also stimulates heavy-chain isotype switching and affinity maturation, which explains why these changes typically are seen in antibody responses to T-dependent protein antigens.

Extrafollicular and Germinal Center Reactions

The initial T-B interaction, which occurs outside the lymphoid follicles, results in the production of low levels of antibodies, which may be of switched isotypes (described next) but are generally of low affinity

Fig. 7.9 The principle of conjugate vaccines: the hapten-carrier concept. In order to generate strong antibody responses against a microbial polysaccharide, the polysaccharide is coupled to a protein (in this case, tetanus toxoid). B cells that recognize the polysaccharide ingest it and present peptides from the protein to helper T cells, which stimulate the polysaccharide-specific B cells. Thus isotype switching, affinity maturation, and long-lived plasma cells and memory cells (all features of responses to proteins) are induced in a response to polysaccharides. (Note that some B cells will also recognize the tetanus toxoid and antibodies will be produced against the carrier protein, but this has no bearing on the antipolysaccharide response.) *Ig,* Immunoglobulin.

(see Fig. 7.7B). The plasma cells that are generated in these extra-follicular foci are typically short-lived and produce antibodies for a few weeks, and few memory B cells are generated.

Many of the events in fully developed antibody responses occur in germinal centers that are formed in lymphoid follicles and require the participation of a specialized type of helper T cell (Fig. 7.11). Some of the activated helper T cells express high levels of the chemokine receptor CXCR5, which draws these cells into the adjacent follicles. The CD4+ T cells that migrate into B cell–rich follicles are called **follicular helper T (Tfh) cells.** The generation and function of Tfh cells are dependent on a receptor of the CD28 family called inducible

Fig. 7.10 Mechanisms of helper T cell–mediated activation of B lymphocytes. Helper T cells recognize peptide antigens presented by B cells on the B cells. The helper T cells are activated to express CD40 ligand *(CD40L)* and secrete cytokines, both of which bind to their receptors on the same B cells and activate the B cells.

Activation of B cells
and migration
into germinal center

B cell proliferation

Somatic mutation
and affinity
maturation;
isotype switching

Exit of high-affinity
antibody-secreting cells,
and memory B cells

Fig. 7.11 The germinal center reaction. B cells that have been activated by T helper cells at the edge of a primary follicle migrate into the follicle and proliferate, forming the dark zone of the germinal center. Germinal center B cells undergo extensive isotype switching and somatic mutation of Ig genes and migrate into the light zone, where B cells with the highest-affinity Ig receptors are selected to survive, and they differentiate into plasma cells or memory cells, which leave the germinal center. The right panel shows the histology of a secondary follicle with a germinal center in a lymph node. The germinal center includes a basal dark zone and an adjacent light zone. The mantle zone is the part of the follicle outside the germinal center.

costimulator (ICOS), which binds to its ligand expressed on B cells and other cells. Inherited mutations in the *ICOS* gene are the cause of some antibody deficiencies (see Chapter 12). Tfh cells may secrete cytokines, such as interferon (IFN)-γ, interleukin (IL)-4, or IL-17, which are characteristic of Th1, Th2, and Th17 subsets; the role of these cytokines in B cell responses is described below. In addition, most Tfh cells secrete the cytokine IL-21, which has an important but incompletely understood role in Tfh cell function.

A few of the activated B cells from the extrafollicular focus migrate back into the lymphoid follicle, together with Tfh cells, and begin to divide rapidly in response to signals from the Tfh cells. It is estimated that these B cells have a doubling time of approximately 6 hours, so one cell may produce several thousand progeny within a week.

The region of the follicle containing these proliferating B cells is the **germinal center**, so named because it was once incorrectly thought that these were the sites where new lymphocytes are generated (germinated). In the germinal center, B cells undergo extensive isotype switching and somatic mutation of Ig genes; both processes are described below. The highest-affinity B cells are the ones that are selected during the germinal center reaction to differentiate into memory B cells and long-lived plasma cells. Proliferating B cells reside in the dark zone of the germinal center (see Fig. 7.11), while selection occurs in the less dense light zone.

Heavy-Chain Isotype (Class) Switching

Helper T cells stimulate the progeny of IgM– and IgD–expressing B lymphocytes to change the heavy-chain

Fig. 7.12 Immunoglobulin *(Ig)* heavy-chain isotype (class) switching. Antigen-stimulated B lymphocytes may differentiate into IgM antibody-secreting cells, or, under the influence of CD40 ligand *(CD40L)* and cytokines, some of the B cells may differentiate into cells that produce different Ig heavy-chain isotypes. The principal effector functions of some of these isotypes are listed; all isotypes may function to neutralize microbes and toxins. B cell–activating factor belonging to the TNF family *(BAFF)* is a cytokine that may be involved in switching to IgA, especially in T-independent responses. Switching to IgG subclasses is stimulated by the cytokine interferon (IFN)-γ in mice, but in humans it is thought to be stimulated by other cytokines. *IL-4,* interleukin-4; *TGF-β,* transforming growth factor β.

isotypes (classes) of the antibodies they produce, without changing their antigen specificities (Fig. 7.12). Different antibody isotypes perform different functions, and therefore the process of isotype switching broadens the functional capabilities of humoral immune responses. For example, an important defense mechanism against the extracellular stages of most bacteria and viruses is to coat (opsonize) these microbes with antibodies and cause them to be phagocytosed by neutrophils and macrophages. This reaction is best mediated by antibody classes, such as IgG1 and IgG3 (in humans), that bind to high-affinity phagocyte Fc receptors specific for the Fc portion of the γ heavy chain (see Chapter 8). Helminths, in contrast, are too large to be phagocytosed, and they are best eliminated by eosinophils. Therefore, defense against these parasites involves coating them with antibodies to which eosinophils bind.

The antibody class that is able to do this is IgE, because eosinophils have high-affinity receptors for the Fc portion of the ε heavy chain. Thus, effective host defense requires that the immune system make different antibody isotypes in response to different types of microbes, even though all naive B lymphocytes specific for all these microbes express antigen receptors of the IgM and IgD isotypes.

Another functional consequence of isotype switching is that the IgG antibodies produced are able to bind to a specialized Fc receptor called the neonatal Fc receptor (FcRn). FcRn expressed in the placenta mediates the transfer of maternal IgG to the fetus, providing protection to the newborn, and FcRn expressed on endothelial cells and phagocytes plays a special role in protecting IgG from intracellular catabolism, thereby prolonging its half-life in the blood (see Chapter 8).

Rearranged DNA in IgM-producing cells

VDJ S_μ C_μ S_γ C_γ

Signals from helper T cells (CD40 ligand, cytokines)

Induction of AID

VDJ S_μ C_μ S_γ C_γ

AID

Recombination of S_μ with S_γ; deletion of intervening C genes

VDJ C_γ

VDJ C_γ

Transcription; RNA splicing

γ RNA   V DJ C_γ AAA

Translation

γ protein

IgG

Fig. 7.13 Mechanism of immunoglobulin heavy-chain isotype switching. In an immunoglobulin (Ig)M-producing B cell, the rearranged VDJ encoding the V region is adjacent to the μ constant region genes *(Cμ)*. Signals from helper T cells (CD40 ligand and cytokines) may induce recombination of switch *(S)* regions such that the rearranged VDJ DNA is moved close to a C gene downstream of Cμ, which are *Cγ* genes in the example shown. The enzyme activation-induced deaminase *(AID)*, which is induced in the B cells by signals from Tfh cells, alters nucleotides in the switch regions so that they can be cleaved by other enzymes and joined to downstream switch regions. Subsequently, when the heavy-chain gene is transcribed, the VDJ exon is spliced onto the exons of the downstream C gene, producing a heavy chain with a new constant region and thus a new class of Ig. Note that although the C region changes, the VDJ region, and thus the specificity of the antibody, is preserved. (Each C region gene consists of multiple exons, but only one is shown for simplicity.)

syndrome is caused by mutations in the *CD40L* gene, which is located on the X chromosome, leading to production of nonfunctional forms of CD40L in males who inherit the mutation. In this disease, much of the serum antibody is IgM, because of defective heavy-chain isotype switching. Patients with this disease also have defective cell-mediated immunity against intracellular microbes, because CD40L is important for T cell–mediated activation of macrophages and for the amplification of T cell responses by dendritic cells (see Chapter 6).

The molecular mechanism of isotype switching, called switch recombination, takes the previously formed VDJ exon encoding the V domain of an Ig μ heavy chain and moves it adjacent to a downstream C region (Fig. 7.13). IgM-producing B cells, which have not undergone switching, contain in their Ig heavy-chain locus a rearranged VDJ exon adjacent to the first constant region cluster, which is Cμ. The heavy-chain mRNA is produced by splicing a VDJ exon to Cμ exons in the initially transcribed RNA, and this mRNA is translated to produce a μ heavy chain, which combines with a light chain to give rise to an IgM antibody. Thus, the first antibody produced by B cells is IgM. In the intron 5′ of each constant region is a guanine-cytosine (GC)-rich sequence called the switch region. Signals from CD40 and cytokine receptors stimulate transcription through one of the constant regions that is downstream of Cμ. During switch recombination, the switch region upstream of Cμ recombines with the switch region adjacent to the transcriptionally active downstream constant region, and the intervening DNA is deleted. An

Heavy-chain isotype switching is induced by a combination of CD40L-mediated signals and cytokines. These signals act on antigen-stimulated B cells and induce switching in some of the progeny of these cells. In the absence of CD40 or CD40L, B cells secrete only IgM and fail to switch to other isotypes, indicating the essential role of this ligand-receptor pair in isotype switching. A disease called the **X-linked hyper-IgM**

enzyme called activation-induced deaminase (AID), which is induced by CD40 signals, plays a key role in this process. AID converts cytosines in the transcribed switch region DNA to uracil (U). The sequential action of other enzymes results in the removal of the U's and the creation of nicks in the DNA. Such a process on both strands leads to double-stranded DNA breaks. When double-stranded DNA breaks in two switch regions are brought together and repaired, the intervening DNA is removed, and the rearranged VDJ exon that was originally close to Cμ may now be brought immediately upstream of the constant region of a different isotype (e.g., IgG, IgA, IgE). The result is that the B cell begins to produce a new heavy-chain isotype (determined by the C region of the antibody) with the same specificity as that of the original B cell, because specificity is determined by the sequence of the VDJ exon, which is not altered.

Cytokines produced by follicular helper T cells determine which heavy-chain isotype is produced (see Fig. 7.12). The production of opsonizing IgG antibodies, which bind to phagocyte Fc receptors, is stimulated by IL-10 and other cytokines in humans and mainly by IFN-γ in mice. In antibody responses, these cytokines are produced by Tfh cells. The IgG antibodies that are produced opsonize microbes and promote their phagocytosis and intracellular killing. By contrast, switching to the IgE class is stimulated by IL-4 produced by Tfh cells. IgE functions to eliminate helminths, acting in concert with eosinophils, which are activated by another Th2 cytokine, IL-5. Predictably, helminths induce strong Th2 and related Tfh cell responses. Thus, the nature of the helper T cell response to a microbe guides the subsequent antibody response, making it optimal for combatting that microbe. These are excellent examples of how different components of the immune system are regulated coordinately and function together in defense against different types of microbes and how helper T cells may function as the master controllers of immune responses.

The antibody isotype produced is also influenced by the site of immune responses. For example, IgA antibody is the major isotype produced in mucosal lymphoid tissues, probably because cytokines such as transforming growth factor (TGF)–β that promote switching to IgA are abundant in these tissues. IgA is the principal antibody isotype that can be actively secreted through mucosal epithelia (see Chapter 8). B-1 cells also appear

Fig. 7.14 Affinity maturation in antibody responses. Early in the immune response, low-affinity antibodies are produced. During the germinal center reaction, somatic mutation of immunoglobulin *(Ig)* V genes and selection of mutated B cells with high-affinity antigen receptors result in the production of antibodies with high affinity for antigen.

to be important sources of IgA antibody in mucosal tissues, especially against nonprotein antigens.

Affinity Maturation

Affinity maturation is the process by which the affinity of antibodies produced in response to a protein antigen increases with prolonged or repeated exposure to that antigen (Fig. 7.14). Because of affinity maturation, the ability of antibodies to bind to a microbe or microbial antigen increases if the infection is persistent or recurrent. This increase in affinity is caused by point mutations in the V regions, and particularly in the antigen-binding hypervariable regions, of the genes encoding the antibodies produced. Affinity maturation is seen only in responses to helper T cell–dependent protein antigens, indicating that helper cells are critical in the process. These findings raise two intriguing questions: how are mutations in Ig genes induced in B cells, and how are the highest affinity (i.e., most useful) B cells selected to become progressively more numerous?

Affinity maturation occurs in the germinal centers of lymphoid follicles and is the result of somatic hypermutation of Ig genes in dividing B cells, followed by the selection of high-affinity B cells by

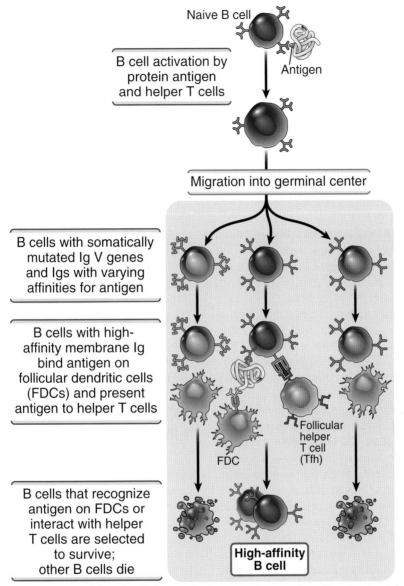

Naive B cell

B cell activation by
protein antigen
and helper T cells

Antigen

Migration into germinal center

B cells with somatically
mutated Ig V genes
and Igs with varying
affinities for antigen

B cells with high-
affinity membrane Ig
bind antigen on
follicular dendritic cells
(FDCs) and present
antigen to helper T cells

Follicular
helper
T cell
(Tfh)

FDC

B cells that recognize
antigen on FDCs or
interact with helper
T cells are selected
to survive;
other B cells die

**High-affinity
B cell**

Fig. 7.15 Selection of high-affinity B cells in germinal centers. Some activated B cells migrate into follicles to form germinal centers, where they undergo rapid proliferation and accumulate mutations in their immunoglobulin *(Ig)* V genes. These B cells produce antibodies with different affinities for the antigen. Follicular dendritic cells *(FDCs)* display the antigen, and B cells that recognize the antigen are selected to survive. FDCs display antigens by utilizing Fc receptors to bind immune complexes or by using C3 receptors to bind immune complexes with attached C3b and C3d complement proteins (not shown). B cells also bind the antigen, process it, and present it to follicular helper T *(Tfh)* cells in the germinal centers, and signals from the Tfh cells promote survival of the B cells. As more antibody is produced, the amount of available antigen decreases, so only the B cells that express receptors with higher affinities can bind the antigen and are selected to survive.

antigen (Fig. 7.15). In the dark zones of germinal centers (where the proliferating B cells are concentrated), numerous point mutations are introduced into the Ig genes of the rapidly dividing B cells. The enzyme AID, which is required for isotype switching, also plays a critical role in somatic mutation. This enzyme, as stated above, converts C into U. The uracils that are produced in Ig V-region DNA are frequently replaced by thymidines during DNA replication, creating C-to-T mutations, or they are removed and repaired by error-prone mechanisms that often lead to introduction of nucleotides other than the original mutated cytosine. The frequency of Ig gene mutations is estimated to be one in 10^3 base pairs per cell division, which is much greater than the mutation rate in most other genes. For this reason, Ig mutation in germinal center B cells is called somatic hypermutation. This extensive mutation results in the generation of different B cell clones whose Ig molecules may bind with widely varying affinities to the antigen that initiated the response. The next step in the process is the selection of B cells with the most useful antigen receptors.

Germinal center B cells undergo apoptosis unless rescued by antigen recognition and T cell help. While somatic hypermutation of Ig genes is taking place in germinal centers, the antibody secreted earlier during the immune response binds residual antigen. The antigen-antibody complexes that are formed may activate complement. These complexes are displayed by **follicular dendritic cells** (FDCs), which reside in the light zone of the germinal center and express receptors for the Fc portions of antibodies and for complement products, both of which help to display the antigen-antibody complexes. B cells that have undergone somatic hypermutation are given a chance to bind antigen either on FDCs or free in the germinal center. These B cells can internalize the antigen, process it, and present peptides to germinal center Tfh cells, which then provide critical survival signals. High-affinity B cells more effectively compete for the antigen and thus are more likely to survive than B cells with Igs that have lower affinities for the antigen, akin to a process of Darwinian survival of the fittest. As the immune response to a protein antigen develops, and also with repeated antigen exposure, the amount of antibody produced increases. As a result, the amount of antigen available in the germinal center decreases. The B cells that are selected to survive must be able to bind antigen at lower and lower concentrations, and therefore these are cells whose antigen receptors are of higher and higher affinity.

Generation of Plasma Cells and Memory B Cells

Activated B cells in germinal centers may differentiate into long-lived plasma cells or memory cells. The antibody-secreting cells enter the circulation and are called **plasmablasts**. From the blood, they tend to migrate to the bone marrow or mucosal tissues, where they may survive for years as plasma cells and continue to produce high-affinity antibodies, even after the antigen is eliminated. It is estimated that more than half of the antibodies in the blood of a normal adult are produced by these long-lived plasma cells; thus, circulating antibodies reflect each individual's history of antigen exposure. These antibodies provide a level of immediate protection if the antigen (microbe or toxin) reenters the body.

A fraction of the activated B cells, which often are the progeny of isotype-switched high-affinity B cells, do not differentiate into active antibody secretors but instead become **memory cells**. Memory B cells do not secrete antibodies, but they circulate in the blood and reside in mucosal and other tissues. They survive for months or years in the absence of additional antigen exposure, undergo slow cycling, and are ready to respond rapidly if the antigen is reintroduced. Therefore, memory from a T-dependent antibody response can last for a lifetime. The requirements for activation of functionally quiescent memory B cells to differentiate into plasma cells, and especially the role of T cell help in this reaction, are not well defined.

ANTIBODY RESPONSES TO T-INDEPENDENT ANTIGENS

Polysaccharides, lipids, and other nonprotein antigens elicit antibody responses without the participation of helper T cells. Recall that these nonprotein antigens cannot bind to MHC molecules, so they cannot be seen by T cells (see Chapter 3). Many bacteria contain polysaccharide-rich capsules, and defense against such bacteria is mediated primarily by antibodies that bind to capsular polysaccharides and target the bacteria for phagocytosis. Antibody responses to T-independent antigens differ from responses to proteins, and most of these differences are attributable to the roles of helper T cells in antibody responses to proteins (Fig. 7.16; see also Fig. 7.2). Extensive cross-linking of BCRs by multivalent antigens may activate the B cells strongly enough to stimulate their proliferation and differentiation without a requirement for T cell help. Polysaccharides also activate the complement system, and many T-independent antigens engage TLRs, thus providing activating signals to the B cells that enhance B cell activation in the absence of T cell help (see Fig. 7.5).

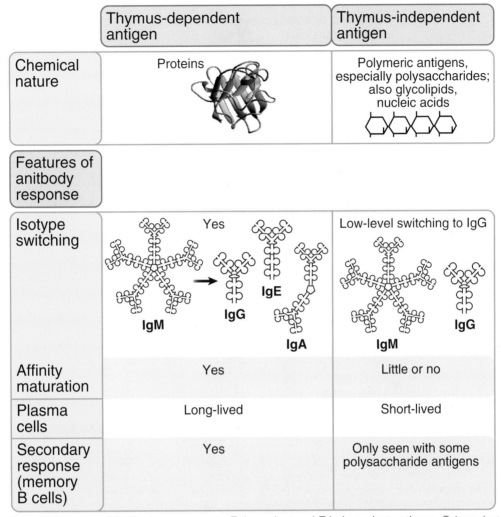

	Thymus-dependent antigen	Thymus-independent antigen
Chemical nature	Proteins	Polymeric antigens, especially polysaccharides; also glycolipids, nucleic acids
Features of anitbody response		
Isotype switching	Yes (IgM → IgG, IgE, IgA)	Low-level switching to IgG (IgM, IgG)
Affinity maturation	Yes	Little or no
Plasma cells	Long-lived	Short-lived
Secondary response (memory B cells)	Yes	Only seen with some polysaccharide antigens

Fig. 7.16 Features of Antibody responses to T-dependent and T-independent antigens. T-dependent antigens (proteins) and T-independent antigens (nonproteins) induce antibody responses with different characteristics, largely reflecting the influence of helper T cells in T-dependent responses to protein antigens and the absence of T cell help in T-independent responses. *Ig*, Immunoglobulin.

REGULATION OF HUMORAL IMMUNE RESPONSES: ANTIBODY FEEDBACK

After B lymphocytes differentiate into antibody-secreting cells and memory cells, a fraction of these cells survive for long periods, but most of the activated B cells probably die by apoptosis. This gradual loss of the activated B cells contributes to the physiologic decline of the humoral immune response. B cells also use a special mechanism for shutting off antibody production. As IgG antibody is produced and circulates throughout the body, the antibody binds to antigen that is still available in the blood and tissues, forming immune complexes. B cells specific for the antigen may bind the antigen part of the immune complex by their Ig receptors. At the same time, the Fc tail of the attached IgG antibody may be recognized by a special type of Fc receptor expressed on B cells (as well as on many myeloid cells) called FcγRIIB (Fig. 7.17). This Fc receptor delivers inhibitory signals that shut off antigen receptor–induced signals, thereby terminating B cell responses. This process, in which antibody bound to antigen inhibits further antibody

Fig. 7.17 Mechanism of antibody feedback. Secreted immunoglobulin *(Ig)*G antibodies form immune complexes (antigen-antibody complexes) with residual antigen (shown here as a virus but more commonly is a soluble antigen). The complexes interact with B cells specific for the antigen, with the membrane Ig antigen receptors recognizing epitopes of the antigen and a certain type of Fc receptor (FcγRIIB) recognizing the bound antibody. The Fc receptors block activating signals from the antigen receptor, terminating B cell activation. The cytoplasmic domain of B cell FcγRIIB contains an ITIM that binds enzymes that inhibit antigen receptor–mediated B cell activation. *ITAM,* immunoreceptor tyrosine-based activation motif; *ITIM,* immunoreceptor tyrosine-based inhibition motif.

production, is called **antibody feedback**. It serves to terminate humoral immune responses once sufficient quantities of IgG antibodies have been produced. Inhibition by the FcγRIIB also functions to limit antibody responses against self antigens, and polymorphisms in the gene encoding this receptor are associated with the autoimmune disease systemic lupus erythematosus (see Chapter 9).

SUMMARY

- Humoral immunity is mediated by antibodies that bind to extracellular microbes and their toxins, which are neutralized or targeted for destruction by phagocytes and the complement system.

- Humoral immune responses to nonprotein antigens are initiated by recognition of the antigens by specific membrane Ig antigen receptors of naive B cells. The binding of multivalent antigen cross-links B cell antigen receptors of specific B cells, and biochemical signals are delivered to the inside of the B cells by Ig-associated signaling proteins. These signals induce B cell clonal expansion and IgM secretion.

- Humoral immune responses to a protein antigen, called T-dependent responses, are initiated by binding of the protein to specific Ig receptors of naive B cells in lymphoid follicles. This results in the generation of signals that prepare the B cell for interaction with activated helper T cells that express CD40L and secrete cytokines. The B cells internalize and process that antigen and present class II MHC–displayed peptides to activated helper T cells specific for the displayed peptide-MHC complex. These helper T cells contribute to early B cell activation at extrafollicular sites.
- The early T-dependent humoral response occurs in extrafollicular foci and generates low levels of antibodies, with little isotype switching, that are produced by short-lived plasma cells.
- Activated B cells induce the further activation of T cells and their differentiation into Tfh cells. The B cells, together with the Tfh cells, migrate into follicles and form germinal centers.
- The full T-dependent humoral response develops in germinal centers and leads to extensive isotype switching and affinity maturation; generation of long-lived plasma cells that secrete antibodies for many years; and development of long-lived memory B cells, which rapidly respond to reencounter with antigen by proliferation and secretion of high-affinity antibodies.
- Heavy-chain isotype switching (or class switching) is the process by which the isotype, but not the

specificity, of the antibodies produced in response to an antigen changes as the humoral response proceeds. Isotype switching is stimulated by the combination of CD40L and cytokines, both expressed by helper T cells. Different cytokines induce switching to different antibody isotypes, enabling the immune system to respond in the most effective way to different types of microbes.

- Affinity maturation is the process by which the affinity of antibodies for protein antigens increases with prolonged or repeated exposure to the antigens. The process is initiated by signals from Tfh cells, resulting in migration of the B cells into follicles and the formation of germinal centers. Here the B cells proliferate rapidly, and their Ig V genes undergo extensive somatic mutation. The antigen may be displayed by FDCs in the germinal centers. B cells that recognize the antigen with high affinity are selected to survive, giving rise to affinity maturation of the antibody response.
- Polysaccharides, lipids, and other nonprotein antigens are called T-independent antigens because they induce antibody responses without T cell help. Most T-independent antigens contain multiple identical epitopes that are able to cross-link many Ig receptors on a B cell, providing signals that stimulate B cell responses even in the absence of helper T cell activation. Antibody responses to T-independent antigens show less heavy-chain class switching and affinity maturation than typical for responses to T-dependent protein antigens.
- Secreted antibodies form immune complexes with residual antigen and shut off B cell activation by engaging an inhibitory Fc receptor on B cells.

REVIEW QUESTIONS

1. What are the signals that induce B cell responses to protein antigens and polysaccharide antigens?
2. What are the major differences between primary and secondary antibody responses to a protein antigen?
3. How do helper T cells specific for an antigen interact with B lymphocytes specific for the same antigen? Where in a lymph node do these interactions mainly occur?
4. What are the signals that induce heavy-chain isotype switching, and what is the importance of this phenomenon for host defense against different microbes?
5. What is affinity maturation? How is it induced, and how are high-affinity B cells selected to survive?
6. What are the characteristics of antibody responses to polysaccharides and lipids? What types of bacteria stimulate mostly these types of antibody responses?

Answers to and discussion of the Review Questions are available at Student Consult.

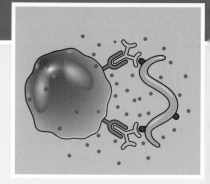

8

Effector Mechanisms of Humoral Immunity
Elimination of Extracellular Microbes and Toxins

Humoral immunity is the type of host defense mediated by secreted antibodies that is necessary for protection against extracellular microbes and their toxins. Antibodies prevent infections by blocking microbes from binding to and entering host cells. Antibodies also bind to microbial toxins and prevent them from damaging host cells. In addition, antibodies function to eliminate microbes, toxins, and infected cells from the body. Although antibodies are a major mechanism of adaptive immunity against extracellular microbes, they cannot reach microbes that live inside cells. However, humoral immunity is vital even for defense against microbes that live inside cells, such as viruses, because antibodies can bind to these microbes before they enter host cells or during passage from infected to uninfected cells, thus preventing spread of infection. Defects in antibody production are associated with increased susceptibility to infections by many bacteria, viruses, and parasites. All the vaccines that are currently in use work by stimulating the production of antibodies.

This chapter describes how antibodies provide defense against infections, addressing the following questions:
- What are the mechanisms used by secreted antibodies to combat different types of infectious agents and their toxins?
- What is the role of the complement system in defense against microbes?
- How do antibodies combat microbes that enter through the gastrointestinal and respiratory tracts?
- How do antibodies protect the fetus and newborn from infections?

Before describing the mechanisms by which antibodies function in host defense, we summarize the features of antibody molecules that are important for these functions.

PROPERTIES OF ANTIBODIES THAT DETERMINE EFFECTOR FUNCTION

Several features of the production and structure of antibodies contribute in important ways to the functions of these molecules in host defense.

Antibodies function in the circulation, in tissues throughout the body, and in the lumens of mucosal organs. Antibodies are produced after stimulation of B lymphocytes by antigens in peripheral (secondary) lymphoid organs (lymph nodes, spleen, mucosal lymphoid tissues) and at tissue sites of inflammation. Many of the antigen-stimulated B lymphocytes differentiate into antibody-secreting plasma cells, some of which remain in lymphoid organs or inflamed tissues and others migrate to and reside in the bone marrow. Different plasma cells synthesize and secrete antibodies of different heavy-chain isotypes (classes). These secreted antibodies enter the blood, from where they may reach any peripheral site of infection, or enter mucosal secretions, where they prevent infections by microbes that try to enter through epithelia.

Protective antibodies are produced during the first (primary) response to a microbe and in larger amounts during subsequent (secondary) responses (see Fig. 7.3 in Chapter 7). Antibody production begins within the first week after infection or vaccination. The plasma cells that migrate to the bone marrow continue to produce antibodies for months or years. If the microbe again tries to infect the host, the continuously secreted antibodies provide immediate protection. At the same time, memory cells that had developed during the initial B cell response rapidly differentiate into antibody-producing cells upon encounter with the antigen, providing a large burst of antibody for more effective defense against the infection. A goal of vaccination is to stimulate the development of long-lived plasma cells and memory cells.

Antibodies use their antigen-binding (Fab) regions to bind to and block the harmful effects of microbes and toxins, and they use their Fc regions to activate diverse effector mechanisms that eliminate these microbes and toxins (Fig. 8.1). This spatial segregation of the antigen recognition and effector functions of antibody molecules was introduced in Chapter 4. Antibodies block the infectivity of microbes and the injurious effects of microbial toxins simply by binding to the microbes and toxins, using only their Fab regions to do so. Other functions of antibodies require the participation of various components of host defense, such as phagocytes and the complement system. The Fc portions of immunoglobulin (Ig) molecules, made up of the heavy-chain constant regions, contain the binding sites for Fc receptors on phagocytes and for complement proteins. The binding of antibodies to Fc receptors and

complement proteins occurs only after several Ig molecules recognize and become attached to a microbe or microbial antigen. Therefore, even the Fc-dependent functions of antibodies require antigen recognition by the Fab regions. This feature of antibodies ensures that they activate effector mechanisms only when needed—that is, when they recognize their target antigens.

Heavy-chain isotype (class) switching and affinity maturation enhance the protective functions of antibodies. Isotype switching and affinity maturation are two changes that occur in the antibodies produced by antigen-stimulated B lymphocytes, especially during responses to protein antigens (see Chapter 7). Heavy-chain isotype switching results in the production of antibodies with distinct Fc regions, capable of different effector functions (see Fig. 8.1). By switching to different antibody isotypes in response to various microbes, the humoral immune system is able to engage diverse host mechanisms that are optimal for combating those microbes. Affinity maturation is induced by prolonged or repeated stimulation with protein antigens, and it leads to the production of antibodies with higher and higher affinities for the antigen, compared to the antibodies initially secreted. This change increases the ability of antibodies to bind to and neutralize or eliminate microbes. The progressive increase in antibody affinity with repeated stimulation of B cells is one of the reasons for the recommended practice of giving multiple rounds of immunizations with the same antigen for generating protective immunity.

Switching to the IgG isotype prolongs the duration that an antibody remains in the blood and therefore increases the functional activity of the antibody. Most circulating proteins have half-lives of hours to days in the blood, but IgG has an unusually long half-life because of a special mechanism involving a particular Fc receptor. The neonatal Fc receptor (FcRn) is expressed in placenta, endothelium, phagocytes, and a few other cell types. In the placenta, the FcRn transports antibodies from the mother's circulation to the fetus (discussed later). In other cell types, the FcRn protects IgG antibodies from intracellular catabolism (Fig. 8.2). FcRn is found in the endosomes of endothelial cells and phagocytes, where it binds to IgG that has been taken up by the cells. Once bound to the FcRn, the IgG is recycled back into the circulation or tissue fluids, thus avoiding lysosomal degradation. This unique mechanism for protecting a blood protein is the reason why IgG antibodies

Fig. 8.1 Effector functions of antibodies. Antibodies are produced by the activation of B lymphocytes by antigens and other signals (not shown). Antibodies of different heavy-chain classes (isotypes) perform different effector functions, as illustrated schematically in (A) and summarized in (B). (Some properties of antibodies are listed in Chapter 4, Fig. 4.3.) *Ig*, Immunoglobulin; *NK*, natural killer.

Fig. 8.2 Neonatal Fc receptor *(FcRn)* contributes to the long half-life of IgG molecules. Circulating or extravascular IgG antibodies (mainly of the IgG1, IgG2, and IgG4 subclasses) are ingested by endothelial cells and phagocytes and bind the FcRn, a receptor present in the acidic environment of endosomes. In these cells, FcRn sequesters the IgG molecules in endosomal vesicles (pH ~4). The FcRn-IgG complexes recycle back to the cell surface, where they are exposed to the neutral pH (~7) of the blood, which releases the bound antibody back into the circulation or tissue fluid. *Ig,* Immunoglobulin.

Fig. 8.3 Antibodies and Fc-containing fusion proteins. An antibody specific for the cytokine tumor necrosis factor *(TNF)* *(left)* can bind to and block the activity of the cytokine and remain in the circulation for a long time (weeks) due to recycling by the neonatal Fc receptor (FcRn). The soluble extracellular domain of the TNF receptor *(right)* can also act as an antagonist of the cytokine, and coupling the soluble receptor to an IgG Fc domain, using a genetic engineering approach, results in a prolonged half-life of the fusion protein in the blood by the same FcRn-dependent mechanism. *Ig,* Immunoglobulin.

NEUTRALIZATION OF MICROBES AND MICROBIAL TOXINS

Antibodies bind to and block, or neutralize, the infectivity of microbes and the interactions of microbial toxins with host cells (Fig. 8.4). Antibodies in mucosal secretions in the gut and airways block the entry of ingested and inhaled microbes (discussed later in the chapter). After microbes enter the host, they use molecules in their envelopes or cell walls to bind to and gain entry into host cells. Antibodies may attach to these microbial surface molecules, thereby preventing the microbes from infecting host cells. The most effective vaccines available today work by stimulating the production of neutralizing antibodies that block initial infection. Microbes that are able to enter host cells may replicate inside the cells and then be released and go on to infect other neighboring cells. Antibodies can neutralize the microbes during their transit from cell to cell and thus also limit the spread of infection. If an infectious microbe does colonize the host, its harmful effects may be caused by endotoxins or exotoxins, which often bind to specific receptors on host cells in order to mediate their effects. Antibodies prevent binding of the toxins to host cells and thus block their harmful effects. Emil von Behring and Shibasaburo Kitasato's demonstration of this type of protection mediated by the administration of antibodies against diphtheria toxin was the first

have a half-life of about 3 weeks, much longer than that of other Ig isotypes and most other plasma proteins. This property of Fc regions of IgG has been exploited to increase the half-life of other proteins by coupling the proteins to an IgG Fc region (Fig. 8.3). One of several therapeutic agents based on this principle is the tumor necrosis factor (TNF) receptor–Fc fusion protein, which functions as an antagonist of TNF and is used to treat various inflammatory diseases. By coupling the extracellular domain of the TNF receptor to the Fc portion of a human IgG molecule using a genetic engineering approach, the half-life of the hybrid protein becomes much greater than that of the soluble receptor by itself.

With this introduction, we proceed to a discussion of the mechanisms used by antibodies to combat infections. Much of the chapter is devoted to effector mechanisms that are not influenced by anatomic considerations; that is, they may be active anywhere in the body. At the end of the chapter, we describe the special features of antibody functions at particular anatomic locations.

Fig. 8.4 Neutralization of microbes and toxins by antibodies. A, Antibodies at epithelial surfaces, such as in the gastrointestinal and respiratory tracts, block the entry of ingested and inhaled microbes, respectively. **B,** Antibodies prevent the binding of microbes to cells, thereby blocking the ability of the microbes to infect host cells. **C,** Antibodies block the binding of toxins to cells, thereby inhibiting the pathologic effects of the toxins.

formal demonstration of therapeutic immunity against a microbe or its toxin, then called serum therapy, and the basis for awarding Behring the first Nobel Prize in Physiology or Medicine in 1901.

OPSONIZATION AND PHAGOCYTOSIS

Antibodies coat microbes and promote their ingestion by phagocytes (Fig. 8.5). The process of coating particles for subsequent phagocytosis is called opsonization, and the molecules that coat microbes and enhance their phagocytosis are called opsonins. When several IgG molecules bind to a microbe, an array of their Fc regions projects away from the microbial surface. If the antibodies belong to certain isotypes (IgG1 and IgG3 in humans), their Fc regions bind to a high-affinity receptor for the Fc regions of γ heavy chains, called FcγRI (CD64), which is expressed on neutrophils and macrophages (Fig. 8.6). The phagocyte extends its plasma membrane around the attached microbe and ingests the microbe into a vesicle called a phagosome, which fuses with lysosomes. The binding of antibody Fc tails to FcγRI also activates the phagocytes, because the FcγRI contains a signaling chain that triggers numerous biochemical pathways in the phagocytes. Large amounts of reactive oxygen species, nitric oxide, and proteolytic enzymes are produced in the lysosomes of the activated neutrophils and macrophages, all of which contribute to the destruction of the ingested microbe.

Fig. 8.5 Antibody-mediated opsonization and phagocytosis of microbes. Antibodies of certain IgG subclasses (IgG1 and IgG3) bind to microbes and are then recognized by Fc receptors on phagocytes. Signals from the Fc receptors promote the phagocytosis of the opsonized microbes and activate the phagocytes to destroy these microbes. *Ig*, Immunoglobulin.

Antibody-mediated phagocytosis is the major mechanism of defense against encapsulated bacteria, such as pneumococci. The polysaccharide-rich capsules of these bacteria protect the organisms from phagocytosis in the absence of antibody, but opsonization by antibody promotes phagocytosis and destruction of the bacteria. The spleen contains large numbers of phagocytes and is an important site of phagocytic clearance of opsonized bacteria. This is why patients who have undergone splenectomy are susceptible to disseminated infections by encapsulated bacteria.

One of the Fcγ receptors, FcγRIIB, does not mediate effector functions of antibodies but rather shuts down antibody production and reduces inflammation. The role of FcγRIIB in feedback inhibition of B cell activation was discussed in Chapter 7 (see Fig. 7.16). FcγRIIB also inhibits activation of macrophages and dendritic cells and may thus serve an antiinflammatory function as well. Pooled IgG from healthy donors is given intravenously to treat various inflammatory diseases. This preparation is called **intravenous immune globulin** (IVIG), and its beneficial effect in these diseases is partly mediated by its binding to FcγRIIB on various cells.

Fc Receptor	Affinity for Ig	Cell distribution	Function
FcγRI (CD64)	High; binds IgG1 and IgG3	Macrophages, neutrophils	Phagocytosis; activation of phagocytes
FcγRIIB (CD32)	Low	B lymphocytes, DCs, mast cells, neutrophils, macrophages	Feedback inhibition of B cells, attenuation of inflammation
FcγRIIIA (CD16)	Low	NK cells	Antibody-dependent cellular cytotoxicity (ADCC)
FcεRI	High; binds IgE	Mast cells, basophils, eosinophils	Activation (degranulation) of mast cells and basophils

Fig. 8.6 Fc receptors. The cellular distribution and functions of different types of human Fc receptors. *DCs,* Dendritic cells; *Ig,* immunoglobulin; *NK,* natural killer.

Fig. 8.7 Antibody-dependent cellular cytotoxicity. Antibodies of certain immunoglobulin G (IgG) subclasses (IgG1 and IgG3) bind to antigens on the surface of infected cells, and their Fc regions are recognized by an Fcγ receptor on natural killer (NK) cells. The NK cells are activated and kill the antibody-coated cells. Ig, Immunoglobulin.

Fig. 8.8 Immunoglobulin E (IgE)- and eosinophil-mediated killing of helminths. IgE antibody binds to helminths and recruits and activates eosinophils via FcεRI, leading to degranulation of the cells and release of toxic mediators. Interleukin-5 (IL-5) secreted by Th2 cells enhances the ability of eosinophils to kill the parasites. Ig, Immunoglobulin.

ANTIBODY-DEPENDENT CELLULAR CYTOTOXICITY

Natural killer (NK) cells bind to antibody-coated cells and destroy these cells (Fig. 8.7). NK cells express an Fcγ receptor called FcγRIII (CD16), which is one of several kinds of NK cell–activating receptors (see Chapter 2). FcγRIII binds to arrays of IgG antibodies attached to the surface of a cell, generating signals that cause the NK cell to discharge its granule proteins, which kill the antibody-coated cell by the same mechanisms that CD8+ cytotoxic T lymphocytes use to kill infected cells (see Chapter 6). This process is called antibody-dependent cellular cytotoxicity (ADCC). Cells infected with enveloped viruses typically express viral glycoproteins on their surface that can be recognized by specific antibodies, and this may facilitate ADCC-mediated destruction of the infected cells. ADCC is also one of the mechanisms by which therapeutic antibodies used to treat cancers eliminate tumor cells.

IMMUNOGLOBULIN E– AND EOSINOPHIL/MAST CELL–MEDIATED REACTIONS

Immunoglobulin E (IgE) antibodies activate mast cell and eosinophil–mediated reactions that provide defense against helminthic parasites and are involved in allergic diseases. Most helminths are too large to be phagocytosed, and their thick integument makes them resistant to many of the microbicidal substances produced by neutrophils and macrophages. The humoral immune response to helminths is dominated by IgE antibodies. IgE binds to the worms and promotes the attachment of eosinophils through the high-affinity Fc receptor for IgE, FcεRI, which is expressed on eosinophils and mast cells. Engagement of FcεRI, together with the cytokine interleukin-5 (IL-5) produced by Th2 helper T cells reacting against the helminths, leads to activation of the eosinophils, which release their granule contents, including proteins that can kill the worms (Fig. 8.8). IgE antibodies also bind to and activate mast cells, which secrete cytokines, including chemokines, that attract more leukocytes that function to destroy the helminths.

This IgE-mediated reaction illustrates how Ig isotype switching optimizes host defense. B cells respond to helminths by switching to IgE, which is useful against helminths, but B cells respond to most bacteria and viruses by switching to IgG antibodies, which promote phagocytosis by FcγRI. As discussed in Chapters 6 and 7, these patterns of isotype switching are determined by the cytokines produced by helper T cells responding to the different types of microbes.

IgE antibodies also are involved in allergic diseases (see Chapter 11).

THE COMPLEMENT SYSTEM

The complement system is a collection of circulating and cell membrane proteins that play important roles in host defense against microbes and in antibody-mediated tissue injury. The term *complement* refers to the ability of these proteins to assist, or complement, the activity of antibodies in destroying (lysing) cells, including microbes. The complement system may be activated by microbes in the absence of antibody, as part of the innate immune response to infection, and by antibodies attached to microbes, as part of adaptive immunity (see Fig. 2.12 in Chapter 2).

The activation of the complement system involves sequential proteolytic cleavage of complement proteins, leading to the generation of effector molecules that participate in eliminating microbes in different ways. This cascade of complement protein activation, like all enzymatic cascades, is capable of achieving tremendous amplification, because even a small number of activated complement molecules produced early in the cascade may generate a large number of effector molecules. Activated complement proteins become covalently attached to the cell surfaces where the activation occurs, ensuring that complement effector functions are limited to the correct sites. Normal host cells possess several regulatory mechanisms that inhibit the activation of complement and the deposition of activated complement proteins, thus preventing complement-mediated damage to healthy cells.

Pathways of Complement Activation

There are three major pathways of complement activation: the alternative and lectin pathways are initiated by microbes in the absence of antibody, and the classical pathway is initiated by certain isotypes of antibodies attached to antigens (Fig. 8.9). Several proteins in each pathway interact in a precise sequence. The most abundant complement protein in the plasma, C3, plays a central role in all three pathways. The early steps of all three pathways function to generate a large number of functionally active fragments of C3 bound to the microbe or cell where the complement pathway was initiated. (By convention, the smaller proteolyic fragment of any complement protein is given the "a" suffix, and the larger piece is the "b" fragment; C2 is an exception.)

- The **alternative pathway** of complement activation is triggered by spontaneous hydrolysis of C3 in plasma at a low level. The breakdown products of C3 are unstable, and, in the absence of infection, are rapidly degraded and lost. However, when a breakdown product of C3 hydrolysis, called C3b, is deposited on the surface of a microbe, it forms stable covalent bonds with microbial proteins or polysaccharides. The microbe-bound C3b binds another protein called Factor B, which is then cleaved by a plasma protease called Factor D to generate the Bb fragment. This fragment remains attached to C3b, and the C3bBb complex functions as a proteolytic enzyme, called

the alternative pathway C3 convertase, that breaks down more C3. The C3 convertase is stabilized by properdin, a positive regulator of the complement system. As a result of this enzymatic activity, many more C3b and C3bBb molecules are produced and become attached to the microbe. Some of the C3bBb molecules bind an additional C3b molecule, and the resulting C3bBb3b complexes function as C5 convertases, to cleave the complement protein C5 and initiate the late steps of complement activation.

- The **classical pathway** of complement activation is triggered when IgM or certain subclasses of IgG (IgG1 and IgG3 in humans) bind to antigens (e.g., on a microbial cell surface). As a result of this binding, adjacent Fc regions of the antibodies become accessible to and bind the C1 complement protein (which is made up of a binding component called C1q and two proteases called C1r and C1s). The attached C1 becomes enzymatically active, resulting in the binding and sequential cleavage of two proteins, C4 and C2. One of the C4 fragments that is generated, C4b, becomes covalently attached to the antibody or to the microbial surface where the antibody is bound, and then binds C2, which is cleaved by active C1 to yield the C4b2a complex. This complex is the classical pathway C3 convertase, which functions to break down C3, and the C3b that is generated again becomes attached to the microbe. Some of the C3b binds to the C4b2a complex, and the resultant C4b2a3b complex functions as a C5 convertase, which cleaves the C5 complement protein.

- The **lectin pathway** of complement activation is initiated not by antibodies but by the attachment of plasma mannose-binding lectin (MBL) to microbes. Serine proteases structurally related to C1s of the classical pathway are associated with MBL and serve to activate C4. The subsequent steps are essentially the same as in the classical pathway.

The net result of these early steps of complement activation is that microbes acquire a coat of covalently attached C3b. Note that the alternative and lectin pathways are effector mechanisms of innate immunity, whereas the classical pathway is a mechanism of adaptive humoral immunity. These pathways differ in their initiation, but once triggered, their late steps are the same.

The late steps of complement activation are initiated by the binding of C5 to the C5 convertase and subsequent proteolysis of C5, generating C5b (Fig. 8.10).

Fig. 8.9 Early steps of complement activation. A, The steps in the activation of the alternative, classical, and lectin pathways. Although the sequence of events is similar, the three pathways differ in their requirement for antibody and the proteins used. Note that C5 is cleaved by the C5 convertase but is not a component of the enzyme.

B

Alternative pathway proteins

Protein	Serum conc. (μg/mL)	Function
C3	640–1660	C3b binds to the surface of microbes, where it functions as an opsonin and as a component of C3 and C5 convertases C3a stimulates inflammation
Factor B	200	Bb is a serine protease and the active enzyme of C3 and C5 convertases
Factor D	1–2	Plasma serine protease that cleaves Factor B when it is bound to C3b

C

Classical and lectin pathway proteins

Protein	Serum conc. (μg/mL)	Function
C1 ($C1qr_2s_2$)		Initiates the classical pathway; C1q binds to Fc portion of antibody; C1r and C1s are proteases that lead to C4 and C2 activation
C4	150–450	C4b covalently binds to surfaces of microbes or cells where antibody is bound and complement is activated C4b binds to C2 for cleavage by C1s C4a stimulates inflammation
C2	20	C2a is a serine protease functioning as an active enzyme of C3 and C5 convertases
Mannose binding lectin (MBL)	0.8–1	Initiates the lectin pathway; MBL binds to terminal mannose residues of microbial carbohydrates. MBL-associated proteases activate C4 and C2, as C1r and C1s do in the classical pathway.

Fig. 8.9, cont'd B, The important properties of the proteins involved in the early steps of the alternative pathway of complement activation. **C,** The important properties of the proteins involved in the early steps of the classical and lectin pathways. Note that C3, which is listed among the alternative pathway proteins **(B),** also is the central component of the classical and lectin pathways.

Fig. 8.10 Late steps of complement activation. **A,** The late steps of complement activation start after the formation of the C5 convertase and are identical in the alternative and classical pathways. Products generated in the late steps induce inflammation (C5a) and cell lysis (membrane attack complex). **B,** Properties of the proteins in the late steps of complement activation.

The remaining components, C6, C7, C8, and C9, bind sequentially to a complex nucleated by C5b. The final protein in the pathway, C9, polymerizes to form a pore in the cell membrane through which water and ions can enter, causing death of the microbe. The C5-9 complex is called the **membrane attack complex** (MAC), and its formation is the end result of complement activation.

Functions of the Complement System

The complement system plays an important role in the elimination of microbes during innate and adaptive immune responses. The main effector functions of the complement system are illustrated in Fig. 8.11.

- **Opsonization.** Microbes coated with C3b are phagocytosed by virtue of C3b being recognized by

Fig. 8.11 The functions of complement. A, C3b opsonizes microbes and is recognized by the type 1 complement receptor (CR1) of phagocytes, resulting in ingestion and intracellular killing of the opsonized microbes. Thus C3b is an opsonin. CR1 also recognizes C4b, which may serve the same function. Other complement products, such as the inactivated form of C3b (iC3b), also bind to microbes and are recognized by other receptors on phagocytes (e.g., type 3 complement receptor, a member of integrin family of proteins). **B,** Membrane attack complex creates pores in cell membranes and induces osmotic lysis of the cells. **C,** Small peptides released during complement activation bind to receptors on neutrophils and other leukocytes and stimulate inflammatory reactions. The peptides that serve this function are mainly C5a and C3a, released by proteolysis of C5 and C3, respectively.

complement receptor type 1 (CR1, or CD35), which is expressed on phagocytes. Thus, C3b functions as an opsonin. Opsonization is probably the most important function of complement in defense against microbes.

- **Cell lysis**. The MAC can induce osmotic lysis of cells, including microbes. MAC-induced lysis is effective only against microbes that have thin cell walls and little or no glycocalyx, such as the *Neisseria* species of bacteria.

- **Inflammation.** The small peptide fragments C3a and C5a, which are produced by proteolysis of C3 and C5, are chemotactic for neutrophils, stimulate the release of inflammatory mediators from various leukocytes, and stimulate movement of leukocytes and plasma proteins across the endothelium into tissues. In this way, complement fragments induce inflammatory reactions that also serve to eliminate microbes.

In addition to its antimicrobial effector functions, the complement system stimulates B cell responses

and antibody production. When C3 is activated by a microbe by the alternative pathway, one of its breakdown products, C3d, is recognized by complement receptor type 2 (CR2) on B lymphocytes. Signals delivered by this receptor enhance B cell responses against the microbe. This process is described in Chapter 7 (see Fig. 7.5A) and is an example of an innate immune response to a microbe (complement activation) enhancing an adaptive immune response to the same microbe (B cell activation and antibody production). Complement proteins bound to antigen-antibody complexes are recognized by follicular dendritic cells in germinal centers, allowing the antigens to be displayed for further B cell activation and selection of high-affinity B cells. This complement-dependent antigen display is another way in which the complement system promotes antibody production.

Inherited deficiencies of complement proteins result in immune deficiencies and, in some cases, increased incidence of autoimmune disease. Deficiency of C3 results in increased susceptibility to bacterial infections that may be fatal early in life. Deficiencies of the early proteins of the classical pathway, C2 and C4, may have no clinical consequence, may result in increased susceptibility to infections, or are associated with an increased incidence of systemic lupus erythematosus, an immune complex-mediated autoimmune disease. The increased incidence of lupus may be because the classical pathway functions to eliminate immune complexes from the circulation, and these complexes accumulate in individuals lacking C2 and C4. In addition, complement deficiencies may lead to defective signaling in B cells and a failure of B cell tolerance (see Chapter 9). Deficiencies of C9 and MAC formation result in increased susceptibility to *Neisseria* infections. Some individuals inherit polymorphisms in the gene encoding MBL, leading to production of a protein that is functionally defective; such defects are associated with increased susceptibility to infections. Inherited deficiency of the alternative pathway protein properdin also causes increased susceptibility to bacterial infection.

Regulation of Complement Activation

Mammalian cells express regulatory proteins that inhibit complement activation, thus preventing complement-mediated damage to host cells (Fig. 8.12). Many such regulatory proteins have been described, and defects in these proteins are associated with clinical syndromes caused by uncontrolled complement activation.

- A regulatory protein called C1 inhibitor (C1 INH) stops complement activation early, at the stage of C1 activation. Deficiency of C1 INH is the cause of a disease called **hereditary angioedema.** C1 INH is a serine protease inhibitor that functions as a major physiologic inhibitor of the cleavage of kallikrein, the precursor of the vasoactive molecule bradykinin. Therefore, C1 INH deficiency results not only in increased complement activation but also increased proteolytic activation of bradykinin, and this is the main reason for the vascular changes that lead to leakage of fluid (edema) in many tissues.

- Decay-accelerating factor (DAF) is a glycolipid-linked cell surface protein that disrupts the binding of Bb to C3b and the binding of C4b to C2a, thus blocking C3 convertase formation and terminating complement activation by both the alternative and the classical pathways. A disease called **paroxysmal nocturnal hemoglobinuria** results from the acquired deficiency in hematopoietic stem cells of an enzyme that synthesizes the glycolipid anchor for several cell-surface proteins, including the complement regulatory proteins DAF and CD59. In these patients, unregulated complement activation occurs on erythrocytes, leading to their lysis.

- A plasma enzyme called Factor I cleaves C3b into inactive fragments, with membrane cofactor protein (MCP) and the plasma protein Factor H serving as cofactors in this enzymatic process. Deficiency of the regulatory proteins Factors H and I results in increased complement activation and reduced levels of C3 because of its consumption, causing increased susceptibility to infection. Mutations in Factor H that compromise its binding to cells are associated with a rare genetic disease called atypical hemolytic uremic syndrome, in which there are clotting, vascular, and renal abnormalities. Certain genetic variants of Factor H are linked to an eye disease called age-related macular degeneration.

These regulatory proteins are made by vertebrate host cells but not by microbes. Because microbes lack these regulatory proteins, the complement system can be activated on microbial surfaces much more effectively than on normal host cells. Even in vertebrate cells, the regulation can be overwhelmed by too much complement activation. For instance, host cells can become targets of complement if they are coated with large amounts of antibodies, as in some hypersensitivity diseases (see Chapter 11).

FUNCTIONS OF ANTIBODIES AT SPECIAL ANATOMIC SITES

The effector mechanisms of humoral immunity described so far may be active at any site in the body to which antibodies gain access. As mentioned previously, antibodies are produced in peripheral lymphoid organs and bone marrow and readily enter the blood, from which they may go anywhere. Antibodies also serve vital protective functions at two special anatomic sites: the mucosal organs and the fetus.

Mucosal Immunity

Immunoglobulin A (IgA) is produced in mucosal lymphoid tissues, transported across epithelia, and binds to and neutralizes microbes in the lumens of the mucosal organs (Fig. 8.13). Microbes often are inhaled or ingested, and antibodies that are secreted into the lumens of the respiratory or gastrointestinal tract bind to these microbes and prevent them from colonizing the host. This type of immunity is called mucosal immunity (or secretory immunity). The principal class of antibody produced in mucosal tissues is IgA. In fact, IgA accounts for about two-thirds of the approximately 3 g of antibody produced daily by a healthy adult, reflecting the vast surface area of the intestines. The propensity of B cells in mucosal epithelial tissues to produce IgA is because the cytokines that induce switching to this isotype, including transforming growth factor β (TGF-β), are produced at high levels in mucosa-associated lymphoid tissues. In addition, IgA-producing B cells that are generated in regional lymph nodes or spleen tend to home to mucosal tissues

Fig. 8.12 Regulation of complement activation. **A,** C1 inhibitor *(C1 INH)* prevents the assembly of the C1 complex, which consists of C1q, C1r, and C1s proteins, thereby blocking complement activation by the classical pathway. **B,** The lipid-linked cell surface protein decay-accelerating factor *(DAF)* and the type 1 complement receptor (CR1) interfere with the formation of the C3 convertase by blocking the binding of Bb (in the alternative pathway) or C2a (in the classical pathway). Membrane cofactor protein (or CD46) and CR1 serve as cofactors for cleavage of C3b by a plasma enzyme called factor I, thus destroying any C3b that may be formed (not shown).

C Plasma proteins

Protein	Plasma concentration	Function
C1 inhibitor (C1 INH)	200 µg/ml	Inhibits C1r and C1s serine protease activity
Factor I	35 µg/ml	Proteolytically cleaves C3b and C4b
Factor H	480 µg/ml	Causes dissociation of alternative pathway C3 convertase subunits Co-factor for Factor I-mediated cleavage of C3b
C4 binding protein (C4BP)	300 µg/ml	Causes dissociation of classical pathway C3 convertase subunits Co-factor for Factor I-mediated cleavage of C4b

Membrane proteins

Protein	Distribution	Function
Membrane co-factor protein (MCP, CD46)	Leukocytes, epithelial cells, endothelial cells	Co-factor for Factor I-mediated cleavage of C3b and C4b
Decay accelerating factor (DAF)	Blood cells, endothelial cells, epithelial cells	Blocks formation of C3 convertase
CD59	Blood cells, endothelial cells, epithelial cells	Blocks C9 binding and prevents formation of the MAC
Type 1 complement receptor (CR1, CD35)	Mononuclear phagocytes, neutrophils, B and T cells, erythrocytes, eosinophils, FDCs	Causes dissociation of C3 convertase subunits Co-factor for Factor I-mediated cleavage of C3b and C4b

Fig. 8.12, cont'd C, The major regulatory proteins of the complement system and their functions. *FDCs,* Follicular dendritic cells; *MAC,* membrane attack complex.

Fig. 8.13 Transport of immunoglobulin A (IgA) through epithelium. In the mucosa of the gastrointestinal and respiratory tracts, IgA is produced by plasma cells in the lamina propria and is actively transported through epithelial cells by an IgA-specific Fc receptor, called the poly-Ig receptor because it recognizes IgM as well. On the luminal surface, the IgA with a portion of the bound receptor is released. Here the antibody recognizes ingested or inhaled microbes and blocks their entry through the epithelium.

in response to chemokines produced in these tissues. Also, some of the IgA is produced by a subset of B cells, called B-1 cells, best studied in rodents, which also have a propensity to migrate to mucosal tissues; these cells secrete IgA in response to nonprotein antigens, without T cell help.

Intestinal mucosal B cells are located in the lamina propria, beneath the epithelial barrier, and IgA is produced in this region. To bind and neutralize microbial pathogens in the lumen before they invade, the IgA must be transported across the epithelial barrier into the lumen. Transport through the epithelium is carried out by a special Fc receptor, the poly-Ig receptor, which is expressed on the basal surface of the epithelial cells. This receptor binds IgA, endocytoses it into vesicles, and transports it to the luminal surface. Here the receptor is cleaved by a protease, and the IgA is released into the lumen still carrying a portion of the bound poly-Ig receptor (the secretory component). The attached secretory component protects the antibody from degradation by proteases in the gut. The antibody can then recognize microbes in the lumen and block their binding to and entry through the epithelium. IgA-mediated mucosal immunity is the mechanism of protection from poliovirus infection that is induced by oral immunization with the attenuated virus.

The gut contains a large number of commensal bacteria that are essential for basic functions such as absorption of food and, therefore, have to be tolerated by the immune system. IgA antibodies are produced mainly against potentially harmful and proinflammatory bacteria, thus blocking their entry through the gut epithelium. Harmless commensals are tolerated by the immune system of the gut by mechanisms that are discussed in Chapter 9.

Neonatal Immunity

Maternal antibodies are transported across the placenta to the fetus and across the gut epithelium of neonates, protecting the newborn from infections. Newborn mammals have incompletely developed immune systems and are unable to mount effective immune responses against many microbes. During their early life, they are protected from infections by antibodies acquired from their mothers. This is an example of naturally occurring passive immunity. Neonates acquire maternal antibodies by two routes. During pregnancy, maternal IgG binds to the FcRn expressed in the placenta, and is transported into the fetal circulation. After birth, infants ingest maternal IgA antibodies that are secreted into their mothers' colostrum and milk. Ingested IgA antibodies provide mucosal immune protection to the neonate. Thus, neonates acquire the antibody profiles of their mothers and are protected from infectious microbes to which the mothers were exposed or vaccinated.

Mechanism of immune evasion	Example(s)	
Antigenic variation	Many viruses (e.g., influenza, HIV) Bacteria (e.g., *Neisseria gonorrhoeae, Escherichia coli*) Protozoa (e.g., *Trypanosoma cruzi*)	
Inhibition of complement activation	Many bacteria	
Blocking by hyaluronic acid capsule	Streptococcus	

Fig. 8.14 Evasion of humoral immunity by microbes. This figure shows some of the mechanisms by which microbes evade humoral immunity, with illustrative examples. *HIV,* Human immunodeficiency virus.

EVASION OF HUMORAL IMMUNITY BY MICROBES

Microbes have evolved numerous mechanisms to evade humoral immunity (Fig. 8.14). Many bacteria and viruses mutate their antigenic surface molecules so that they can no longer be recognized by antibodies produced in response to the original microbe. Antigenic variation typically is seen in viruses, such as influenza virus, human immunodeficiency virus (HIV), and rhinovirus. HIV mutates its genome at a high rate, and therefore different strains contain many variant forms of the major antigenic surface glycoprotein of HIV, called gp120. As a result, antibodies against exposed determinants on gp120 in any one HIV subtype may not protect against other virus subtypes that appear in infected individuals. This is one reason why gp120 vaccines are not effective in protecting people from HIV infection. Bacteria such as *Escherichia coli* vary the antigens contained in their pili and thus evade antibody-mediated defense. The trypanosome that causes sleeping sickness expresses new surface glycoproteins whenever it encounters antibodies against the original glycoprotein. As a result, infection with

this protozoan parasite is characterized by waves of parasitemia, each wave consisting of an antigenically new parasite that is not recognized by antibodies produced against the parasites in the preceding wave. Other microbes inhibit complement activation, or resist opsonization and phagocytosis by concealing surface antigens under a hyaluronic acid capsule.

VACCINATION

Now that we have discussed the mechanisms of host defense against microbes, including cell-mediated immunity in Chapter 6 and humoral immunity in this chapter, it is important to consider how these adaptive immune responses can be induced with prophylactic vaccines.

Vaccination is the process of stimulating protective adaptive immune responses against microbes by exposure to nonpathogenic forms or components of the microbes. The development of vaccines against infections has been one of the great successes of immunology. The only human disease to be intentionally eradicated from the earth is smallpox, and this was achieved by a worldwide program

Type of vaccine	Examples	Form of protection
Live attenuated, or killed, bacteria	BCG, cholera	Antibody response
Live attenuated viruses	Polio, rabies	Antibody response; cell-mediated immune response
Subunit (antigen) vaccines	Tetanus toxoid, diphtheria toxoid	Antibody response
Conjugate vaccines	*Haemophilus influenzae, Streptococcus pneumoniae* (pneumococcus)	Helper T cell–dependent antibody response to polysaccharide antigens
Synthetic vaccines	Hepatitis virus (recombinant proteins)	Antibody response
Viral vectors	Clinical trials have been done	Cell-mediated and humoral immune responses
DNA vaccines	Clinical trials ongoing for several infections	Cell-mediated and humoral immune responses

Fig. 8.15 Vaccination strategies. A summary of different types of vaccines in use or tried, as well as the nature of the protective immune responses induced by these vaccines. *BCG,* Bacille Calmette-Guérin; *HIV,* human immunodeficiency virus.

of vaccination. Polio is likely to be the second such disease, and as mentioned in Chapter 1, many other diseases have been largely controlled by vaccination (see Fig. 1.2).

Several types of vaccines are in use and being developed (Fig. 8.15).

- Some of the most effective vaccines are composed of attenuated microbes, which are treated to abolish pathogenicity while retaining their infectivity and antigenicity. Immunization with these attenuated microbes stimulates the production of neutralizing antibodies against microbial antigens that protect vaccinated individuals from subsequent infections. For some infections, such as polio, the vaccines are given orally to stimulate mucosal IgA responses that protect individuals from natural infection, which occurs by the oral route.
- Vaccines composed of microbial proteins and polysaccharides, called subunit vaccines, work in the same way. Some microbial polysaccharide antigens (which cannot stimulate T cell help) are chemically coupled to proteins so that helper T cells are activated and high-affinity antibodies are produced against the polysaccharides.

These are called conjugate vaccines, and they are excellent examples of the practical application of our knowledge of helper T cell–B cell interactions (see Chapter 7). Immunization with inactivated microbial toxins and with microbial proteins synthesized in the laboratory stimulates antibodies that bind to and neutralize the native toxins and the microbes, respectively.

One of the continuing challenges in vaccination is to develop vaccines that stimulate cell-mediated immunity against intracellular microbes. Injected or orally administered antigens are extracellular antigens, and they induce mainly antibody responses. Many newer approaches are being tried to stimulate cell-mediated immunity by vaccination. One of these approaches is to incorporate microbial antigens into viral vectors, which will infect host cells and produce the antigens inside the cells. Another technique is to immunize individuals with DNA encoding a microbial antigen in a bacterial plasmid. The plasmid is ingested by host APCs, and the antigen is produced inside the cells. Many of these strategies have been successfully tested in animal models, but few have shown clinical efficacy to date.

SUMMARY

- Humoral immunity is the type of adaptive immunity that is mediated by antibodies. Antibodies prevent infections by blocking the ability of microbes to invade host cells, and they eliminate microbes by activating several effector mechanisms.
- In antibody molecules, the antigen-binding (Fab) regions are spatially separate from the effector (Fc) regions. The ability of antibodies to neutralize microbes and toxins is entirely a function of the antigen-binding regions. Even Fc-dependent effector functions are activated only after antibodies bind antigens.
- Antibodies are produced in lymphoid tissues and bone marrow, but they enter the circulation and are able to reach any site of infection. Heavy-chain isotype switching and affinity maturation enhance the protective functions of antibodies.
- Antibodies neutralize the infectivity of microbes and the pathogenicity of microbial toxins by binding to and interfering with the ability of these microbes and toxins to attach to host cells.
- Antibodies coat (opsonize) microbes and promote their phagocytosis by binding to Fc receptors on phagocytes. The binding of antibody Fc regions to Fc receptors also stimulates the microbicidal activities of phagocytes.
- The complement system is a collection of circulating and cell surface proteins that play important roles in host defense. The complement system may be activated on microbial surfaces without antibodies (alternative and lectin pathways, mechanisms of innate immunity) and after the binding of antibodies to antigens (classical pathway, a mechanism of adaptive humoral immunity).
- Complement proteins are sequentially cleaved, and active components, in particular C4b and C3b, become covalently attached to the surfaces on which complement is activated. The late steps of complement activation lead to the formation of the cytolytic MAC.
- Different products of complement activation promote phagocytosis of microbes, induce cell lysis, and stimulate inflammation. Mammals express cell surface and circulating regulatory proteins that prevent inappropriate complement activation on host cells.
- IgA antibody is produced in the lamina propria of mucosal organs and is actively transported by a special Fc receptor across the epithelium into the lumen, where it blocks the ability of microbes to invade the epithelium.
- Neonates acquire IgG antibodies from their mothers through the placenta, using the FcRn to capture and transport the maternal antibodies. Infants also acquire IgA antibodies from the mother's colostrum and milk by ingestion.
- Microbes have developed strategies to resist or evade humoral immunity, such as varying their antigens and becoming resistant to complement and phagocytosis.
- Most vaccines in current use work by stimulating the production of neutralizing antibodies.

REVIEW QUESTIONS

1. What regions of antibody molecules are involved in the functions of antibodies?
2. How do heavy-chain isotype (class) switching and affinity maturation improve the ability of antibodies to combat infectious pathogens?
3. In what situations does the ability of antibodies to neutralize microbes protect the host from infections?
4. How do antibodies assist in the elimination of microbes by phagocytes?
5. How is the complement system activated?
6. Why is the complement system effective against microbes but does not react against host cells and tissues?
7. What are the functions of the complement system, and what components of complement mediate these functions?
8. How do antibodies prevent infections by ingested and inhaled microbes?
9. How are neonates protected from infection before their immune system has reached maturity?

Answers to and discussion of the Review Questions are available at Student Consult.

Immunologic Tolerance and Autoimmunity
Self–Nonself Discrimination in the Immune System and Its Failure

CHAPTER OUTLINE

One of the remarkable properties of the normal immune system is that it can react to an enormous variety of microbes but does not react against the individual's own (self) antigens. This unresponsiveness to self antigens, also called **immunologic tolerance**, is maintained despite the fact that the molecular mechanisms by which lymphocyte receptor specificities are generated are not biased to exclude receptors for self antigens. In other words, lymphocytes with the ability to recognize self antigens are constantly being generated during the normal process of lymphocyte maturation. Furthermore, many self antigens have ready access to the immune system, so unresponsiveness to these antigens cannot be maintained simply by concealing them from lymphocytes. The process by which antigen-presenting cells (APCs) display antigens to T cells does not distinguish between foreign and self proteins, so self antigens are normally seen by lymphocytes. It follows that there must exist mechanisms that prevent immune responses to self antigens. These mechanisms are responsible for one of the cardinal features of the immune system—namely, its ability to discriminate between self and nonself (usually microbial) antigens. If these mechanisms fail, the immune system may attack the individual's own cells and tissues. Such reactions are called **autoimmunity**, and the diseases they cause are called autoimmune diseases. In addition to tolerating the presence of self antigens, the immune system has to coexist with many commensal microbes that live on the epithelial barriers of their human hosts, often in a state of symbiosis, and the immune system of a pregnant female has to accept the presence of a fetus that expresses antigens derived from the father. Unresponsiveness to commensal microbes and the fetus is maintained by many of the same mechanisms involved in unresponsiveness to self.

In this chapter we address the following questions:

- How does the immune system maintain unresponsiveness to self antigens?
- What are the factors that may contribute to the loss of self-tolerance and the development of autoimmunity?
- How does the immune system maintain unresponsiveness to commensal microbes and the fetus?

This chapter begins with a discussion of the important principles and features of self-tolerance. Then we discuss the different mechanisms that maintain tolerance to self antigens, as well as commensal microbes and the fetus, and how tolerance may fail, resulting in autoimmunity.

IMMUNOLOGIC TOLERANCE: GENERAL PRINICIPLES AND SIGNIFICANCE

Immunologic tolerance is a lack of response to antigens that is induced by exposure of lymphocytes to these antigens. When lymphocytes with receptors for a particular antigen encounter this antigen, any of several outcomes is possible. The lymphocytes may be activated to proliferate and to differentiate into effector and memory cells, leading to a productive immune response; antigens that elicit such a response are said to be **immunogenic**. The lymphocytes may be functionally inactivated or killed, resulting in tolerance; antigens that induce tolerance are said to be **tolerogenic**. In some situations, the antigen-specific lymphocytes may not react in any way; this phenomenon has been called immunologic ignorance, implying that the lymphocytes simply ignore the presence of the antigen. Normally, microbes are immunogenic and self antigens are tolerogenic.

The choice between lymphocyte activation and tolerance is determined largely by the nature of the antigen and the additional signals present when the antigen is displayed to the immune system. In fact, the same antigen may be administered in different ways to induce an immune response or tolerance. This experimental observation has been exploited to analyze what factors determine whether activation or tolerance develops as a consequence of encounter with an antigen.

The phenomenon of immunologic tolerance is important for several reasons. First, as we stated at the outset, self antigens normally induce tolerance, and failure of self-tolerance is the underlying cause of autoimmune diseases. Second, if we learn how to induce tolerance in lymphocytes specific for a particular antigen, we may be able to use this knowledge to prevent or control unwanted immune reactions. Strategies for inducing tolerance are being tested to treat allergic and autoimmune diseases and to prevent the rejection of organ transplants. The same strategies may be valuable in gene therapy to prevent immune responses against the products of newly expressed genes or vectors and even for stem cell transplantation if the stem cell donor is genetically different from the recipient.

Immunologic tolerance to different self antigens may be induced when developing lymphocytes encounter these antigens in the generative (central) lymphoid organs, a process called central tolerance, or when mature lymphocytes encounter self-antigens in peripheral (secondary) lymphoid organs or peripheral tissues, called peripheral tolerance (Fig. 9.1). Central tolerance is a mechanism of tolerance only to self antigens that are present in the generative lymphoid organs—namely, the bone marrow and thymus. Tolerance to self antigens that are not present in these organs must be induced and maintained by peripheral mechanisms. We have only limited knowledge of which self antigens induce central or peripheral tolerance or are ignored by the immune system.

With this brief background, we proceed to a discussion of the mechanisms of immunologic tolerance and how the failure of each mechanism may result in autoimmunity. Tolerance in T cells, particularly CD4+ helper T lymphocytes, is discussed first because many of the mechanisms of self-tolerance were defined by studies of these cells. In addition, CD4+ helper T cells orchestrate virtually all immune responses to protein antigens, so tolerance in these cells may be enough to prevent both cell-mediated and humoral immune responses against self proteins. Conversely, failure of tolerance in helper T cells may result in autoimmunity manifested by T cell–mediated attack against tissue self antigens or by the production of autoantibodies against self proteins.

CENTRAL T LYMPHOCYTE TOLERANCE

The principal mechanisms of central tolerance in T cells are death of immature T cells and the generation of CD4+ regulatory T cells (Fig. 9.2). The lymphocytes

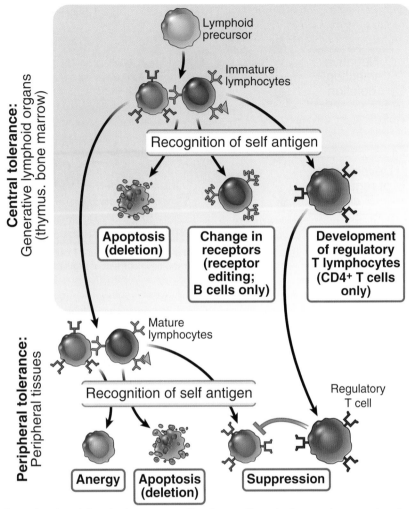

Fig. 9.1 Central and peripheral tolerance to self antigens. Central tolerance: Immature lymphocytes specific for self antigens may encounter these antigens in the generative (central) lymphoid organs and are deleted; B lymphocytes may change their specificity (receptor editing); and some T lymphocytes develop into regulatory T cells. Some self-reactive lymphocytes may complete their maturation and enter peripheral tissues. Peripheral tolerance: mature self-reactive lymphocytes may be inactivated or deleted by encounter with self antigens in peripheral tissues or suppressed by regulatory T cells.

that develop in the thymus consist of cells with receptors capable of recognizing many antigens, both self and foreign. If a lymphocyte that has not completed its maturation interacts strongly with a self antigen, displayed as a peptide bound to a self major histocompatibility complex (MHC) molecule, that lymphocyte receives signals that trigger apoptosis. Thus, the self-reactive cell dies before it can become functionally competent. This process, called **negative selection** (see Chapter 4), is a major mechanism of central tolerance. The process of

negative selection affects self-reactive CD4+ T cells and CD8+ T cells, which recognize self peptides displayed by class II MHC and class I MHC molecules, respectively. Why immature lymphocytes die upon receiving strong T cell receptor (TCR) signals in the thymus, while mature lymphocytes that get strong TCR signals in the periphery are activated, is not fully understood.

Some immature CD4+ T cells that recognize self antigens in the thymus with high affinity do not die but develop into regulatory T cells and enter peripheral

Fig. 9.2 Central T cell tolerance. Strong recognition of self antigens by immature T cells in the thymus may lead to death of the cells (negative selection, or deletion), or the development of regulatory T cells that enter peripheral tissues.

tissues (see Fig. 9.2). The functions of regulatory T cells are described later in the chapter. What determines whether a thymic CD4⁺ T cell that recognizes a self antigen will die or become a regulatory T cell is also not established.

Immature lymphocytes may interact strongly with an antigen if the antigen is present at high concentrations in the thymus and if the lymphocytes express receptors that recognize the antigen with high affinity. Antigens that induce negative selection may include proteins that are abundant throughout the body, such as plasma proteins and common cellular proteins.

Surprisingly, many self proteins that are normally present only in certain peripheral tissues, called tissue-restricted antigens, are also expressed in some of the epithelial cells of the thymus. A protein called **AIRE** (autoimmune regulator) is responsible for the thymic expression of these peripheral tissue antigens. Mutations in the *AIRE* gene are the cause of a rare disorder called autoimmune polyendocrine syndrome. In this disorder, several tissue antigens are not expressed in the thymus because of a lack of functional AIRE protein, so immature T cells specific for these antigens are not eliminated and do not develop into regulatory cells. These cells mature into functionally competent T cells that enter the peripheral immune system and are capable of reacting harmfully against the tissue-restricted antigens, which are expressed normally in the appropriate peripheral tissues even in the absence of AIRE. Therefore, T cells specific for these

antigens emerge from the thymus, encounter the antigens in the peripheral tissues, and attack the tissues and cause disease. It is not clear why endocrine organs are the most frequent targets of this autoimmune attack. Although this rare syndrome illustrates the importance of negative selection in the thymus for maintaining self-tolerance, it is not known if defects in negative selection contribute to common autoimmune diseases.

Central tolerance is imperfect, and some self-reactive lymphocytes mature and are present in healthy individuals. As discussed next, peripheral mechanisms may prevent the activation of these lymphocytes.

PERIPHERAL T LYMPHOCYTE TOLERANCE

Peripheral tolerance is induced when mature T cells recognize self antigens in peripheral tissues, leading to functional inactivation (anergy) or death, or when the self-reactive lymphocytes are suppressed by regulatory T cells (Fig. 9.3). Each of these mechanisms of peripheral T cell tolerance is described in this section. Peripheral tolerance is clearly important for preventing T cell responses to self antigens that are not present in the thymus, and it also may provide backup mechanisms for preventing autoimmunity in situations where central tolerance to antigens that are expressed in the thymus is incomplete.

Antigen recognition without adequate costimulation results in T cell anergy or death or makes T cells

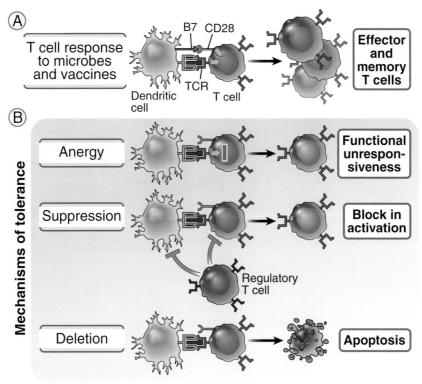

Fig. 9.3 Peripheral T cell tolerance. A, Normal T cell responses require antigen recognition and costimulation. **B,** Three major mechanisms of peripheral T cell tolerance are illustrated: cell-intrinsic anergy, suppression by regulatory T cells, and deletion (apoptotic cell death). *TCR,* T cell receptor.

sensitive to suppression by regulatory T cells. As noted in previous chapters, naive T lymphocytes need at least two signals to induce their proliferation and differentiation into effector and memory cells: Signal 1 is always antigen, and signal 2 is provided by costimulators that are expressed on APCs, typically as part of the innate immune response to microbes (or to damaged host cells) (see Chapter 5, Fig. 5.6). It is believed that dendritic cells in normal uninfected tissues and peripheral lymphoid organs are in a resting (or immature) state, in which they express little or no costimulators, such as B7 proteins (see Chapter 5). These dendritic cells constantly process and display the self antigens that are present in the tissues. T lymphocytes with receptors for the self antigens are able to recognize the antigens and thus receive signals from their antigen receptors (signal 1), but the T cells do not receive strong costimulation because there is no accompanying innate immune response. Thus, the presence or absence of costimulation is a major factor determining whether T cells are activated or tolerized.

Anergy

Anergy in T cells refers to long-lived functional unresponsiveness that is induced when these cells recognize self antigens (Fig. 9.4). Self antigens are normally displayed with low levels of costimulators, as discussed earlier. Antigen recognition without adequate costimulation is thought to be the basis of anergy induction, by mechanisms that are described later. Anergic cells survive but are incapable of responding to the antigen.

The two best-defined mechanisms responsible for the induction of anergy are abnormal signaling by the TCR complex and the delivery of inhibitory signals from receptors other than the TCR complex.

- When T cells recognize antigens without costimulation, the TCR complex may lose its ability to transmit activating signals. In some cases, this is related to the activation of enzymes (ubiquitin ligases) that modify signaling proteins and target them for intracellular destruction by proteases.

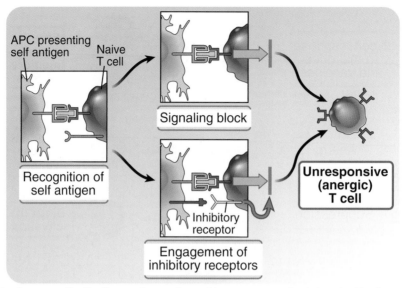

Fig. 9.4 T cell anergy. If a T cell recognizes antigen without strong costimulation, the T cell receptors may lose their ability to deliver activating signals, or the T cell may engage inhibitory receptors, such as cytotoxic T lymphocyte–associated protein 4 (CTLA-4) and programmed cell death protein 1 (PD-1), that block activation. *APC,* Antigen-presenting cells.

- On recognition of self antigens, T cells also may preferentially use one of the inhibitory receptors of the CD28 family, cytotoxic T lymphocyte–associated antigen 4 (CTLA-4, or CD152) or programmed cell death protein 1 (PD-1, CD279), which were introduced in Chapter 5. Anergic T cells may express higher levels of these inhibitory receptors, which will inhibit responses to subsequent antigen recognition. The functions and mechanisms of action of these receptors are described in more detail below.

Regulation of T Cell Responses by Inhibitory Receptors

Immune responses are influenced by a balance between engagement of activating and inhibitory receptors. This idea is established for B and T lymphocytes and natural killer (NK) cells. In T cells, the main activating receptors are the TCR complex and costimulatory receptors such as CD28 (see Chapter 5), and the best-defined inhibitory receptors, also called coinhibitors, are CTLA-4 and PD-1. The functions and mechanisms of action of these inhibitors are complementary (Fig. 9.5).

- **CTLA-4.** CTLA-4 is expressed transiently on activated $CD4^+$ T cells and constitutively on regulatory T cells (described later). It functions to suppress the activation of responding T cells. CTLA-4 works by blocking and removing B7 molecules from the surface of APCs, thus reducing costimulation by CD28 and preventing the activation of T cells (see Fig. 9-5A). The choice between engagement of CTLA-4 or CD28 is determined by the affinity of these receptors for B7 and the level of B7 expression. CTLA-4 has a higher affinity for B7 molecules than does CD28, so it binds B7 tightly and prevents the binding of CD28. This competition is especially effective when B7 levels are low (as would be expected normally when APCs are displaying self and probably tumor antigens); in these situations, the receptor that is preferentially engaged is the high-affinity blocking receptor CTLA-4. However, when B7 levels are high (as in infections), not all the ligands will be occupied by CTLA-4 and some B7 will be available to bind to the low-affinity activating receptor CD28, leading to T cell costimulation.

- **PD-1.** PD-1 is expressed on $CD8^+$ and $CD4^+$ T cells after antigen stimulation. Its cytoplasmic tail has inhibitory signaling motifs with tyrosine residues that are phosphorylated upon recognition of its ligands PD-L1 or PD-L2. Once phosphorylated, these tyrosines bind a tyrosine phosphatase that inhibits kinase-dependent activating signals from CD28 and the TCR complex (see Fig. 9-5B). Because the expression of PD-1 on T cells is increased upon chronic T cell activation and

	CTLA-4	PD-1
Major site of action	Secondary lymphoid organs	Peripheral tissues
Stage of immune response that is inhibited	Induction (priming)	Effector phase
Cell type that is inhibited	CD4+ same as or more than CD8+	CD8+ > CD4+
Cellular expression	Tregs, activated T cells	Mainly activated T cells
Main signals inhibited	Competitive inhibitor of CD28 costimulation by binding to B7 with high affinity and removing B7 from APCs	Signaling inhibitor of CD28 and TCR: inhibits kinase-depending signals by activating phosphatase
Role in Treg-mediated suppression of immune responses	Yes	No

Fig. 9.5 Mechanisms of action and properties of cytotoxic T lymphocyte–associated protein 4 (CTLA-4) and programmed cell death protein 1 (PD-1). A, CTLA-4 is a competitive inhibitor of the B7-CD28 interaction. B, PD-1 activates a phosphatase that inhibits signals from the TCR complex and CD28. C, Some of the major differences between these checkpoint molecules are summarized. *APC,* Antigen-presenting cells; *TCR,* T cell receptor.

expression of the ligands is increased by cytokines produced during prolonged inflammation, this pathway is most active in situations of chronic or repeated antigenic stimulation. This may happen in responses to chronic infections, tumors, and self antigens, when PD-1–expressing T cells encounter the ligand on infected cells, tumor cells, or APCs.

One of the most impressive therapeutic applications of our understanding of these inhibitory receptors is treatment of cancer patients with antibodies that block these receptors. Such treatment leads to enhanced antitumor immune responses and tumor regression in a significant fraction of the patients (see Chapter 10). This type of therapy has been termed **checkpoint blockade**, because the inhibitory receptors impose checkpoints in immune responses, and the treatment blocks these checkpoints ("removes the brakes" on immune responses). Predictably, patients treated with checkpoint blockade often develop autoimmune reactions, consistent with the idea that the inhibitory receptors are constantly functioning to keep autoreactive T cells in check. Rare patients with mutations in one of their two copies of the *CTLA4* gene, which reduce expression of the receptor, also develop multiorgan inflammation (and a profound, as yet unexplained, defect in antibody production).

Several other receptors on T cells other than CTLA-4 and PD-1 have been shown to inhibit immune responses and are currently being tested as targets of checkpoint blockade therapy. Some of these receptors are members of the tumor necrosis factor (TNF) receptor family or other protein families. Their role in maintaining tolerance to self antigens is not clearly established.

Immune Suppression by Regulatory T Cells

Regulatory T cells develop in the thymus or peripheral tissues on recognition of self antigens and suppress the activation of potentially harmful lymphocytes specific for these self antigens (Fig. 9.6). The majority

Fig. 9.6 Development and function of regulatory T cells. CD4+ T cells that recognize self antigens may differentiate into regulatory cells in the thymus or peripheral tissues, in a process that is dependent on the transcription factor FoxP3. (The *larger arrow* from the thymus, compared with the one from peripheral tissues, indicates that most of these cells probably arise in the thymus.) These regulatory cells inhibit the activation of naive T cells and their differentiation into effector T cells by contact-dependent mechanisms or by secreting cytokines that inhibit T cell responses. The generation and maintenance of regulatory T cells also require interleukin-2 (not shown). *DC,* Dendritic cell; *NK,* natural killer.

of self-reactive regulatory T cells probably develop in the thymus (see Fig. 9.2), but they may also arise in peripheral lymphoid organs. Most regulatory T cells are CD4+ and express high levels of CD25, the α chain of the interleukin-2 (IL-2) receptor. They also express a transcription factor called FoxP3, which is required for the development and function of the cells. Mutations of the gene encoding FoxP3 in humans or in mice cause a systemic, multiorgan autoimmune disease, demonstrating the importance of FoxP3+ regulatory T cells for the maintenance of self-tolerance. The human disease is known by the acronym **IPEX,** for immune dysregulation, polyendocrinopathy, enteropathy, X-linked syndrome.

The survival and function of regulatory T cells are dependent on the cytokine IL-2. This role of IL-2 accounts for the severe autoimmune disease that develops in mice in which IL-2 or IL-2 receptor genes are deleted and in humans with homozygous mutations in the α or β chain of the IL-2 receptor. Recall that we introduced IL-2 in Chapter 5 as a cytokine made by antigen-activated T cells that stimulates proliferation of these cells. Thus, IL-2 is an example of a cytokine that serves two opposite roles: it promotes immune responses by stimulating T cell proliferation, and it inhibits immune responses by maintaining functional regulatory T cells. Numerous clinical trials are testing the ability of IL-2 to promote regulation and control harmful immune reactions, such as inflammation in autoimmune diseases and graft rejection.

The cytokine transforming growth factor β (TGF-β) also plays a role in the generation of regulatory T cells, perhaps by stimulating expression of the FoxP3 transcription factor. Many cell types can produce TGF-β, but the source of TGF-β for inducing regulatory T cells in the thymus or peripheral tissues is not defined.

Regulatory T cells may suppress immune responses by several mechanisms.
- Some regulatory cells produce cytokines (e.g., IL-10, TGF-β) that inhibit the activation of lymphocytes, dendritic cells, and macrophages.
- Regulatory cells express CTLA-4, which, as discussed earlier, may block or remove B7 molecules made by APCs and make these APCs incapable of providing costimulation via CD28 and activating T cells.
- Regulatory T cells, by virtue of the high level of expression of the IL-2 receptor, may bind and consume this

essential T cell growth factor, thus reducing its availability for responding T cells.

The great interest in regulatory T cells has in part been driven by the hypothesis that the underlying abnormality in some autoimmune diseases in humans is defective regulatory T cell function or the resistance of pathogenic T cells to regulation. There is also growing interest in cellular therapy with regulatory T cells to treat graft-versus-host disease, graft rejection, and autoimmune disorders.

Deletion: Apoptosis of Mature Lymphocytes

Recognition of self antigens may trigger pathways of apoptosis that result in elimination (deletion) of the self-reactive lymphocytes (Fig. 9.7). There are two likely mechanisms of death of mature T lymphocytes induced by self antigens:
- Antigen recognition induces in T cells the production of proapoptotic proteins that cause mitochondrial proteins, such as cytochrome c, to leak out and activate cytosolic enzymes called caspases that induce apoptosis. In normal immune responses, the activity of these proapoptotic proteins is counteracted by antiapoptotic proteins that are induced by costimulation and by growth factors produced during the responses. However, self antigens, which are recognized without strong costimulation, do not stimulate production of antiapoptotic proteins, and the relative deficiency of survival signals induces death of the cells that recognize these antigens.
- Recognition of self antigens may lead to the coexpression of death receptors and their ligands. This ligand-receptor interaction generates signals through the death receptor that culminate in the activation of caspases and apoptosis. The best-defined death receptor–ligand pair involved in self-tolerance is a protein called Fas (CD95), which is expressed on many cell types, and Fas ligand (FasL), which is expressed mainly on activated T cells.

Evidence from genetic studies supports the role of apoptosis in self-tolerance. Eliminating the mitochondrial pathway of apoptosis in mice results in a failure of deletion of self-reactive T cells in the thymus and also in peripheral tissues. Mice with mutations in the *fas* and *fasl* genes and children with mutations in *FAS* all develop autoimmune diseases with lymphocyte accumulation. Children with mutations in the genes encoding caspase-8 or -10, which are downstream of FAS signaling, also have similar autoimmune diseases. The human diseases, collectively called the **autoimmune**

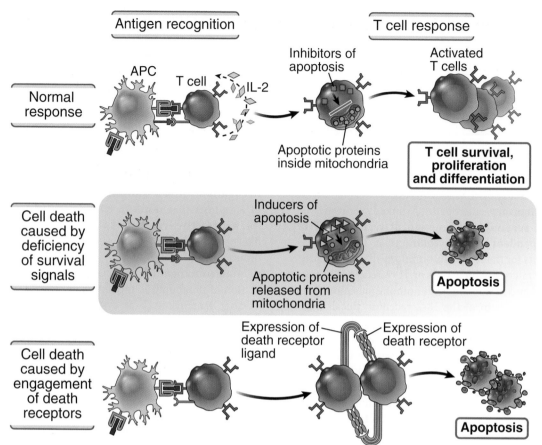

Fig. 9.7 Mechanisms of apoptosis of T lymphocytes. T cells respond to antigen presented by normal antigen-presenting cells (APCs) by secreting interleukin-2 (IL-2), expressing antiapoptotic (prosurvival) proteins, and undergoing proliferation and differentiation. The antiapoptotic proteins prevent the release of mediators of apoptosis from mitochondria. Self antigen recognition by T cells without costimulation may lead to relative deficiency of intracellular antiapoptotic proteins, and the excess of proapoptotic proteins causes cell death by inducing release of mediators of apoptosis from mitochondria (death by the mitochondrial [intrinsic] pathway of apoptosis). Alternatively, self antigen recognition may lead to expression of death receptors and their ligands, such as Fas and Fas ligand (FasL), on lymphocytes, and engagement of the death receptor leads to apoptosis of the cells by the death receptor (extrinsic) pathway.

lymphoproliferative syndrome (ALPS), are rare and are the only known examples of defects in apoptosis causing an autoimmune disorder.

From this discussion of the mechanisms of T cell tolerance, it should be clear that self antigens differ from foreign microbial antigens in several ways, which contribute to the choice between tolerance induced by the former and activation by the latter (Fig. 9.8).

- Self antigens are present in the thymus, where they induce deletion and generate regulatory T cells; by contrast, most microbial antigens tend to be excluded from the thymus because they are typically captured from their sites of entry and transported into peripheral lymphoid organs (see Chapter 3).

- Self antigens are displayed by resting (costimulator-deficient) APCs in the absence of innate immunity, thus favoring the induction of T cell anergy or death, or suppression by regulatory T cells. By contrast, microbes elicit innate immune reactions, leading to the expression of costimulators and cytokines that promote T cell proliferation and differentiation into effector cells.

- Self antigens are present throughout life and may therefore cause prolonged or repeated TCR engagement, again promoting anergy, apoptosis, and the development of regulatory T cells.

Feature of antigen	Tolerogenic self antigens	Immunogenic foreign antigens
	Tissue	Microbe
Location of antigens	Presence in generative organs (some self antigens) induces negative selection and other mechanisms of central tolerance	Presence in blood and peripheral tissues (most microbial antigens) permits concentration in peripheral lymphoid organs
Accompanying costimulation	Deficiency of costimulators may lead to T cell anergy or apoptosis, development of Treg, or sensitivity to suppression by Treg	Expression of costimulators, typically seen with microbes, promotes lymphocyte survival and activation
Duration of antigen exposure	Long-lived persistence (throughout life); prolonged TCR engagement may induce anergy and apoptosis	Short exposure to microbial antigen reflects effective immune response

Fig. 9.8 Features of protein antigens that influence the choice between T cell tolerance and activation. This figure summarizes some of the characteristics of self and foreign (e.g., microbial) protein antigens that determine why the self antigens induce tolerance and microbial antigens stimulate T cell–mediated immune responses. *TCR,* T cell receptor; *Treg,* T regulatory cells.

B LYMPHOCYTE TOLERANCE

Self polysaccharides, lipids, and nucleic acids are T-independent antigens that are not recognized by T cells. These antigens must induce tolerance in B lymphocytes to prevent autoantibody production. Self proteins may not elicit autoantibody responses because of tolerance in helper T cells and in B cells. It is suspected that diseases associated with autoantibody production, such as systemic lupus erythematosus (SLE), are caused by defective tolerance in both B lymphocytes and helper T cells.

Central B Cell Tolerance

When immature B lymphocytes interact strongly with self antigens in the bone marrow, the B cells either change their receptor specificity (receptor editing) or are killed (deletion) (Fig. 9.9).

- **Receptor editing.** Immature B cells are at a stage of maturation in the bone marrow when they have rearranged their immunoglobulin (Ig) genes, express IgM with a heavy chain and light chain, and have shut off the *RAG* genes that encode the recombinase. If these B cells recognize self antigens in the bone marrow,

they may reexpress *RAG* genes, resume light-chain gene recombination, and express a new Ig light chain (see Chapter 4). The heavy chain gene cannot recombine because some segments are lost during the initial recombination. The new light chain associates with the previously expressed Ig heavy chain to produce a new antigen receptor that may no longer recognize the self antigen. This process of changing receptor specificity, called **receptor editing,** reduces the chance that potentially harmful self-reactive B cells will leave the marrow. It is estimated that 25% to 50% of mature B cells in a normal individual may have undergone receptor editing during their maturation. (There is no evidence that developing T cells can undergo receptor editing.)

- **Deletion.** If editing fails, immature B cells that strongly recognize self antigens receive death signals and die by apoptosis. This process of deletion is similar to negative selection of immature T lymphocytes. As in the T cell compartment, negative selection of B cells eliminates lymphocytes with high-affinity receptors for abundant, and usually widely expressed, cell membrane or soluble self antigens.

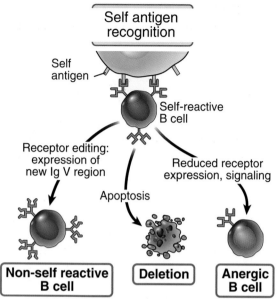

Fig. 9.9 Central tolerance in immature B lymphocytes. An immature B cell that recognizes self antigen in the bone marrow changes its antigen receptor (receptor editing), dies by apoptosis (negative selection, or deletion), or reduces antigen receptor expression and becomes functionally unresponsive. *Ig*, Immunoglobulin.

- **Anergy.** Some self antigens, such as soluble proteins, may be recognized in the bone marrow with low avidity. B cells specific for these antigens survive, but antigen receptor expression is reduced, and the cells become functionally unresponsive (anergic).

Peripheral B Cell Tolerance

Mature B lymphocytes that encounter self antigens in peripheral lymphoid tissues become incapable of responding to that antigen (Fig. 9.10). According to one hypothesis, if B cells recognize a protein antigen but do not receive T cell help (because helper T cells have been eliminated or are tolerant), the B cells become anergic because of a block in signaling from the antigen receptor. Anergic B cells may leave lymphoid follicles and are subsequently excluded from the follicles. These excluded B cells may die because they do not receive necessary survival stimuli. B cells that recognize self antigens in the periphery may also undergo apoptosis, or inhibitory receptors on the B cells may be engaged, thus preventing activation. As mentioned earlier, regulatory T cells may also contribute to B cell tolerance.

Fig. 9.10 Peripheral tolerance in B lymphocytes. A mature B cell that recognizes a self-antigen without T cell help is functionally inactivated and becomes incapable of responding to that antigen (anergy), or it dies by apoptosis (deletion), or its activation is suppressed by engagement of inhibitory receptors.

TOLERANCE TO COMMENSAL MICROBES AND FETAL ANTIGENS

Before concluding our discussion of the mechanisms of immunologic tolerance, it is useful to consider two other types of antigens that are not self but are produced by cells or tissues that have to be tolerated by the immune system. These are products of commensal microbes that live in symbiosis with humans and paternally derived antigens in the fetus. Coexistence with these antigens is dependent on many of the same mechanisms that are used to maintain peripheral tolerance to self antigens.

Tolerance to Commensal Microbes in the Intestines and Skin

The microbiome of healthy humans consists of approximately 10^{14} bacteria and viruses (which is estimated to be almost 10 times the number of nucleated human cells, prompting microbiologists to point out that we are only 10% human and 90% microbial!). These microbes reside in the intestinal and respiratory tracts and on the skin, where they serve many essential functions. For instance, in the gut, the normal bacteria aid in digestion and absorption of foods and prevent overgrowth of potentially harmful organisms. Mature lymphocytes in these tissues are capable of recognizing the organisms but do not react against them, so the microbes are not eliminated, and harmful inflammation is not triggered.

In the gut, several mechanisms account for the inability of the healthy immune system to react against commensal microbes. These mechanisms include an abundance of IL-10–producing regulatory T cells, and an unusual property of intestinal dendritic cells such that signaling from some Toll-like receptors leads to inhibition rather than activation. In addition, many commensal bacteria are physically separated from the intestinal immune system by the epithelium. The mechanisms that maintain tolerance to commensal bacteria in the skin are not as well defined.

Tolerance to Fetal Antigens

The evolution of placentation in eutherian mammals allowed the fetus to mature before birth but created the problem that paternal antigens expressed in the fetus, which are foreign to the mother, have to be tolerated by the immune system of the pregnant mother. One mechanism of this tolerance is the generation of peripheral FoxP3+ regulatory T cells specific for these paternal antigens. In fact, during mammalian evolution, placentation is strongly correlated with the ability to generate stable peripheral regulatory T cells. It is unclear whether women who suffer recurrent pregnancy losses have a defect in the generation or maintenance of these regulatory T cells. Other mechanisms of fetal tolerance include exclusion of inflammatory cells from the pregnant uterus, poor antigen presentation in the placenta, and an inability to generate harmful Th1 responses in the healthy pregnant uterus.

Now that we have described the principal mechanisms of immunologic tolerance, we consider the consequences of the failure of self-tolerance—namely, the development of autoimmunity.

AUTOIMMUNITY

Autoimmunity is defined as an immune response against self (autologous) antigens. It is an important cause of disease, estimated to affect 5% to 10% of the population in developed countries, and the prevalence of several autoimmune diseases is increasing. Different autoimmune diseases may be organ-specific, affecting only one or a few organs, or systemic, with widespread tissue injury and clinical manifestations. Tissue injury in autoimmune diseases may be caused by antibodies against self antigens or by T cells reactive with self antigens (see Chapter 11).

Pathogenesis

The principal factors in the development of autoimmunity are the inheritance of susceptibility genes and environmental triggers, such as infections (Fig. 9.11). It is postulated that susceptibility genes interfere with pathways of self-tolerance and lead to the persistence of self-reactive T and B lymphocytes. Environmental stimuli may cause cell and tissue injury and inflammation and activate these self-reactive lymphocytes, resulting in the generation of effector T cells and autoantibodies that are responsible for the autoimmune disease.

Despite our growing knowledge of the immunologic abnormalities that may result in autoimmunity, we still do not know the etiology of common human autoimmune diseases. This lack of understanding results from several factors: autoimmune diseases in humans usually are heterogeneous and multifactorial; the self antigens that are the inducers and targets of the autoimmune reactions often are unknown; and the diseases may manifest clinically long after the autoimmune reactions have been initiated. Recent advances, including the identification of disease-associated genes and better techniques for studying immune responses in humans, hold promise for providing answers to the enigma of autoimmunity.

Genetic Factors

Inherited risk for most autoimmune diseases is attributable to multiple gene loci, of which the largest contribution is made by MHC genes. If an autoimmune disease develops in one of two twins, the same disease is more likely to develop in the other twin than in an unrelated member of the general population. Furthermore, this increased incidence is greater among monozygotic (identical) twins than among dizygotic twins. These findings prove the importance of genetics in the susceptibility to autoimmunity. Genome-wide association studies have revealed some of the common variations (polymorphisms) of genes that may contribute to different autoimmune diseases. Emerging results suggest that different polymorphisms are more frequent (predisposing) or less frequent (protective) in patients than in healthy controls. The likelihood of a particular autoimmune disease in people with versus without a particular HLA allele is expressed as the odds ratio or relative risk. The importance of these polymorphisms is reinforced by the finding that many of them affect genes involved in immune responses, and the same genetic

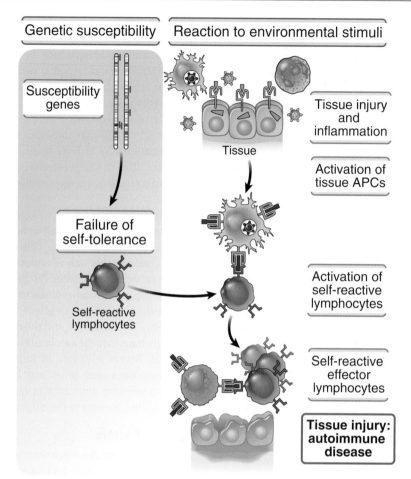

Fig. 9.11 Postulated mechanisms of autoimmunity. In this proposed model of organ-specific T cell–mediated autoimmunity, various genetic loci may confer susceptibility to autoimmunity, probably by influencing the maintenance of self-tolerance. Environmental triggers, such as infections and other inflammatory stimuli, promote the influx of lymphocytes into tissues and the activation of antigen-presenting cells (APCs) and subsequently of self-reactive T cells, resulting in tissue injury.

polymorphism may be associated with more than one autoimmune disease. However, these polymorphisms are frequently present in healthy individuals, and the individual contribution of each of these genes to the development of autoimmunity is very small, so many risk alleles together are needed to cause the disease.

Many autoimmune diseases in humans and inbred animals are linked to particular MHC alleles (Fig. 9.12). The association between human leukocyte antigen (HLA) alleles and autoimmune diseases in humans was recognized many years ago and was one of the first indications that T cells played an important role in these disorders (because the only known function of MHC molecules is to present peptide antigens to T cells). The incidence of numerous autoimmune diseases is greater among individuals who inherit particular HLA allele(s) than in the general population. Most of these disease associations are with class II HLA alleles (HLA-DR and HLA-DQ), perhaps because class II MHC molecules control the action of CD4+ T cells, which are involved in both cell-mediated and humoral immune responses to proteins as well in regulating immune responses. It is important to point out that, although an HLA allele may increase the risk of developing a particular autoimmune disease, the HLA allele is not, by itself, the cause of the disease. In fact, the disease never develops in the vast majority of people who inherit an HLA allele that does confer increased risk of the disease. Despite the clear association of MHC alleles with several autoimmune diseases, how these alleles contribute to the development of the diseases remains

Disease	MHC allele	Relative risk
Ankylosing spondylitis	HLA-B27	90
Rheumatoid arthritis	HLA-DRB1*01/*04/*10	4-12
Type 1 diabetes mellitus	HLA-DRB1*0301/0401	35
Pemphigus vulgaris	HLA-DR4	14

Fig. 9.12 Association of autoimmune diseases with alleles of the major histocompatibility complex (MHC) locus. Family and linkage studies show a greater likelihood of developing certain autoimmune diseases in persons who inherit particular human leukocyte antigen (HLA) alleles than in persons who lack these alleles (odds ratio or relative risk). Selected examples of HLA disease associations are listed. For instance, in people who have the HLA-B27 allele, the risk of development of ankylosing spondylitis, an autoimmune disease of the spine, is 90 to 100 times higher than in B27-negative people; other diseases show various degrees of association with other HLA alleles. The asterisks indicate HLA alleles identified by molecular (DNA-based) typing instead of the older serologic (antibody-based) methods.

unknown. Some hypotheses are that particular MHC alleles may be especially effective at presenting pathogenic self peptides to autoreactive T cells or that they are inefficient at displaying certain self antigens in the thymus, leading to defective negative selection of T cells.

Polymorphisms in non-HLA genes are associated with various autoimmune diseases and may contribute to failure of self-tolerance or abnormal activation of lymphocytes (Fig. 9.13A). Many such disease-associated genetic variants have been described:
- Polymorphisms in the gene encoding the tyrosine phosphatase PTPN22 (protein tyrosine phosphatase N22) may lead to uncontrolled activation of both B and T cells and are associated with numerous autoimmune diseases, including rheumatoid arthritis, SLE, and type 1 diabetes mellitus.
- Variants of the innate immune cytoplasmic microbial sensor NOD-2 that cause reduced resistance to intestinal microbes are associated with Crohn disease, an inflammatory bowel disease, in some ethnic populations.
- Other polymorphisms associated with multiple autoimmune diseases include genes encoding the IL-2 receptor α chain (CD25), believed to influence the balance of effector and regulatory T cells; the receptor for the cytokine IL-23, which promotes the development of proinflammatory Th17 cells; and CTLA-4, a key inhibitory receptor in T cells discussed earlier. Surprisingly, many of these polymorphisms are in the regulatory regions of the genes (promoters and enhancers) and not in the coding sequences, suggesting that they influence expression of the genes.

Some rare autoimmune disorders are Mendelian in origin, caused by mutations in single genes that have high penetrance and lead to autoimmunity in most individuals who inherit these mutations, although the pattern of inheritance varies. These genes, alluded to earlier, include *AIRE*, *FOXP3*, *FAS*, and *CTLA4* (see Fig. 9.13B). Mutations in these genes have been valuable for identifying key molecules and pathways involved in self-tolerance. However, these Mendelian forms of autoimmunity are exceedingly rare, and common autoimmune diseases are not caused by mutations in any of these known genes.

Role of Infections and Other Environmental Influences

Infections may activate self-reactive lymphocytes, thereby triggering the development of autoimmune diseases. Clinicians have recognized for many years that the clinical manifestations of autoimmunity sometimes are preceded by infectious prodromes. This association between infections and autoimmune tissue injury has been formally established in animal models.

Infections may contribute to autoimmunity in several ways (Fig. 9.14):
- An infection in a tissue may induce a local innate immune response, which may lead to increased production of costimulators and cytokines by tissue APCs. These activated tissue APCs may be able to stimulate self-reactive T cells that encounter self antigens in the tissue. In other words, infection may break T cell tolerance and promote the activation of self-reactive lymphocytes. This may lead to disease if it occurs in people who are already genetically at risk

A Genes that may contribute to genetically complex autoimmune diseases

Gene(s)	Disease association	Mechanism
PTPN22	RA, several others	Abnormal tyrosine phosphatase regulation of T cell selection and activation?
NOD2	Crohn disease	Defective resistance or abnormal responses to intestinal microbes?
IL23R	IBD, PS, AS	Component of IL-23 receptor; role in generation and maintenance of Th17 cells
CTLA4	T1D, RA	Inhibitory receptor of T cells, effector molecule of regulatory T cells
CD25 (IL-2Rα)	MS, type 1 diabetes, others	Abnormalities in effector and/or regulatory T cells?
C2, C4 (Complement proteins)	SLE	Defects in clearance of immune complexes or in B cell tolerance?
FCGRIIB (FCγRIIb)	SLE	Defective feedback inhibition of B cells

B Single-gene defects that cause autoimmunity (Mendelian diseases)

Gene(s)	Disease association	Mechanism
AIRE	Autoimmune polyendocrine syndrome (APS-1)	Reduced expression of peripheral tissue antigens in the thymus, leading to defective elimination of self-reactive T cells
CTLA4	Autosomal dominant immune dysregulation syndrome	Impaired regulatory T cell function leading to loss of B and T cell homeostasis
FOXP3	Immune dysregulation, X-linked polyendocrinopathy and enteropathy (IPEX)	Deficiency of regulatory T cells
FAS	Autoimmune lymphoproliferative syndrome (ALPS)	Defective apoptosis of self-reactive T and B cells in the periphery

Fig. 9.13 Roles of non–MHC genes in autoimmunity. A, Select examples of variants (polymorphisms) of genes that confer susceptibility to autoimmune diseases but individually have small or no effects. **B,** Examples of genes whose mutations result in autoimmunity. These are rare examples of autoimmune diseases with Mendelian inheritance. The pattern of inheritance varies in the different diseases. APS-1 is autosomal recessive, and in most patients, both alleles of the gene *(AIRE)* have to be abnormal to cause the disease. IPEX is X-linked, so mutation in one allele of the gene *(FOXP3)* is sufficient to cause a defect in boys. ALPS is autosomal dominant with highly variable penetrance, because FAS and FASL are trimeric proteins and mutations in one of the alleles of either gene result in reduced expression of intact trimers. The disease caused by *CTLA4* mutations is also autosomal dominant, perhaps because mutation in one allele reduces the expression of the protein enough to impair its function. *AS,* Ankylosing spondylitis; *IBD,* inflammatory bowel disease; *IL,* interleukin; *MS,* multiple sclerosis; *PS,* psoriasis; *RA,* rheumatoid arthritis; *SLE,* systemic lupus erythematosus; *T1D,* type 1 diabetes.

Fig. 9.14 Mechanisms by which microbes may promote autoimmunity. A, Normally, an encounter of mature T cells with self antigens presented by resting tissue antigen-presenting cells *(APCs)* results in peripheral tolerance. **B,** Microbes may activate the APCs to express costimulators, and when these APCs present self antigens, the specific T cells are activated, rather than being rendered tolerant. **C,** Some microbial antigens may cross-react with self antigens (mimicry). Therefore, immune responses initiated by the microbes may become directed at self cells and self tissues. This figure illustrates concepts as they apply to T cells; molecular mimicry also may apply to self-reactive B lymphocytes.

for developing autoimmunity. One cytokine produced in innate immune responses to viruses is type I interferon (IFN). Excessive production of type I IFN has been associated with the development of several autoimmune diseases, notably lupus. It may activate APCs or lymphocytes, but what stimulates its production and how it contributes to autoimmunity is not well understood.

- Some infectious microbes may produce peptide antigens that are similar to, and cross-react with, self antigens. Immune responses to these microbial peptides may result in an immune attack against self antigens. Such cross-reactions between microbial

and self antigens are termed **molecular mimicry.** Although the contribution of molecular mimicry to autoimmunity has fascinated immunologists, its actual significance in the development of most autoimmune diseases remains unknown. In some disorders, antibodies produced against a microbial protein bind to self proteins. For example, in rheumatic fever, a fairly common disease before the widespread use of antibiotics, antibodies against streptococci cross-react with a myocardial antigen and cause heart disease.

- The innate response to infections may alter the chemical structure of self antigens. For example, some periodontal bacterial infections are associated with rheumatoid arthritis. It is postulated that the inflammatory responses to these bacteria lead to enzymatic conversion of arginines to citrullines in self proteins, and the citrullinated proteins are recognized as nonself and elicit adaptive immune responses.

- Infections also may injure tissues and release antigens that normally are sequestered from the immune system. For example, some sequestered antigens (e.g., in testis and eye) normally are not seen by the immune system and are ignored. Release of these antigens (e.g., by trauma or infection) may initiate an autoimmune reaction against the tissue.
- The abundance and composition of normal commensal microbes in the gut, skin, and other sites (the microbiome) may also influence the health of the immune system and the maintenance of self-tolerance. This possibility has generated a great deal of interest, but normal variations in the microbiome of humans related to

environmental exposure and diet make it difficult to define the relationship between particular microbes and the development of autoimmune diseases.

Paradoxically, some infections appear to confer protection from autoimmune diseases. This conclusion is based on epidemiologic data and limited experimental studies. The basis of this protective effect of infections is unknown.

Several other environmental and host factors may contribute to autoimmunity. Many autoimmune diseases are more common in women than in men, but how gender might affect immunologic tolerance or lymphocyte activation remains unknown. Exposure to sunlight is a trigger for the development of the autoimmune disease SLE, in which autoantibodies are produced against self nucleic acids and self nucleoproteins. It is postulated that these nuclear antigens may be released from cells that die by apoptosis as a consequence of exposure to ultraviolet radiation in sunlight.

SUMMARY

- Immunologic tolerance is specific unresponsiveness to an antigen induced by exposure of lymphocytes to that antigen. All individuals are tolerant of (unresponsive to) their own (self) antigens. Tolerance against antigens may be induced by administering that antigen in particular ways, and this strategy may be useful for treating immunologic diseases and for preventing the rejection of transplants.
- Central tolerance is induced in immature lymphocytes that encounter antigens in the generative lymphoid organs. Peripheral tolerance results from the recognition of antigens by mature lymphocytes in peripheral tissues.
- Central tolerance of T cells is the result of strong recognition of antigens in the thymus due to an abundance of antigen or a high affinity of TCRs. Some of these self-reactive T cells die (negative selection), thus eliminating the potentially most dangerous T cells, which express high-affinity receptors for self antigens. Other T cells of the CD4 lineage develop into regulatory T cells that suppress self-reactivity in the periphery.
- Peripheral tolerance in T cells is induced by multiple mechanisms. Anergy (functional inactivation) results from the recognition of antigens without costimulators (second signals). The mechanisms of

anergy include a block in TCR signaling and engagement of inhibitory receptors such as CTLA-4 and PD-1. Self-reactive regulatory T cells suppress potentially pathogenic T cells. Deletion (death by apoptosis) may occur when T cells encounter self antigens.

- In B lymphocytes, central tolerance occurs when immature cells recognize self antigens in the bone marrow. Some of the cells change their receptors (receptor editing), and others die by apoptosis (negative selection, or deletion). Peripheral tolerance is induced when mature B cells recognize self antigens without T cell help, which results in anergy and death of the B cells, or engagement of inhibitory receptors.
- Autoimmune diseases result from a failure of self-tolerance. Multiple factors contribute to autoimmunity, including the inheritance of susceptibility genes and environmental triggers such as infections.
- Many genes contribute to the development of autoimmunity. The strongest associations are between HLA genes and various T cell–dependent autoimmune diseases.
- Infections predispose to autoimmunity by causing inflammation and stimulating the expression of costimulators or because of cross-reactions between microbial and self antigens.

REVIEW QUESTIONS

1. What is immunologic tolerance? Why is it important?
2. How is central tolerance induced in T lymphocytes and B lymphocytes?
3. Where do regulatory T cells develop, and how do they protect against autoimmunity?
4. How is functional anergy induced in T cells? How may this mechanism of tolerance fail to give rise to autoimmune disorders?
5. What are the mechanisms that prevent immune responses against commensal microbes and fetuses?
6. What are some of the genes that contribute to autoimmunity? How may MHC genes play a role in the development of autoimmune diseases?
7. What are some possible mechanisms by which infections promote the development of autoimmunity?

Answers to and discussion of the Review Questions are available at Student Consult.

10

Immunology of Tumors and Transplantation
Immune Responses to Cancer Cells and Normal Foreign Cells

CHAPTER OUTLINE

Cancer and organ transplantation are two situations in which the immune response to human cells that are genetically distinct from the normal self has important clinical consequences. In order for cancers to grow, they have to evade host immunity, and effective methods of enhancing patients' immune responses against tumors, called cancer immunotherapy, have transformed clinical oncology. In organ transplantation, the situation is the reverse: immune responses against grafted tissues from other people are a major barrier to successful transplantation, and suppressing these responses is a central focus of transplantation medicine. Because of the importance of the immune system in host responses to tumors and transplants, tumor immunology and transplantation immunology have become subspecialties in which researchers and clinicians come together to address both fundamental and clinical questions.

Immune responses against tumors and transplants share several characteristics. These are situations in which the immune system is not responding to microbes, as it usually does, but to noninfectious cells that are perceived as foreign. The antigens that mark tumors and transplants as foreign may be expressed in virtually any cell type that is the target of malignant transformation or is grafted from one individual to another. Therefore, immune responses against tumors and transplants may be directed against diverse cell types. Also, the immune system uses the same major mechanism, the activation of cytotoxic T lymphocytes (CTLs), to kill both tumor cells and the cells of tissue transplants.

In this chapter we focus on the following questions:
- What are the antigens in tumors and tissue transplants that are recognized as foreign by the immune system?
- How does the immune system recognize and react to tumors and transplants?
- How can immune responses to tumors and grafts be manipulated to enhance tumor rejection and inhibit graft rejection?

We discuss tumor immunity first and then transplantation, and we point out the principles common to both.

Evidence	Conclusion
Lymphocytic infiltrates around some tumors and enlargement of draining lymph nodes correlate with better prognosis	Immune responses against tumors inhibit tumor growth
Transplants of tumors between syngeneic animals are rejected, and more rapidly if the animals have been previously exposed to the tumors; immunity to tumor transplants can be transferred by lymphocytes from a tumor bearing animal	Tumor rejection shows features of adaptive immunity (specificity, memory) and is mediated by lymphocytes
Immunodeficient individuals have an increased incidence of some types of tumors	The immune system protects against the growth of tumors
Therapeutic blockade of T cell inhibitory receptors such as PD-1 and CTLA-4 leads to tumor remission	Tumors evade immune surveillance in part by engaging inhibitory receptors on T cells

Fig. 10.1 Evidence supporting the concept that the immune system reacts against tumors. Several lines of clinical and experimental evidence indicate that defense against tumors is mediated by reactions of the adaptive immune system. *CTLA-4*, Cytotoxic T-lymphocyte-associated protein 4; *PD-1*, programmed cell death protein 1.

IMMUNE RESPONSES AGAINST TUMORS

For over a century scientists have proposed that a physiologic function of the adaptive immune system is to prevent the outgrowth of transformed cells and to destroy these cells before they become harmful tumors. Control and elimination of malignant cells by the immune system is called tumor **immune surveillance**. Several lines of evidence support the idea that immune surveillance against tumors is important for preventing tumor growth (Fig. 10.1). However, the fact that common malignant tumors develop in immunocompetent individuals indicates that tumor immunity is often incapable of preventing tumor growth or is easily overwhelmed by rapidly growing tumors. Furthermore, biologists now consider the ability to evade immune destruction as a fundamental feature ("hallmark") of cancers. This has led to the growing realization that the immune response to tumors is often dominated by tolerance or regulation, not by effective immunity. The field of tumor immunology has focused on defining the types of tumor antigens against which the immune system reacts, understanding the nature of the immune responses to tumors and mechanisms by which tumors evade them, and developing strategies for maximally enhancing antitumor immunity.

Tumor Antigens

Malignant tumors express various types of molecules that may be recognized by the immune system as foreign antigens (Fig. 10.2). Protein antigens that elicit CTL responses are the most relevant for protective antitumor immunity. These tumor antigens have to be present in the cytosol of tumor cells in order to be recognized by CD8+ CTLs. The tumor antigens that elicit immune responses can be classified into several groups:

- **Neoantigens encoded by randomly mutated genes.** Recent sequencing of tumor genomes has revealed that common human tumors harbor a large number of mutations in diverse genes, reflecting the genetic instability of malignant cells. These mutations usually play no role in tumorigenesis and are called passenger mutations. Many of these mutations result in expression of mutated proteins, called neoantigens because they are newly expressed in the tumor cells but not in the normal cells of origin of the tumor. Because T cells only recognize peptides bound to major histocompatibility complex (MHC) molecules, mutated tumor proteins can be recognized only if peptides carrying the mutated amino acid sequences can bind to the patients' MHC alleles. Tumor neoantigens may not induce tolerance because

Fig. 10.2 Types of tumor antigens recognized by T cells. Tumor antigens that are recognized by tumor-specific CD8+ T cells may be mutated forms of various self-proteins that do not contribute to malignant behavior of the tumor; products of oncogenes or tumor suppressor genes; self-proteins whose expression is increased in tumor cells; and products of oncogenic viruses. Cancer/testis antigens are proteins that are normally expressed in the testis and are also expressed in some tumors. Tumor antigens also may be recognized by CD4+ T cells, but less is known about the role that CD4+ T cells play in tumor immunity. *EBV*, Epstein-Barr virus.

they are not present in normal cells, and are the most common targets of tumor-specific adaptive immune responses. In fact, the number of these mutations in human cancers correlates with the strength of the antitumor immune responses patients mount and the effectiveness of immunotherapies that enhance those responses. In experimental tumors induced by chemical carcinogens or radiation, the tumor antigens are also mainly random mutants of normal cellular proteins.

- **Products of oncogenes or mutated tumor suppressor genes.** Some tumor antigens are products of mutations, called driver mutations, in genes that are involved in the process of malignant transformation. The driver mutations that encode tumor antigens may be amino acid substitutions, deletions, or new sequences generated by gene translocations, all of which can be seen as foreign.

- **Aberrantly or overexpressed expressed structurally normal proteins.** In several human tumors, antigens that elicit immune responses are normal (unmutated) proteins whose expression is dysregulated in the tumors, sometimes as a consequence of epigenetic changes such as demethylation of the promoters in genes encoding these proteins, and sometimes by gene amplification. These structurally normal self antigens would not be expected to elicit immune responses, but their aberrant expression may be enough to make them immunogenic. For example, self proteins that are expressed only in embryonic tissues may not induce tolerance in adults, and the same proteins expressed in tumors may be recognized as foreign by the immune system.

- **Viral antigens.** In tumors caused by oncogenic viruses, the tumor antigens may be products of the viruses.

Immune Mechanisms of Tumor Rejection

The principal immune mechanism of tumor eradication is killing of tumor cells by CTLs specific for tumor antigens. The majority of tumor neoantigens that elicit immune responses in tumor-bearing individuals are endogenously synthesized cytosolic or nuclear proteins that are processed by proteasomes and displayed as class I MHC–associated peptides. Therefore, these antigens are recognized by class I MHC–restricted CD8+ CTLs, whose function is to kill cells producing the antigens. The role of CTLs in tumor rejection has been established in animal models: tumors can be destroyed by transferring tumor-reactive CD8+ T cells into the tumor-bearing animals. Studies of many human tumors indicate that abundant CTL infiltration predicts a more favorable clinical course compared with tumors with sparse CTLs.

CTL responses against tumors are initiated by recognition of tumor antigens on host antigen-presenting cells (APCs). The APCs ingest tumor cells or their antigens and present the antigens to naive CD8+ T cells in draining lymph nodes (Fig. 10.3). Tumors may arise from virtually any nucleated cell type in any tissue, and, like all nucleated cells, they usually express class I MHC molecules, but often they do not express costimulators or class II MHC molecules. We know, however, that the activation of naive CD8+ T cells to proliferate and differentiate into active CTLs requires recognition of antigen (class I MHC–associated peptide) on dendritic cells in secondary lymphoid organs and also costimulation and/or help from class II MHC–restricted CD4+ T cells (see Chapter 5). How, then, can tumors of different cell types stimulate CTL responses? The likely answer is that tumor cells or their proteins are ingested by the host's dendritic cells, transported to lymph nodes draining the site of the tumor, and the protein antigens of the tumor cells are processed and displayed by class I MHC molecules on the host dendritic cells. This process, called **cross-presentation** or cross-priming, was introduced in Chapter 3 (see Fig. 3.16). Dendritic cells can also present peptides derived from ingested tumor antigens on class II MHC molecules. Thus, tumor antigens may be recognized by CD8+ T cells and by CD4+ T cells.

At the same time that dendritic cells are presenting tumor antigens, they may express costimulators that provide signals for the activation of the T cells. It is not known how tumors induce the expression of costimulators on APCs because, as discussed in Chapter 5, the physiologic stimuli for the induction of costimulators are usually microbes, and tumors are generally sterile. A likely possibility is that tumor cells die if their growth outstrips their blood and nutrient supply, and adjacent normal tissue cells may be injured and die due to the invasive tumor. These dying cells release products (damage-associated molecular patterns; see Chapter 2) that stimulate innate responses. The activation of APCs to express costimulators is part of these responses.

Once naive CD8+ T cells have differentiated into effector CTLs, they are able to migrate back to any site where the tumor is growing, and kill tumor cells expressing the relevant antigens without a requirement for costimulation or T cell help.

Immune mechanisms in addition to CTLs may play a role in tumor rejection. Antitumor CD4+ T cell responses have been detected in patients, and increased numbers of CD4+ effector T cells, especially Th1 cells, in tumor infiltrates are associated with good prognosis. Antitumor

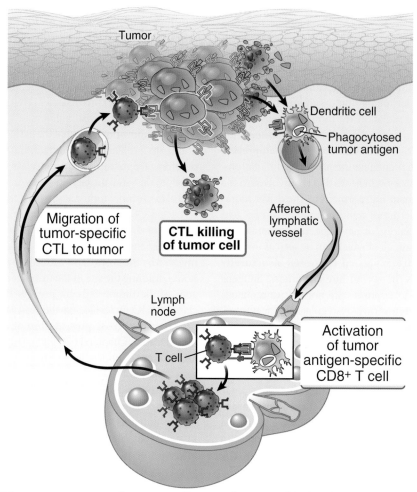

Fig. 10.3 Immune response against tumors. Tumor antigens are picked up by host dendritic cells and responses are initiated in peripheral (secondary) lymphoid organs. Tumor-specific CTLs migrate back to the tumor and kill tumor cells. Other mechanisms of tumor immunity are not shown. *CTL*, Cytotoxic T lymphocyte.

antibodies are also detectable in some cancer patients, but whether these antibodies protect individuals against tumor growth has not been established. Experimental studies have shown that activated macrophages and natural killer (NK) cells are capable of killing tumor cells, and Th1 responses work largely by activating macrophages, but the protective role of these effector mechanisms in tumor-bearing patients is not clearly established.

Evasion of Immune Responses by Tumors

Immune responses often fail to check tumor growth because cancers evade immune recognition or resist immune effector mechanisms. The immune system faces daunting challenges in combating malignant tumors, because immune responses must kill all the tumor cells in order to be effective, and tumors can grow rapidly. Often, the growth of the tumor simply outstrips immune defenses. Not surprisingly, tumor cells that evade the host immune response are selected to survive and grow. Tumors use several mechanisms to avoid destruction by the immune system (Fig. 10.4):

- Some tumors stop expressing class I MHC molecules or molecules involved in antigen processing or MHC assembly, so they cannot display antigens to CD8+ T cells. Mutations affecting class I MHC–associated antigen presentation are likely more effective at immune evasion than loss of tumor neoantigens because any tumor may express many immunogenic antigens, all

Fig. 10.4 How tumors evade immune responses. Antitumor immunity develops when T cells recognize tumor antigens and are activated. Tumor cells may evade immune responses by losing expression of antigens or major histocompatibility complex *(MHC)* molecules or by producing immunosuppressive cytokines or ligands such as PD-L1 for inhibitory receptors on T cells. Tumors may also create an immunosuppressive microenvironment with regulatory T cells and antiinflammatory myeloid cells. *CTL,* Cytotoxic T lymphocyte, *MDSC,* myeloid derived suppressor cell.

of which would have to be mutated or lost, whereas mutation in any component of antigen presentation will lead to failure to present all antigens.

- Tumors engage pathways that inhibit T cell activation. For example, many tumors express PD-L1, a ligand for the T cell inhibitory receptor programmed cell death protein 1 (PD-1). Furthermore, tumors, being persistent, cause repeated stimulation of T cells specific for tumor antigens. The result is that the T cells develop an exhausted state, in which they express high levels of PD-1, cytotoxic T lymphocyte–associated antigen 4 (CTLA-4), and other inhibitory molecules, and become unresponsive to antigen.

- Factors in the tumor microenvironment may impair the ability of dendritic cells to induce strong antitumor immune responses. For example, dendritic cells that capture tumor antigens often express only low levels of B7 costimulators, resulting in preferential engagement of the inhibitory receptor CTLA-4 on naive T cells in the draining lymph nodes, rather than the stimulatory receptor CD28 (see Chapter 9). Some tumors may induce regulatory T cells, which also suppress antitumor immune responses. Myeloid-derived suppressor cells, which are developmentally related to neutrophils and monocytes but have mainly antiinflammatory functions, are abundant in tumors, and are believed to contribute to immunosuppression.

- Some tumors may secrete immunosuppressive cytokines, such as transforming growth factor β.

Cancer Immunotherapy

The main strategies for cancer immunotherapy currently in practice include introduction of antitumor antibodies and autologous T cells that recognize tumor antigens and enhancing patients' own antitumor immune responses with antibodies that block immune checkpoints and vaccination. Until recently, most treatment protocols for disseminated cancers, which cannot be cured surgically, relied on chemotherapy and irradiation, both of which damage normal nontumor tissues and are associated with serious toxicities. Because the immune response is highly specific, it has long been hoped that tumor-specific immunity may be used to selectively eradicate tumors without injuring the patient. Only recently has the promise of cancer immunotherapy been realized in patients. The history of cancer immunotherapy illustrates how the initial, often empirical, approaches have been largely supplanted by rational strategies based on our improved understanding of immune responses (Fig. 10.5).

Passive Immunotherapy With Monoclonal Antibodies

A strategy for tumor immunotherapy which has been in practice for a limited number of tumors for decades relies on the injection of monoclonal antibodies which target cancer cells for immune destruction or inhibition of growth (Fig. 10.6A). Monoclonal antibodies against various tumor antigens have been used in many cancers. The antibodies bind to antigens on the surface of the tumors (not the neoantigens produced inside cells) and activate

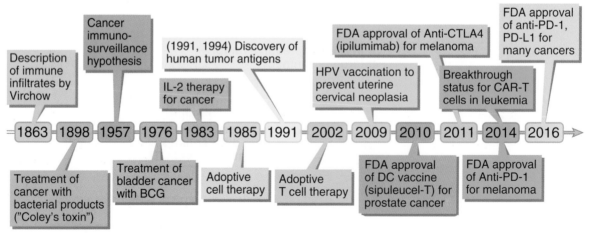

Fig. 10.5 History of cancer immunotherapy. Some of the important discoveries in the field of cancer immunotherapy are summarized. *BCG*, Bacillus Calmette-Guerin; *CAR*, chimeric antigen receptor; *CTLA-4*, cytotoxic T-lymphocyte-associated protein 4; *DC*, dendritic cell; *FDA*, Federal Drug Administration; *HPV*, human papillomavirus; *IL-2*, interleukin-2; *PD-1*, programmed cell death protein 1. (Modified from Lesterhuis WJ, Haanen JB, Punt CJ: Cancer immunotherapy—revisited, *Nature Reviews Drug Discovery* 10:591–600, 2011.)

A Passive immunity by transfer of autologous T cells or monoclonal antibodies

B Adoptive T cell therapy with CAR-T cells

Fig. 10.6 Tumor immunotherapy by adoptive transfer of antibodies and T cells. **A,** Passive immunotherapy with tumor specific T cells or monoclonal antibodies. **B,** Adoptive T cell therapy with CAR-T cells: T cells isolated from the blood of a patient are expanded by culture with anti-CD3 and anti-CD28, genetically modified to express recombinant chimeric antigen receptors *(CARs)* (see Fig. 10-7), and transferred back into the patient.

host effector mechanisms, such as phagocytes, NK cells, or the complement system, that destroy the tumor cells. For example, an antibody specific for CD20, which is expressed on B cells, is used to treat B cell tumors, usually in combination with chemotherapy. Although normal B cells are also depleted, their function can be replaced by administration of pooled immunoglobulin from normal donors. Because CD20 is not expressed by hematopoietic stem cells, normal B cells are replenished after the antibody treatment is stopped. Other monoclonal antibodies that are used in cancer therapy may work by blocking growth factor signaling (e.g., anti-Her2/Neu for breast cancer and anti–EGF-receptor antibody for various tumors) or by inhibiting angiogenesis (e.g., antibody against the vascular endothelial growth factor for colon cancer and other tumors).

Adoptive T Cell Therapy

Tumor immunologists have attempted to enhance antitumor immunity by removing T cells from cancer patients, activating the cells ex vivo so there are more of them

and they are more potent effector cells, and transferring the cells back into the patient. Many variations of this approach, called adoptive T cell therapy, have been tried.

- **Adoptive therapy with autologous tumor-specific T cells.** T cells specific for tumor antigens can be detected in the circulation and among tumor-infiltrating lymphocytes of cancer patients. T cells can be isolated from the blood or tumor biopsies of a patient, expanded by culture with growth factors, and injected back into the same patient (see Fig. 10-6A). Presumably, this expanded T cell population contains activated tumor-specific CTLs, which migrate into the tumor and destroy it. This approach, which has been combined with administration of T cell-stimulating cytokines such as interleukin-2 (IL-2) and traditional chemotherapy, has shown inconsistent results among different patients and tumors. One likely reason is that the frequency of tumor-specific T cells is too low to be effective in these lymphocyte populations.
- **Chimeric antigen receptor (CAR) expressing T cells.** In a more recent modification of adoptive T cell

therapy, blood T cells from cancer patients are transduced with viral vectors that express a chimeric antigen receptor (CAR), which recognizes a tumor antigen and provides potent signals to activate the T cells (see Fig. 10-6B). The CARs currently in use have a single chain antibody-like extracellular portion with both heavy- and light-chain variable domains, which together form the binding site for a tumor antigen (Fig. 10-7). The specificity of the endogenous T cell receptors (TCRs) of the transduced T cells is irrelevant to the effectiveness of this approach. The use of this antibody-based antigen recognition structure avoids the limitations of MHC restriction of TCRs and permits the use of the same CAR in many different patients, regardless of the human leukocyte antigen (HLA) alleles they express. Furthermore, tumors cannot evade CAR-T cells by downregulating MHC expression. In order to work in T cells, the CARs have intracellular signaling domains of both TCR complex proteins, for example the ITAMs of the TCR complex ζ protein, and the signaling domains of costimulatory receptors such as CD28 and CD137. Therefore, upon antigen binding, these receptors provide both antigen recognition (via the extracellular immunoglobulin [Ig] domain) and activating signals (via the introduced cytoplasmic domains). CAR-expressing T cells are expanded ex vivo and transferred back into the patient, where they recognize the antigen on the tumor cells and become activated to kill the cells. CAR-T cell therapy targeting the B cell protein CD19, and more recently CD20, has shown remarkable efficacy in treating and even curing B cell-derived leukemias and lymphomas that are refractory to other therapies. CARs with other specificities for different tumors are in development and clinical trials. The most serious toxicity associated with CAR-T cell therapy is a cytokine release syndrome, mediated by massive amounts of inflammatory cytokines, including IL-6, interferon-γ, and others, that are released because all of the injected T cells recognize and are activated by the patients' tumor cells. These cytokines cause high fever, hypotension, tissue edema, neurologic derangements, and multi-organ failure. The severity of the syndrome can be mitigated by treatment with anticytokine antibodies. CAR-T cell therapy may also be complicated by on-target, off-tumor toxicities, if the CAR-T cells are specific for an antigen present on normal cells as well as tumors. In the case of CD19- or CD20-specific CARs, the therapy results in depletion of normal B

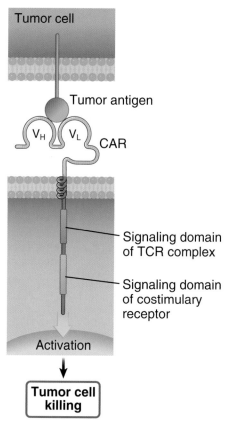

Fig. 10.7 Chimeric antigen receptor. The receptor that is expressed in T cells consists of an extracellular Ig part that recognizes a surface antigen on tumor cells and intracellular signaling domains from the TCR complex and costimulatory receptors that provide the signals that activate the killing function of the T cells.

cells, requiring antibody replacement therapy to prevent immunodeficiency. Such replacement may not be feasible for other tissues that are destroyed because of the reactivity of the CAR. Although CAR-T cell therapy is effective against leukemias and tumors in the blood (to which the injected T cells have ready access), it has so far not been successful in solid tumors because of difficulties in getting T cells into the tumor sites and the challenge of selecting optimal tumor antigens to target without injuring normal tissues.

Immune Checkpoint Blockade

Blocking inhibitory receptors on T cells or their ligands stimulates antitumor immune responses. The realization that tumors evade immune attack by engaging regulatory mechanisms that suppress immune responses has led to a novel and remarkably effective new strategy for

A **Induction of anti-tumor immune response in lymph node**

Tumor peptide-MHC
CD8+ T cell
TCR
Dendritic cell
B7
CTLA-4
CD28

No costimulation

B7
CD28
CTLA-4
Anti-CTLA-4

Costimulation

Primed CTL capable of killing tumor cells

B **CTL-mediated killing of tumor cells**

Tumor peptide-MHC
Inhibited CTL
TCR
Tumor cell
PD-L1
PD-1

T cell inhibition

Activated CTL
PD-L1
PD-1
Anti-PD-L1
Anti-PD-1

No T cell inhibition

Dead tumor cell

Fig. 10.8 Tumor immunotherapy by immune checkpoint blockade. Tumor patients often mount ineffective T cell responses to their tumors because of the upregulation of inhibitory receptors such as CTLA-4 and PD-1 on the tumor specific T cells, and expression of the ligand PD-L1 on the tumor cells. Blocking anti-CTLA4 antibodies (**A**) or anti-PD-1 or anti-PD-L1 antibodies (**B**) are highly effective in treating several types of advanced tumors by releasing the inhibition of tumor-specific T cells by these molecules. Anti-CTLA-4 may work by blocking CTLA-4 on responding T cells (shown) or on Treg. *CTL*, Cytotoxic T lymphocyte; *CTLA-4*, cytotoxic T lymphocyte-associated antigen 4; *MHC*, major histocompatibility complex; *PD-1*, programmed cell death protein 1; *TCR*, T cell receptors.

tumor immunotherapy. The principle of this strategy is to boost host immune responses against tumors by blocking normal inhibitory signals for T cells, thus removing the brakes (checkpoints) on the immune response (Fig. 10.8). This has been accomplished with blocking monoclonal antibodies specific for the T cell inhibitory molecules CTLA-4 and PD-1, first approved for treating metastatic melanoma in 2011 and 2014, respectively. Since then, the use of anti-PD-1 or anti-PD-L1 antibodies has expanded to many different cancer types. The most remarkable feature of these therapies is that they have dramatically improved the chances of survival of patients with advanced, widely metastatic tumors, which previously were almost 100% lethal within months to a few years.

The efficacy of antibodies specific for other T cell inhibitory molecules, such as LAG-3 and TIM-3, are being tested in clinical trials. There are several novel features of immune checkpoint blockade and limitations that still need to be overcome to enhance their usefulness.

- Although the efficacy of checkpoint blockade therapies for many advanced tumors is superior to any previous form of therapy, only a subset of patients (25% to 40% at most) respond to this treatment. The reasons for this poor response are not well understood. Nonresponding tumors may induce T cell expression of checkpoint molecules other than the ones being targeted therapeutically, or they may rely on evasion mechanisms other than engaging these inhibitory receptors. Oncologists and immunologists are currently investigating which biomarkers will predict responsiveness to different checkpoint blockade approaches.

- One of the most reliable indictors that a tumor will respond to checkpoint blockade therapy is if it carries a high number of mutations, which correlates with high numbers of neoantigens and host T cells that can respond to those antigens. In fact, tumors that have deficiencies in mismatch repair enzymes, which normally correct errors in DNA replication that lead to point mutations, have the highest mutation burdens of all cancers, and these cancers are the most likely to respond to checkpoint blockade therapy. Remarkably, anti-PD-1 therapy is now approved for any recurrent or metastatic tumor with mismatch repair deficiencies, regardless of the cell of origin or histologic type of tumor. This is a paradigm shift in how cancer treatments are chosen.

- The combined use of different checkpoint inhibitors, or one inhibitor with other modes of therapy, will likely be necessary to achieve higher rates of therapeutic success. The first approved example of this is the combined use of anti-CTLA-4 and anti-PD-1 to treat melanomas, which was shown to be more effective than anti-CTL-4 alone. This reflects the fact that the mechanisms by which CTLA-4 and PD-1 inhibit T cell activation are different (see Fig. 10.8). There are numerous ongoing or planned clinical trials using combinations of checkpoint blockade together with other strategies, such as small molecule kinase inhibitors, oncolytic viral infection of tumors, and other immune stimulants.

- The most common toxicities associated with checkpoint blockade are autoimmune damage to organs. This is predictable, because the physiologic function of the inhibitory receptors targeted is to maintain tolerance to self antigens (see Chapter 9). A wide range of organs may be affected, including colon, lungs, endocrine organs, heart, and skin, each requiring different clinical interventions, sometimes including cessation of the life-saving tumor immunotherapy.

Stimulation of Host Antitumor Immune Responses by Vaccination With Tumor Antigens

One way of stimulating active immunity against tumors is to vaccinate patients with their own tumor cells or with antigens from these cells. Unlike standard antimicrobial vaccines, which are prophylactic in that they prevent infections, tumor vaccines are meant to be therapeutic, in that they stimulate immune responses to attack cancers that have already developed. An important reason for defining tumor antigens is to produce and use these antigens to vaccinate individuals against their own tumors. Most tumor vaccines tried to date have used antigens that are shared by the same type of cancers in different patients. These antigens are usually differentiation antigens that identify cells of a particular lineage, both normal and neoplastic. Vaccines incorporating such antigens have had little success, perhaps because the antigens are expressed at some level in normal cells and tend to induce tolerance that has to be overcome for induction of effective antitumor immunity.

More recently, there has been interest in developing personalized cancer vaccines tailored for each patient's tumor. As we discussed earlier, the most common antigens that induce immune responses in cancer patients are neoantigens generated by passenger mutations affecting random cellular proteins, and the mutations must be within peptides that can bind to the patient's HLA molecules in order to recognized by T cells. A current focus of the tumor vaccination field is to use DNA sequencing technologies to determine all the mutations in the protein-coding DNA sequences (exosomes) of an individual's cancer cell genome. HLA-binding prediction algorithms are then applied to identify mutant peptides that are most likely to bind to the HLA alleles of the patient. After these peptides are defined, personalized tumor vaccines are created using several of the neoantigen peptides. This approach is promising, but it also has significant challenges. The vaccines have to be customized for each patient; effective CTLs have to be generated by the vaccination (which has been difficult to do so far with most vaccines, which work by stimulating production of antibodies); tumors may evolve under the selection pressure of the vaccine-induced immune response and lose MHC molecules or the target antigens; and because these are therapeutic vaccines given to tumor-bearing patients, they have to overcome the immune evasion mechanisms that tumors may have established in the patient.

Tumor-specific vaccines may be administered as a mixture of the antigen with adjuvants, just like antimicrobial vaccines. In another approach, a tumor patient's dendritic cells are expanded in vitro from blood precursors, the dendritic cells are exposed to tumor cells or tumor antigens, and these tumor-antigen–pulsed dendritic cells are used as vaccines. The dendritic cells bearing tumor antigens will theoretically mimic the normal

Evidence	Conclusion
Prior exposure to donor MHC molecules leads to accelerated graft rejection	Graft rejection shows memory and specificity, two cardinal features of adaptive immunity
The ability to reject a graft rapidly can be transferred to a naive individual by lymphocytes from a sensitized individual	Graft rejection is mediated by lymphocytes
Depletion or inactivation of T lymphocytes by drugs or antibodies results in reduced graft rejection	Graft rejection requires T lymphocytes

Fig. 10.9 Evidence indicating that the rejection of tissue transplants is an immune reaction. Clinical and experimental evidence indicates that rejection of grafts is a reaction of the adaptive immune system. *MHC*, Major histocompatibility complex.

pathway of cross-presentation and will generate CTLs against the tumor cells. The success of checkpoint blockade therapies, described previously, has raised hopes that vaccination used in combination with therapies to block immune regulation will have added benefits.

Tumors caused by oncogenic viruses can be prevented by vaccinating against these viruses. Two such vaccines that are proving to be remarkably effective are against hepatitis B virus (the cause of a form of liver cancer) and human papillomavirus (the cause of cervical cancer and some types of oropharyngeal cancer). These are prophylactic vaccines given to individuals before they are infected, and thus prevent infections by the tumor-causing viruses.

IMMUNE RESPONSES AGAINST TRANSPLANTS

Some of the earliest attempts to replace damaged tissues by transplantation were during World War II as a way of treating pilots who had received severe skin burns in airplane crashes. It was soon realized that individuals reject tissue grafts from other individuals. Rejection results from inflammatory reactions that damage the transplanted tissues. Studies since the 1940s and 1950s established that graft rejection is mediated by the adaptive immune system because it shows specificity and memory and it is dependent on lymphocytes (Fig. 10.9). Much of the knowledge about the immunology of transplantation came from experiments with inbred strains of rodents, particularly mice. All members of an inbred strain are genetically identical to one another and

different from the members of other strains. The experimental studies showed that grafts among members of one inbred strain are accepted and grafts from one strain to another are rejected, firmly establishing rejection as a process controlled by the animals' genes. Later experiments defined the nature of the genes that control graft rejection and showed that the products of many of these genes are expressed in all tissues.

As mentioned in Chapter 3, the genes that contributed the most to the rejection of grafts exchanged between mice of different inbred strains are called **major histocompatibility complex (MHC)** genes. The language of transplantation immunology evolved from the experimental studies. The individual who provides the graft is called the **donor**, and the individual in whom the graft is placed is the **recipient** or **host**. Animals that are identical to one another (and grafts exchanged among these animals) are said to be **syngeneic**; animals (and grafts) of one species that differ from other animals of the same species are said to be **allogeneic**; and animals (and grafts) of different species are **xenogeneic**. Allogeneic and xenogeneic grafts, also called **allografts** and **xenografts**, are always rejected by a recipient with a normal immune system. The antigens that serve as the targets of rejection are called alloantigens and xenoantigens, and the antibodies and T cells that react to these antigens are alloreactive and xenoreactive, respectively. In the clinical situation, transplants are exchanged between allogeneic individuals who are members of an outbred species who differ from one another (except for identical twins). Most of the following discussion focuses on immune responses to allografts.

Transplantation Antigens

The antigens of allografts that serve as the principal targets of rejection are proteins encoded in the MHC. Homologous MHC genes and molecules are present in all mammals; the human MHC is called the **human leukocyte antigen (HLA)** complex. It took more than 20 years after the discovery of the MHC to show that the physiologic function of MHC molecules is to display peptide antigens for recognition by T lymphocytes (see Chapter 3). Recall that every person expresses six class I HLA alleles (one allele of HLA-A, -B, and -C from each parent) and usually six or seven class II HLA alleles (one allele of HLA-DQ and HLA-DP and one or two of HLA-DR from each parent). MHC genes are highly polymorphic, with over 12,000 HLA alleles among all humans, encoding about 2800 HLA-A proteins, 3500 HLA-B proteins, 2500 HLA-C proteins, 1800 HLA-DRβ proteins, 800 DQβ proteins, and 700 DPβ proteins. Because of this tremendous polymorphism, two unrelated individuals are very likely to express several HLA proteins that are different from, and therefore appear foreign to, each other. Because the genes in the HLA locus are tightly linked, all the HLA genes from each parent are inherited together, as a haplotype, in a Mendelian pattern, and therefore the chance that two siblings will have the same MHC alleles is 1 in 4.

The reaction to allogeneic MHC antigens on another individual's cells is one of the strongest immune responses known. T cell receptors (TCRs) for antigens have evolved to recognize MHC molecules, which is essential for surveillance of cells harboring infectious microbes. As a result of positive selection of developing T cells in the thymus, mature T cells that have some affinity for self MHC molecules survive, and many of these will have high affinity for self MHC displaying foreign peptides. Allogeneic MHC molecules containing peptides derived from the allogeneic cells may look like self MHC molecules plus bound foreign peptides (Fig. 10.10). Therefore, recognition of allogeneic MHC molecules in allografts is an example of an immunologic cross-reaction.

There are several reasons why recognition of allogeneic MHC molecules results in strong T cell reactions. Many clones of T cells, including memory T cells generated from prior infections, that are specific for different foreign peptides bound to the same self MHC molecule may cross-react with any one allogeneic MHC molecule, regardless of the bound peptide, as long as the allogeneic MHC molecule resembles complexes of self MHC plus foreign peptides. As a result, many self MHC–restricted T cells specific for different peptide antigens may recognize any one allogeneic MHC molecule. Also, the process of negative selection in the thymus eliminates cells that strongly recognize self MHC, but there is no mechanism for selectively eliminating T cells whose TCRs have a high affinity for allogeneic MHC molecules because these are never present in the thymus. Furthermore, a single allogeneic graft cell will express thousands of MHC molecules, every one of which may be recognized as foreign by a graft recipient's T cells. By contrast, in the case of an infected cell, only a small fraction of the self MHC molecules on the cell surface will carry a foreign microbial peptide recognized by the host's T cells. The net result of these features of allorecognition is that the frequency of alloreactive T cells in any individual is about 1000-fold greater than the frequency of T cells that recognize any one microbial antigen.

Although MHC proteins are the major antigens that stimulate graft rejection, other polymorphic proteins also may play a role in rejection. Non-MHC antigens that induce graft rejection are called minor histocompatibility antigens, and most are normal cellular proteins that differ in sequence between donor and recipient. These polymorphic proteins yield peptides that are presented by the recipient's MHC molecules and trigger a T cell response. The rejection reactions that minor histocompatibility antigens elicit usually are not as strong as reactions against foreign MHC proteins.

Induction of Immune Responses Against Transplants

In order to elicit antigraft immune responses, alloantigens from the graft are transported by dendritic cells to draining lymph nodes, where they are recognized by alloreactive T cells (Fig. 10.11). The dendritic cells that present alloantigens also provide costimulators and can stimulate helper T cells as well as alloreactive CTLs. The effector T cells that are generated circulate back to the transplant and mediate rejection.

T cells in allograft recipients may recognize unprocessed donor MHC molecules on the surface of graft cells, or they may recognize peptides derived from donor MHC molecules bound to recipient MHC molecules on the surface of recipient APCs (Fig. 10.12). These two pathways of presentation of graft antigens have different features and names.

(A) Normal

T cell receptor

Foreign peptide

Self MHC

> **Self MHC molecule presents foreign peptide to T cell selected to recognize self MHC weakly, but may recognize self MHC-foreign peptide complexes well**

(B) Allorecognition

Self peptide

Allogeneic MHC

> **The self MHC-restricted T cell recognizes the allogeneic MHC molecule whose structure resembles a self MHC-foreign peptide complex**

(C) Allorecognition

Self peptide

Allogeneic MHC

> **The self MHC-restricted T cell recognizes a structure formed by both the allogeneic MHC molecule and the bound peptide**

Fig. 10.10 Recognition of allogeneic major histocompatibility complex (MHC) molecules by T lymphocytes. Recognition of allogeneic MHC molecules may be thought of as a cross-reaction in which a T cell specific for a self MHC molecule–foreign peptide complex (A) also recognizes an allogeneic MHC molecule whose structure resembles that of the self MHC molecule–foreign peptide complex (B and C). Peptides derived from the graft or recipient (labeled self peptide) may not contribute to allorecognition (B), or they may form part of the complex that the T cell recognizes (C). The type of T cell recognition depicted in B and C is direct allorecognition.

Fig. 10.11 Immune response against transplants. Graft antigens that are expressed on donor dendritic cells or captured by recipient dendritic cells are transported to peripheral lymphoid organs where alloantigen-specific T cells are activated (the sensitization step). The T cells migrate back into the graft and destroy graft cells (rejection). Antibodies are also produced against graft antigens and can contribute to rejection (not shown). The example shown is that of a kidney graft, but the same general principles apply to all organ grafts.

- **Direct allorecognition**. Most tissues contain dendritic cells, and when the tissues are transplanted, the dendritic cells in the graft may migrate to secondary lymphoid organs of the recipient. When naïve T cells in the recipient recognize donor allogeneic MHC molecules on these graft-derived dendritic cells, the T cells are activated; this process is called **direct recognition** (or direct presentation) of alloantigens. Direct recognition stimulates the development of alloreactive T cells (e.g., CTLs) that can then directly recognize the allogeneic MHC molecules on cells of the graft and destroy the graft.
- **Indirect allorecognition**. Graft cells (or alloantigens) may be ingested by recipient dendritic cells and transported to draining lymph nodes. Here, donor alloantigens are processed and presented by self MHC molecules on the recipient APCs. This process is called **indirect recognition** (or indirect presentation) and is similar to the cross-presentation of tumor antigens to CD8+ T cells, discussed earlier. If alloreactive CTLs are induced by the indirect pathway, these CTLs are specific for donor alloantigens displayed by the recipient's self MHC molecules on the recipient's APCs, so they cannot recognize and kill cells in the graft (which, of course, express donor MHC molecules). When graft alloantigens are recognized by the indirect pathway, the subsequent rejection of the graft likely is mediated mainly by alloreactive CD4+ T cells. These T cells may enter the graft together with host APCs, recognize graft antigens that are picked up and displayed by those APCs, and secrete cytokines that injure the graft by an inflammatory reaction. Indirect allorecognition by host CD4+ T cells also contributes to stimulating production of host antibodies that bind to graft MHC molecules, as discussed later.

A Direct allorecognition

Allogeneic MHC

Allogeneic antigen-presenting cell (dendritic cell)

Alloreactive T cell

> **T cell recognizes unprocessed allogeneic MHC molecule on graft APCs**

B Indirect allorecognition

Allogeneic MHC

Dendritic cell in recipient

Alloreactive T cell

Self MHC

Uptake and processing of allogeneic MHC molecules by recipient APC

Peptide derived from allogeneic MHC molecule

Allogeneic tissue cell

> **T cell recognizes processed peptide of allogeneic MHC molecule bound to self MHC molecule on host APC**

Fig. 10.12 Direct and indirect recognition of alloantigens. A, Direct alloantigen recognition occurs when T cells bind directly to intact allogeneic major histocompatibility complex *(MHC)* molecules on antigen-presenting cells *(APCs)* in a graft, as illustrated in Fig. 10.8. **B,** Indirect alloantigen recognition occurs when allogeneic MHC molecules from graft cells are taken up and processed by recipient APCs, and peptide fragments of the allogeneic MHC molecules are presented by recipient (self) MHC molecules. Recipient APCs also may process and present graft proteins other than allogeneic MHC molecules.

We do not know the relative importance of the direct and indirect pathways of allorecognition in T cell–mediated rejection of allografts. The direct pathway may be most important for CTL-mediated acute rejection, and the indirect pathway may play a greater role in chronic rejection, as described later.

T cell responses to allografts require costimulation, but which stimuli in grafts enhance the expression of costimulators on APCs is unclear. As with tumors, graft cells may undergo necrosis, perhaps in the period of ischemia before the transplant is done, and substances released from the injured and dead cells activate APCs by innate immune mechanisms. As we discuss later, blocking costimulation is one therapeutic strategy for promoting graft survival.

The **mixed lymphocyte reaction** (MLR) is an in vitro model of T cell recognition of alloantigens. In this model, T cells from one individual are cultured with leukocytes of another individual, and the responses of the T cells are assayed. The magnitude of this response is proportional to the extent of the MHC differences between these individuals and is a rough predictor of the outcomes of grafts exchanged between these individuals.

Although much of the emphasis on allograft rejection has been on the role of T cells, it is clear that alloantibodies also contribute to rejection. Most of these antibodies are helper T cell–dependent high-affinity antibodies. In order to produce alloantibodies, recipient B cells recognize donor alloantigens and then process and present peptides derived from these antigens to helper T cells (that may have been previously activated by recipient dendritic cells presenting the same donor alloantigen), thus initiating the process of antibody production. This is a good example of indirect presentation of alloantigens, in this case by B lymphocytes.

Immune Mechanisms of Graft Rejection

Graft rejection is classified into hyperacute, acute, and chronic, on the basis of clinical and pathologic features (Fig. 10.13). This historical classification was devised by clinicians based on rejection of kidney allografts, and it has stood the test of time remarkably well. It also has become apparent that each type of rejection is mediated by a particular type of immune response.

- **Hyperacute rejection** occurs within minutes of transplantation and is characterized by thrombosis of graft vessels and ischemic necrosis of the graft. Hyperacute rejection is mediated by circulating antibodies that are specific for antigens on graft endothelial cells and that are present before transplantation. These preformed antibodies may be natural IgM antibodies specific for blood group antigens (discussed later in this chapter), or they may be antibodies specific for allogeneic MHC molecules that were induced by previous exposure to allogeneic cells due to blood transfusions, pregnancy, or prior organ transplantation. Almost immediately after transplantation, the antibodies bind to antigens on the graft vascular endothelium and activate the complement and clotting systems, leading to injury to the endothelium and thrombus formation. Hyperacute rejection is not a common problem in clinical transplantation, because every donor and recipient are matched for blood type and potential recipients are tested for antibodies against the cells of the prospective donor. (The test for antibodies is called a cross-match.) However, hyperacute rejection is a major barrier to xenotransplantation, as discussed later.

- **Acute rejection** occurs within days or weeks after transplantation and is the principal cause of early graft failure. Acute rejection is mediated by T cells and antibodies specific for alloantigens in the graft. The T cells may be CD8+ CTLs that directly destroy graft cells or CD4+ cells that secrete cytokines and induce inflammation, which destroys the graft. T cells may also react against cells in graft vessels, leading to vascular damage. Antibodies contribute especially to the vascular component of acute rejection. Antibody-mediated injury to graft vessels is caused mainly by complement activation by the classical pathway. Current immunosuppressive therapy is designed to prevent and reduce acute rejection by blocking the activation of alloreactive T cells.

- **Chronic rejection** is an indolent form of graft damage that occurs over months or years, leading to progressive loss of graft function. Chronic rejection may be manifested as fibrosis of the graft and by gradual narrowing of graft blood vessels, called graft arteriosclerosis. In both lesions, the culprits are believed to be T cells that react against graft alloantigens and secrete cytokines, which stimulate the proliferation and activities of fibroblasts and vascular smooth muscle cells in the graft. Alloantibodies may also contribute to chronic rejection. Although treatments to prevent or curtail acute rejection have steadily improved, leading to better 1-year survival of transplants, chronic rejection is refractory to most of these therapies and is becoming the principal cause of graft failure.

Prevention and Treatment of Graft Rejection

The mainstay of preventing and treating the rejection of organ transplants is immunosuppression, using drugs that deplete T cells or inhibit T cell activation and effector functions (Fig. 10.14). The development of immunosuppressive drugs launched the modern era of organ transplantation because these drugs made it feasible to transplant organs from donors that were not HLA-matched with recipients, especially in situations when such matching was impractical, such as transplantation of heart, lung, and liver.

One of the first and still most useful classes of immunosuppressive drugs used in clinical transplantation are the calcineurin inhibitors, including cyclosporine and tacrolimus (FK506), which function by blocking the protein phosphatase calcineurin. This enzyme is required to activate the transcription factor NFAT (nuclear factor of activated T cells), and blocking its activity inhibits the transcription of cytokine genes in the T cells. Another widely used drug is rapamycin, which inhibits a kinase called mTOR (mammalian target of rapamycin) required for T cell activation. Many other immunosuppressive agents are now used as adjuncts to or instead of calcineurin and mTOR inhibitors (see Fig. 10.14).

All of these immunosuppressive drugs carry the problem of nonspecific immunosuppression (i.e., the drugs inhibit responses to more than the graft). Therefore, patients receiving these drugs as part of their post-transplantation treatment regimen become susceptible to infections, particularly by intracellular microbes, and the patients have an increased risk of developing cancers, especially skin cancers and others caused by oncogenic viruses.

The matching of donor and recipient HLA alleles by tissue typing had an important role in minimizing graft rejection before cyclosporine became available for clinical use. Although MHC matching is critical for the success of transplantation of some types of tissues (e.g., hematopoietic stem cell transplants) and improves survival of other types of organ grafts (e.g., renal allografts), modern immunosuppression is so effective that HLA matching is not considered necessary for many types of organ transplants (e.g., heart and liver), mainly because the number of donors is limited and the recipients often are too sick to wait for well-matched organs to become available.

The long-term goal of transplant immunologists is to induce immunological tolerance specifically for the graft alloantigens. If this is achieved, it will allow graft acceptance without shutting off other immune responses in the host. However, many years of experimental and

A Hyperacute rejection

Endothelial cell

Blood vessel

Complement activation, endothelial damage, inflammation and thrombosis

Circulating alloantigen-specific antibody

Alloantigen (e.g., blood group antigen)

B Acute rejection

Alloantigen-specific CD8+ T cell

Parenchymal cell damage, interstitial inflammation

Parenchymal cells

Alloreactive antibody

Endothelialitis

Endothelial cell

C Chronic rejection

Macrophage

Cytokines

APC

Chronic inflammatory reaction in vessel wall, intimal smooth muscle cell proliferation, vessel occlusion

Cytokines

Alloantigen-specific CD4+ T cell

Vascular smooth muscle cell

Fig. 10.13 Mechanisms and histopathology of graft rejection. A representative histologic appearance of each type of rejection is shown on the right. **A,** In hyperacute rejection, preformed antibodies react with alloantigens on the vascular endothelium of the graft, activate complement, and trigger rapid intravascular thrombosis and necrosis of the vessel wall. **B,** In acute rejection, CD8+ T lymphocytes reactive with alloantigens on graft endothelial cells and parenchymal cells or antibodies reactive with endothelial cells cause damage to these cell types. Inflammation of the endothelium is called endothelialitis. The histology shows acute cellular rejection in *i* and humoral (antibody-mediated) rejection in *ii*. **C,** In chronic rejection with graft arteriosclerosis, T cells reactive with graft alloantigens may produce cytokines that induce inflammation and proliferation of intimal smooth muscle cells, leading to luminal occlusion. *APC*, Antigen-presenting cells.

Drug	Mechanism of action
Cyclosporine and tacrolimus	Blocks T cell cytokine production by inhibiting the phosphatase calcineurin and thus blocking activation of the NFAT transcription factor
Mycophenolate mofetil	Blocks lymphocyte proliferation by inhibiting guanine nucleotide synthesis in lymphocytes
Rapamycin (sirolimus)	Blocks lymphocyte proliferation by inhibiting mTOR and IL-2 signaling
Corticosteroids	Reduce inflammation by effects on multiple cell types
Antithymocyte globulin	Binds to and depletes T cells by promoting phagocytosis or complement-mediated lysis (used to treat acute rejection)
Anti-IL-2 receptor (CD25) antibody	Inhibits T cell proliferation by blocking IL-2 binding; may also opsonize and help eliminate activated IL-2R-expressing T cells
CTLA4-Ig (belatacept)	Inhibits T cell activation by blocking B7 costimulator binding to T cell CD28
Anti-CD52 (alemtuzumab)	Depletes lymphocytes by complement-mediated lysis

Fig. 10.14 Treatments for graft rejection. Agents used to treat rejection of organ grafts and their mechanisms of action. Like cyclosporine, tacrolimus (FK506) is a calcineurin inhibitor. *CTLA4-Ig*, Cytotoxic T lymphocyte–associated protein 4–immunoglobulin (fusion protein), not widely used; *IL*, interleukin; *mTOR*, mammalian target of rapamycin; *NFAT*, nuclear factor of activated T cells.

clinical attempts to induce graft-specific tolerance have not yet resulted in clinically practical methods.

A major problem in transplantation is the shortage of suitable donor organs. **Xenotransplantation** has been considered a possible solution for this problem. Experimental studies show that hyperacute rejection is a frequent cause of xenotransplant loss. The reasons for the high incidence of hyperacute rejection of xenografts are that individuals often contain antibodies that cross-react

with cells from other species and the xenograft cells lack regulatory proteins that can inhibit human complement activation. These antibodies, similar to antibodies against blood group antigens, are called natural antibodies because their production does not require prior exposure to the xenoantigens. It is thought that these antibodies are produced against bacteria that normally inhabit the gut and that the antibodies cross-react with cells of other species. Xenografts also are subject to acute rejection, much like allografts but often even more severe than rejection of allografts. Because of the problem of rejection, and difficulty in procuring organs from animals that are evolutionarily close to humans, clinical xenotransplantation remains a distant goal.

Transplantation of Blood Cells and Hematopoietic Stem Cells

Transfer of blood cells between humans, called transfusion, is the oldest form of transplantation in clinical medicine. The major barrier to transfusion is the presence of allogeneic blood group antigens, the prototypes of which are the ABO antigens (Fig. 10.15). These antigens are expressed on red blood cells, endothelial cells, and many other cell types. ABO antigens are carbohydrates on membrane glycoproteins or glycosphingolipids; they contain a core glycan that may be enzymatically modified by addition of either of two types of terminal sugar residues. There are three alleles of the gene encoding the enzyme that adds these sugars: one encodes an enzyme that adds N-acetylgalactosamine, one that adds galactose, and one that is inactive and cannot add either. Therefore, depending on the alleles inherited, an individual may be one of four different ABO blood groups: Blood group A individuals have N-acetylgalactosamine added to the core glycan; blood group B individuals have a terminal galactose; blood group AB individuals express both terminal sugars on different glycolipid or glycoprotein molecules; and individuals with blood group O express the core glycan without either of the terminal sugars.

Individuals are tolerant of the blood group antigens they express, but make antibodies specific for the antigens they do not express. Thus, type A individuals make anti-B antibodies, type B individuals make anti-A antibodies, O group individuals make both anti-A and anti-B, and type AB individuals do not make anti-A or anti-B antibodies. These antibodies are called natural antibodies because they are made in the absence of the antigen. They are likely produced by B cells in response to antigens of intestinal microbes, and the antibodies cross-react with ABO blood group antigens. Because the blood group antigens are sugars, they do not elicit T cell responses that drive isotype switching, and the antibodies specific for A or B antigens are largely IgM. The preformed antibodies react against transfused blood cells expressing the target antigens and activate complement, which lyses the red cells; the result may be a severe **transfusion reaction**, characterized by a strong systemic inflammatory response, intravascular thrombosis, and kidney damage. This problem is avoided by matching blood donors and recipients so there are no antigens on the donor cells that can be recognized by preformed antibodies in the recipient, a standard practice in medicine.

Blood group antigens other than the ABO antigens also are involved in transfusion reactions, and these usually are less severe. One important example is the RhD antigen, which is a red cell membrane protein expressed by about 90% of people. Pregnant women who are RhD-negative can be immunized by exposure to RhD-expressing red cells from the baby during childbirth if the baby inherited the RhD gene from the father. The mother will produce anti-RhD antibodies that can cross the placenta during subsequent pregnancies and attack Rh-positive fetal cells, causing hemolytic disease of the fetus and newborn.

Hematopoietic stem cell transplantation is being used increasingly to correct hematopoietic defects, to restore bone marrow cells damaged by irradiation and chemotherapy for cancer, and to treat leukemias. Either bone marrow cells or, more often, hematopoietic stem cells mobilized in a donor's blood are injected into the circulation of a recipient, and the cells home to the marrow. The transplantation of hematopoietic stem cells poses many special problems. Before transplantation, some of the bone marrow of the recipient has to be destroyed to create space to receive the transplanted stem cells, and this depletion of the recipient's marrow inevitably causes deficiency of blood cells, including immune cells, resulting in potentially serious immune deficiencies before the transplanted stem cells generate enough replacement blood cells. The immune system reacts strongly against allogeneic hematopoietic stem cells, so successful transplantation requires careful HLA matching of donor and recipient. HLA matching also prevents rejection of transplanted stem cells by NK cells, which are inhibited by recognition of self MHC molecules (see Chapter 2). If mature allogeneic T cells are transplanted with the stem cells, these mature T cells can attack the recipient's tissues, resulting in a clinical reaction called **graft-versus-host disease**. When the donor is an HLA-identical sibling (as in about 80% of cases), this reaction is directed against minor histocompatibility antigens. The same reaction is exploited to kill leukemia cells (so-called graft-versus-leukemia effect), and hematopoietic stem cell transplantation is now commonly used to treat leukemias resistant to chemotherapy. NK cells in the marrow inoculum may also contribute to the destruction of leukemia cells.

Despite these problems, hematopoietic stem cell transplantation is a successful therapy for a wide variety of diseases affecting the hematopoietic and lymphoid systems.

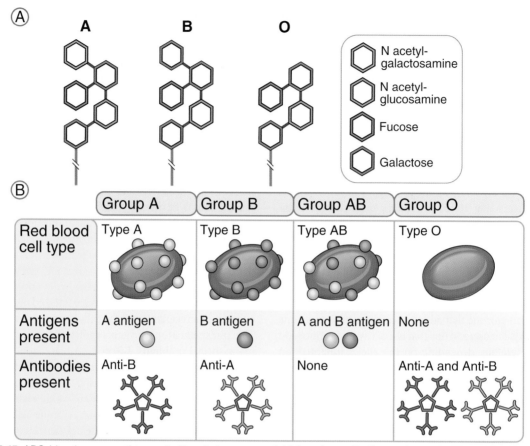

Fig. 10.15 ABO blood group antigens. **A,** Chemical structure of ABO antigens. **B,** Figure shows the antigens and antibodies present in people with the major ABO blood groups.

SUMMARY

- The adaptive immune system is able to eradicate or prevent the growth of tumors.
- Tumors may induce antibody, CD4⁺ T cell, and CD8⁺ T cell responses, but CD8⁺ CTL killing of tumor cells appears to be the most important antitumor effector mechanism.
- Most cancer antigens that induce T cell responses are neoantigens encoded by randomly mutated genes (passenger mutations), which do not contribute to the malignant phenotype of the cancer cells. Other tumor antigens include products of oncogenes and tumor suppressor genes, overexpressed or aberrantly expressed structurally normal molecules, and products of oncogenic viruses.
- CTLs recognize mutant peptides derived from tumor antigens displayed by class I MHC molecules. The

induction of CTL responses against tumor antigens involves ingestion of tumor cells or their antigens by dendritic cells, cross-presentation of the antigens to naïve CD8⁺ T cells, activation of the T cells and differentiation into CTLs, CTL migration from the blood into tumors, CTL recognition of the tumor antigens on the tumor cells, and killing of the tumor cells.
- Tumors may evade immune responses by losing expression of their antigens, shutting off expression of MHC molecules or molecules involved in antigen processing, expressing ligands for T cell inhibitory receptors, and inducing regulatory T cells or secreting cytokines that suppress immune responses.

- CAR-T cell immunotherapy is another breakthrough approach now in clinical practice. CAR-T cells are generated in vitro by transducing a cancer patient's T cells to express a recombinant receptor with an antibody-like binding site for a tumor antigen and a cytoplasmic tail with potent signaling functions. Adoptive transfer of CAR-T cells back into patients has been successful in treating B-cell–derived leukemias and lymphomas.

- Immune checkpoint blockade is the major cancer immunotherapy strategy in current practice. Monoclonal antibodies that block the function of T cell inhibitory molecules, such as CTLA-4 and PD-1, are injected into the patient, which enhances the activation of tumor-specific T cells by tumor antigens. This approach has been highly successful in treating patients with many kinds of advanced cancers, but more than 50% of patients do not respond, and many patients develop autoimmune side effects.

- Personalized neoantigen vaccines are now in clinical trials. The creation of these vaccines relies on cancer genome sequencing to identify neoantigen peptides unique to an individual patient's tumor, which bind to that patient's MHC molecules.

- Organ and tissue transplantation from one individual to another is widely used to treat many diseases, but a major barrier to successful transplantation of foreign tissues is rejection by adaptive immune responses, including CD8$^+$ CTLs, CD4$^+$ helper T cells, and antibodies.

- The most important antigens that stimulate graft rejection are allogeneic MHC molecules, which resemble peptide-loaded self MHC molecules that the graft recipient's T cells can recognize. Allogeneic MHC molecules are either presented by graft APCs without processing to recipient T cells (direct presentation), or are processed and presented as peptides bound to self MHC by host APCs (indirect presentation).

- Grafts may be rejected by different mechanisms. Hyperacute rejection is mediated by preformed antibodies to blood group antigens or HLA molecules, which cause endothelial injury and thrombosis of blood vessels in the graft. Acute rejection is mediated by T cells, which injure graft cells and endothelium, and by antibodies that bind to the endothelium. Chronic rejection is caused by T cells that produce cytokines that stimulate growth of vascular smooth muscle cells and tissue fibroblasts.

- Treatment for graft rejection is designed to suppress T cell responses and inflammation. The mainstay of treatment has been immunosuppressive drugs, including corticosteroids and calcineurin inhibitors, mTOR inhibitors, antimetabolites, and many others.

- Blood cell transfusion is the oldest and most widely used form of transplantation and requires ABO blood group compatibility of donor and recipient. ABO blood group antigens are sugars expressed on the surfaces of red blood cells, endothelial cells, and other cells, and people produce natural antibodies specific for the ABO antigens they do not express.

- Hematopoietic stem cell transplants are widely used to treat cancers of blood cells and to replace defective components of the immune or hematopoietic system. These cell transplants elicit strong rejection reactions, carry the risk of graft-versus-host disease, and often lead to temporary immunodeficiency in recipients.

▌ REVIEW QUESTIONS

1. What are the main types of tumor antigens that the immune system reacts against?
2. What is the evidence that tumor rejection is an immunologic phenomenon?
3. How do naive CD8$^+$ T cells recognize tumor antigens, and how are these cells activated to differentiate into effector CTLs?
4. What are some of the mechanisms by which tumors may evade the immune response?
5. What are some strategies for enhancing host immune responses to tumor antigens?
6. Why do normal T cells, which recognize foreign peptide antigens bound to self MHC molecules, react strongly against the allogeneic MHC molecules of a graft?
7. What are the principal mechanisms of rejection of allografts?
8. How is the likelihood of graft rejection reduced in clinical transplantation?
9. What are some of the problems associated with the transplantation of hematopoietic stem cells?

Answers to and discussion of the Review Questions are available at Student Consult.

Hypersensitivity
Disorders Caused by Immune Responses

The concept that the immune system is required for defending the host against infections has been emphasized throughout this book. However, immune responses are themselves capable of causing tissue injury and disease. Injurious, or pathologic, immune reactions are called **hypersensitivity reactions**. An immune response to an antigen may result not only in protective immunity but also a detectable reaction to challenge with that antigen, called sensitivity, and therefore hypersensitivity is a reflection of excessive or aberrant immune responses. Hypersensitivity reactions may occur in two situations. First, responses to foreign antigens (microbes and noninfectious environmental antigens) may cause tissue injury, especially if the reactions are repetitive or poorly controlled. Second, the immune responses may be directed against self (autologous) antigens, as a result of

the failure of self-tolerance (see Chapter 9). Responses against self antigens are termed **autoimmunity**, and disorders caused by such responses are called **autoimmune diseases**.

This chapter describes the important features of hypersensitivity reactions and the resulting diseases, focusing on their pathogenesis. Their clinicopathologic features are described only briefly and can be found in other medical textbooks. The following questions are addressed:

- What are the mechanisms of different types of hypersensitivity reactions?
- What are the major clinical and pathologic features of diseases caused by these reactions?
- What principles underlie treatment of such diseases?

TYPES OF HYPERSENSITIVITY REACTIONS

Hypersensitivity reactions are classified on the basis of the principal immunologic mechanism that is responsible for tissue injury and disease (Fig. 11.1). We will use the informative descriptive classifications throughout this chapter, but we will also indicate the numerical designations for each type since they are widely used.

- Immediate hypersensitivity, or type I hypersensitivity, is a type of pathologic reaction that is caused by the release of mediators from mast cells. This reaction most often depends on the production of immunoglobulin E (IgE) antibody against environmental antigens and the binding of IgE to mast cells in various tissues.
- Antibodies that are directed against cell or tissue antigens can damage these cells or tissues or can impair their function. These diseases are said to be antibody mediated or type II hypersensitivity.
- Antibodies against soluble antigens in the blood may form complexes with the antigens, and the immune complexes may deposit in blood vessels in various tissues, causing inflammation and tissue injury. Such disorders are called immune complex diseases or type III hypersensitivity.
- Some diseases result from the reactions of T lymphocytes specific for self antigens or microbes in tissues. These are T cell–mediated diseases or type IV hypersensitivity.

This classification scheme is useful because it distinguishes the mechanisms of immune-mediated tissue injury. In many human immunologic diseases, however, the damage may result from a combination of antibody-mediated and T cell–mediated reactions, so it is often difficult to classify these diseases neatly into one type of hypersensitivity.

IMMEDIATE HYPERSENSITIVITY

Immediate hypersensitivity is an IgE antibody– and mast cell–mediated reaction to certain antigens that causes rapid vascular leakage and mucosal secretions, often followed by inflammation. Disorders in which IgE-mediated immediate hypersensitivity is prominent are also called **allergy**, or **atopy**, and individuals with a propensity to develop these reactions are said to be atopic. Immediate hypersensitivity may affect various tissues and may be of varying severity in different individuals. Common types of allergies include hay fever, food allergies, asthma, and anaphylaxis. Allergies are the most frequent disorders of the immune system, estimated to affect 10% to 20% of people, and the incidence of allergic diseases has been increasing, especially in industrialized societies.

The sequence of events in the development of immediate hypersensitivity reactions includes: activation of Th2 and IL-4–secreting follicular helper T (Tfh) cells, which stimulate the production of IgE antibodies in response to an antigen; binding of the IgE to IgE-specific Fc receptors of mast cells; on subsequent exposure to the antigen, cross-linking of the bound IgE by the antigen, leading to activation of the mast cells and release of various mediators (Fig. 11.2). Some mast cell mediators cause a rapid increase in vascular permeability and smooth muscle contraction, resulting in many of the symptoms of these reactions (Fig. 11.3). This vascular and smooth muscle reaction may occur within minutes of reintroduction of antigen into a previously sensitized individual, hence the name immediate hypersensitivity. Other mast cell mediators are cytokines that recruit neutrophils and eosinophils to the site of the reaction over several hours. This inflammatory component is called the **late-phase reaction**, and it is mainly responsible for the tissue injury that results from repeated bouts of immediate hypersensitivity.

With this background, we proceed to a discussion of the steps in immediate hypersensitivity reactions.

Activation of Th2 Cells and Production of IgE Antibody

In individuals who are prone to allergies, exposure to some antigens results in the activation of Th2 cells and IL-4–secreting Tfh cells, and the production of IgE antibody (see Fig. 11.2). Most individuals do not mount strong Th2 responses to environmental antigens. For unknown reasons, when some individuals encounter certain antigens, such as proteins in pollen, certain foods, insect venoms, or animal dander, or if they are treated with certain drugs such as penicillin, there is a strong Th2 response. Immediate hypersensitivity develops as a consequence of the activation of Th2 and IL-4-secreting Tfh cells in response to protein antigens or chemicals that bind to proteins. Antigens that elicit immediate hypersensitivity (allergic) reactions often are called allergens.

Type of hypersensitivity	Pathologic immune mechanisms	Mechanisms of tissue injury and disease
Immediate hypersensitivity (Type I)	Th2 cells, IgE antibody, mast cells, eosinophils Mast cell — IgE — Allergen — Mediators	Mast cell–derived mediators (vasoactive amines, lipid mediators, cytokines) Cytokine-mediated inflammation (eosinophils, neutrophils)
Antibody-mediated diseases (Type II)	IgM, IgG antibodies against cell surface or extracellular matrix antigens Fc receptor — Inflammatory cell — Complement — Antibody	Complement- and Fc receptor–mediated recruitment and activation of leukocytes (neutrophils, macrophages) Opsonization and phagocytosis of cells Abnormalities in cellular function, e.g., hormone or neurotransmitter receptor signaling
Immune complex–mediated diseases (Type III)	Immune complexes of circulating antigens and IgM or IgG antibodies deposited in vascular basement membrane Blood vessel wall — Neutrophils — Antigen-antibody complex	Complement- and Fc receptor–mediated recruitment and activation of leukocytes
T cell-mediated diseases (Type IV)	1. CD4+ T cells (cytokine-mediated inflammation) 2. CD8+ CTLs (T cell–mediated cytolysis) Macrophage — CD8+ T cell — CD4+ T cell — Cytokines	1. Macrophage activation, cytokine-mediated inflammation 2. Direct target cell lysis, cytokine-mediated inflammation

Fig. 11.1 Types of hypersensitivity reactions. In the four major types of hypersensitivity reactions, different immune effector mechanisms cause tissue injury and disease. *CTLs,* Cytotoxic T lymphocytes; *Ig,* immunoglobulin.

First exposure to allergen

Antigen activation of Tfh cells and stimulation of IgE class switching in B cells

Production of IgE

Binding of IgE to FcεRI on mast cells

Repeat exposure to allergen

Activation of mast cell: release of mediators

Allergen

B cell

Tfh cell

IgE

IgE-secreting plasma cell

FcεRI

Mast cell

Mediators

Vasoactive amines, lipid mediators

Cytokines

Immediate hypersensitivity reaction (minutes after repeat exposure to allergen)

Late-phase reaction (6–24 hours after repeat exposure to allergen)

Fig. 11.2 The sequence of events in immediate hypersensitivity. Immediate hypersensitivity reactions are initiated by the introduction of an allergen, which stimulates Th2 and IL-4/IL-13–producing Tfh cells and immunoglobulin E *(IgE)* production. IgE binds to Fc receptors *(FcεRI)* on mast cells, and subsequent exposure to the allergen activates the mast cells to secrete the mediators that are responsible for the pathologic reactions of immediate hypersensitivity.

Any atopic individual may be allergic to one or more of these antigens. It is not understood why only a small subset of common environmental antigens elicit Th2-mediated reactions and IgE production, or what characteristics of these antigens are responsible for their behavior as allergens.

In secondary lymphoid organs, IL-4 secreted by Tfh cells stimulates B lymphocytes to switch to IgE-producing plasma cells. Therefore, atopic individuals produce large amounts of IgE antibody in response to antigens that do not elicit IgE responses in other people. IL-4 and IL-13 secreted by Th2 cells induce some of the responses of tissues in allergic reactions, such as intestinal motility and excess mucus secretions. Th2 cells also secrete IL-5, which promotes eosinophilic inflammation that is characteristic of tissues affected by allergic diseases. Because the majority of Th2 cells migrate to peripheral tissues, whereas Tfh cells remain in secondary lymphoid organs, they likely serve different roles in allergic responses. Switching to IgE occurs mainly in the lymphoid organs and therefore helper function is provided by Tfh cells. Th2 cells may contribute to any isotype switching that occurs in peripheral sites of allergic reactions, and, more importantly, are responsible for inflammation and eosinophil activation at these sites.

The propensity toward differentiation of IL-4 and IL-5 producing T cells, and resulting atopic diseases such as asthma, has a strong genetic basis. A major known risk for developing allergies is a family history of atopic disease, and gene association studies indicate that many different genes play contributory roles. Some of these genes encode cytokines or receptors known to be involved in T and B lymphocyte responses, including IL-4, IL-5, and IL-13, and IL-4 receptor; how these gene variants contribute to atopic diseases is not known. Mutations of filaggrin, a protein required for barrier function of skin, increases risk for atopic dermatitis in early childhood, and subsequent allergic diseases including asthma.

Various environmental factors besides exposure to allergens, including air pollution and exposure to microbes, have a profound influence on the propensity to develop allergies, and this may be one reason why the incidence of allergic diseases, especially asthma, is increasing in industrialized societies.

Fig. 11.3 Immediate hypersensitivity. **A,** Kinetics of the immediate and late-phase reactions. The immediate vascular and smooth muscle reaction to allergen develops within minutes after challenge (allergen exposure in a previously sensitized individual), and the late-phase reaction develops 2 to 24 hours later. **B,** Morphology of the immediate reaction is characterized by vasodilation, congestion, and edema. **C,** The late-phase reaction is characterized by an inflammatory infiltrate rich in eosinophils, neutrophils, and T cells. (Micrographs courtesy Dr. Daniel Friend, Department of Pathology, Brigham and Women's Hospital, Boston.)

Activation of Mast Cells and Secretion of Mediators

IgE antibody produced in response to an allergen binds to high-affinity Fc receptors, specific for the ε heavy chain, that are expressed on mast cells (see Fig. 11.2). Thus, in an atopic individual, mast cells are coated with IgE antibody specific for the antigen(s) to which the individual is allergic. This process of coating mast cells with IgE is called sensitization, because it makes the mast cells sensitive to activation by subsequent encounter with that antigen. In normal individuals, by contrast, mast cells may carry IgE molecules of many different specificities because many antigens may elicit small IgE responses, and the amount of IgE specific for any one antigen is not enough to cause immediate hypersensitivity reactions upon exposure to that antigen.

Mast cells are present in all connective tissues, especially under epithelia, and they are usually located adjacent to blood vessels. Which of the body's mast cells are activated by binding of an allergen often depends on the route of entry of the allergen. For example, inhaled allergens activate mast cells in the submucosal tissues of the bronchus, whereas ingested allergens activate mast cells in the wall of the intestine. Allergens that enter the blood via absorption from the intestine or by direct injection may be delivered to all tissues, resulting in systemic mast cell activation.

The high-affinity receptor for IgE, called FcεRI, consists of three polypeptide chains, one of which binds the Fc portion of the ε heavy chain very strongly, with a K_d

of approximately 10^{-11} M. (The concentration of IgE in the plasma is approximately 10^{-9} M, which explains why even in normal individuals, mast cells are always coated with IgE bound to FcεRI.) The other two chains of the receptor are signaling proteins. The same FcεRI is also present on basophils, which are circulating cells with many of the features of mast cells, but normally the number of basophils in the blood is very low and they are not present in tissues, so their role in immediate hypersensitivity is not as well established as the role of mast cells.

When mast cells sensitized by IgE are exposed to the allergen, they are activated to secrete inflammatory mediators (Fig. 11.4). Mast cell activation results from binding of the allergen to two or more IgE antibodies on the cell. When this happens, the FcεRI molecules that are carrying the IgE are cross-linked, triggering biochemical signals from the signal-transducing chains of FcεRI. The signals lead to the release of inflammatory mediators.

The most important mediators produced by mast cells are vasoactive amines and proteases stored in and released from granules, newly generated and secreted products of arachidonic acid metabolism, and cytokines (see Fig. 11.4). These mediators have different actions. The major amine, histamine, causes increased vascular permeability and vasodilation, leading to the leak of fluid and plasma proteins into tissues, and stimulates the transient contraction of bronchial and intestinal

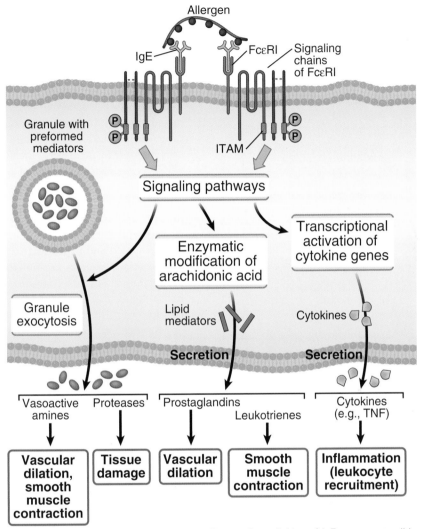

Fig. 11.4 Production and actions of mast cell mediators. Cross-linking of IgE on a mast cell by an allergen stimulates phosphorylation of immunoreceptor tyrosine-based activation motifs *(ITAMs)* in the signaling chains of the IgE Fc receptor *(FcεRI)*, which then initiates multiple signaling pathways. These signaling pathways stimulate the release of mast cell granule contents (amines, proteases), the synthesis of arachidonic acid metabolites (prostaglandins, leukotrienes), and the synthesis of various cytokines. *TNF,* Tumor necrosis factor.

smooth muscle. Proteases may cause damage to local tissues. Arachidonic acid metabolites include prostaglandins, which cause vascular dilation, and leukotrienes, which stimulate prolonged bronchial smooth muscle contraction. Cytokines induce local inflammation (the late-phase reaction, described next). Thus, mast cell mediators are responsible for acute vascular and smooth muscle reactions and more prolonged inflammation, the hallmarks of immediate hypersensitivity.

Cytokines produced by mast cells stimulate the recruitment of leukocytes, which cause the late-phase reaction. The principal leukocytes involved in this reaction are eosinophils, neutrophils, and Th2 cells. Mast cell–derived tumor necrosis factor (TNF) and IL-4 promote neutrophil- and eosinophil-rich inflammation. Chemokines produced by mast cells and by epithelial cells in the tissues also contribute to leukocyte recruitment. Eosinophils and neutrophils

Clinical syndrome	Clinical and pathological manifestations
Allergic rhinitis, sinusitis (hay fever)	Increased mucus secretion; inflammation of upper airways, sinuses
Food allergies	Increased peristalsis due to contraction of intestinal muscles
Asthma	Airway obstruction caused by bronchial smooth muscle hyperactivity; inflammation and tissue injury
Anaphylaxis (may be caused by drugs, bee sting, food)	Fall in blood pressure (shock) caused by vascular dilation; airway obstruction due to laryngeal edema

Fig. 11.5 Clinical manifestations of immediate hypersensitivity reactions. Immediate hypersensitivity may be manifested in many other ways, as in development of skin lesions (e.g., urticaria, eczema).

liberate proteases, which cause tissue damage, and Th2 cells may exacerbate the reaction by producing more cytokines. Eosinophils are prominent in many allergic reactions and are an important cause of tissue injury in these reactions. These cells are activated by the cytokine IL-5, which is produced by Th2 cells and innate lymphoid cells.

Clinical Syndromes and Therapy

Immediate hypersensitivity reactions have diverse clinical and pathologic features, all of which are attributable to mediators produced by mast cells in different amounts and in different tissues (Fig. 11.5).

- Some mild manifestations, such as allergic rhinitis and sinusitis, which are common in **hay fever**, are reactions to inhaled allergens, such as a protein of ragweed pollen. Mast cells in the nasal mucosa produce histamine, and Th2 cells produce IL-13, and these two mediators cause increased production of mucus. Late-phase reactions may lead to more prolonged inflammation.

- In **food allergies**, ingested allergens trigger mast cell degranulation, and the released histamine and other mediators causes increased peristalsis, resulting in vomiting and diarrhea.

- **Asthma** is a clinical syndrome characterized by difficulty in breathing, cough, and wheezing, related to intermittent obstruction of expiratory airflow. The most common cause of asthma is respiratory allergy in which inhaled allergens stimulate bronchial mast cells to release mediators, including leukotrienes, which cause repeated bouts of bronchial constriction and airway obstruction. In chronic asthma, large numbers of eosinophils accumulate in the bronchial mucosa, excessive secretion of mucus occurs in the airways, and the bronchial smooth muscle becomes hypertrophied and hyperreactive to various stimuli. Some cases of asthma are not associated with IgE production and may be triggered by cold or exercise; how either of these causes bronchial hyperreactivity is unknown.

- The most severe form of immediate hypersensitivity is **anaphylaxis**, a systemic reaction characterized by edema in many tissues, including the larynx, accompanied by a fall in blood pressure (anaphylactic shock) and bronchoconstriction. Some of the most frequent inducers of anaphylaxis include bee stings, injected or ingested penicillin-family antibiotics, and ingested nuts or shellfish. The reaction is caused by widespread mast cell degranulation in response to the systemic distribution of the antigen, and it is life threatening because of the sudden fall in blood pressure and airway obstruction.

The therapy for immediate hypersensitivity diseases is aimed at inhibiting mast cell degranulation, antagonizing the effects of mast cell mediators, and reducing inflammation (Fig. 11.6). Common drugs include antihistamines for hay fever, inhaled beta-adrenergic agonists and corticosteroids that relax bronchial smooth muscles and reduce airway inflammation in asthma, and epinephrine in anaphylaxis. Many patients benefit from repeated administration of small doses of allergens, called desensitization or allergen-specific immunotherapy. This treatment may work by changing the T cell response away from Th2 dominance or the antibody response away from IgE, by inducing tolerance in allergen-specific T cells, or by stimulating regulatory T cells (Tregs). Antibodies that block various cytokines or their receptors, including IL-4 and IL-5, are now approved for

Syndrome	Therapy	Mechanism of action
Anaphylaxis	Epinephrine	Causes vascular smooth muscle cell contraction, increases cardiac output (to counter shock), and inhibits bronchial smooth muscle cell contraction
Asthma	Corticosteroids	Reduce inflammation
	Leukotriene antagonists	Relax bronchial smooth muscle and reduce inflammation
	Beta adrenergic receptor antagonists	Relax bronchial smooth muscles
Various allergic diseases	Desensitization (repeated administration of low doses of allergens)	Unknown; may inhibit IgE production and increase production of other Ig isotypes; may induce T cell tolerance
	Anti-IgE antibody	Neutralizes and eliminates IgE
	Antihistamines	Block actions of histamine on vessels and smooth muscles
	Cromolyn	Inhibits mast cell degranulation
	Antibodies that block cytokines and their receptors: anti-IL-5 and anti-IL-5R (asthma), anti-IL-4R (atopic dermatitis)	Block actions of cytokines

Fig. 11.6 Treatment of immediate hypersensitivity reactions. The figure summarizes the principal mechanisms of action of the various drugs used to treat allergic disorders. *Ig*, Immunoglobulin.

the treatment of some forms of asthma and atopic dermatitis, and other cytokine antagonists are being tested in patients.

Before concluding the discussion of immediate hypersensitivity, it is important to address the question of why evolution has preserved an IgE antibody– and mast cell–mediated immune response whose major effects are pathologic. There is no definitive answer to this puzzle, but immediate hypersensitivity reactions likely evolved to protect against pathogens or toxins. It is known that IgE antibody and eosinophils are important mechanisms of defense against helminthic infections, and mast cells play a role in innate immunity against

some bacteria and in destroying venomous toxins produced by arachnids and snakes.

DISEASES CAUSED BY ANTIBODIES SPECIFIC FOR CELL AND TISSUE ANTIGENS

Antibodies, typically of the IgG class, may cause disease, called type II hypersensitivity disorders, by binding to their target antigens in different tissues (Fig. 11.7A). Antibody-mediated hypersensitivity reactions have long been recognized as the basis of many chronic immunologic diseases in humans. Antibodies against

Fig. 11.7 Types of antibody-mediated diseases. Antibodies (other than IgE) may cause tissue injury and disease by: **A**, Binding directly to their target antigens on cells (not shown) and in the extracellular matrix (type II hypersensitivity); or **B**, By forming immune complexes that deposit mainly in blood vessels (type III hypersensitivity).

cells or extracellular matrix components may deposit in any tissue that expresses the relevant target antigen; thus, diseases caused by such antibodies usually are specific for a particular tissue. The antibodies that cause disease are most often autoantibodies against self antigens. The production of autoantibodies results from a failure of self-tolerance. In Chapter 9 we discussed the mechanisms by which self-tolerance may fail, but why this happens in any human autoimmune disease is still not understood.

Mechanisms of Antibody-Mediated Tissue Injury and Disease

Antibodies specific for cell and tissue antigens may deposit in tissues and cause injury by inducing local inflammation, they may induce phagocytosis and destruction of cells, or they interfere with normal cellular functions (Fig. 11.8).

- **Inflammation**. Antibodies against tissue antigens induce inflammation by attracting and activating leukocytes. IgG antibodies of the IgG1 and IgG3 subclasses bind to neutrophil and macrophage Fc receptors and activate these leukocytes, resulting in inflammation (see Chapter 8). The same antibodies, as well as IgM, activate the complement system by the classical pathway, resulting in the production of complement by-products that recruit leukocytes and induce inflammation. When leukocytes are activated at sites of antibody deposition, these cells release reactive oxygen species and lysosomal enzymes that damage the adjacent tissues.

- **Opsonization and phagocytosis**. If antibodies bind to cells, such as erythrocytes, neutrophils, and platelets, the cells are opsonized and may be ingested and destroyed by host phagocytes.

Fig. 11.8 Effector mechanisms of antibody-mediated diseases. Antibodies cause disease by **A,** Inducing inflammation at the site of deposition; **B,** Opsonizing cells (such as red cells) for phagocytosis; and **C,** Interfering with normal cellular functions, such as hormone receptor signaling. All three mechanisms are seen with antibodies that bind directly to their target antigens, but immune complexes cause disease mainly by inducing inflammation (**A**). *TSH,* Thyroid-stimulating hormone.

• **Abnormal cellular responses.** Some antibodies may cause disease without directly inducing tissue injury. For example, in pernicious anemia, autoantibodies specific for a protein required for absorption of vitamin B12 cause a multisystem disease due to B12 deficiency. In some cases of myasthenia gravis, antibodies against the acetylcholine receptor inhibit neuromuscular transmission, causing paralysis. Other antibodies may directly activate receptors, mimicking their physiologic ligands. The only known example is a form of hyperthyroidism called Graves disease, in which antibodies against the receptor for thyroid-stimulating hormone activate thyroid cells even in the absence of the hormone.

Antibody-mediated disease	Target antigen	Mechanisms of disease	Clinicopathologic manifestations
Autoimmune hemolytic anemia	Erythrocyte membrane proteins (Rh blood group antigens, I antigen)	Opsonization and phagocytosis of erythrocytes	Hemolysis, anemia
Autoimmune (idiopathic) thrombocytopenic purpura	Platelet membrane proteins (gpIIb/IIIa integrin)	Opsonization and phagocytosis of platelets	Bleeding
Goodpasture syndrome	Collagen in basement membranes of kidney glomeruli and lung alveoli	Complement and Fc receptor–mediated inflammation	Nephritis, lung hemorrhage
Graves disease (hyperthyroidism)	Thyroid stimulating hormone (TSH) receptor	Antibody-mediated stimulation of TSH receptors	Hyperthyroidism
Myasthenia gravis	Acetylcholine receptor	Antibody inhibits acetycholine binding, down-modulates receptors	Muscle weakness, paralysis
Pemphigus vulgaris	Proteins in intercellular junctions of epidermal cells (epidermal cadherin)	Antibody-mediated disruption of intercellular adhesions	Skin blisters (bullae)
Pernicious anemia	Intrinsic factor of gastric parietal cells	Neutralization of intrinsic factor, decreased absorption of vitamin B_{12}	Anemia due to abnormal erythropoiesis, nerve damage
Rheumatic fever	Streptococcal cell wall antigen; antibody cross-reacts with myocardial antigen	Inflammation, macrophage activation	Myocarditis, arthritis

Fig. 11.9 Human antibody-mediated diseases (type II hypersensitivity). The figure lists examples of human diseases caused by antibodies. In most of these diseases, the role of antibodies is inferred from the detection of antibodies in the blood or the lesions, and in some cases by similarities with experimental models in which the involvement of antibodies can be formally established by transfer studies.

Examples and Treatment of Diseases Caused by Cell- or Tissue-Specific Antibodies

Antibodies specific for cell and tissue antigens are the cause of many human diseases, involving blood cells, heart, kidney, lung, and skin (Fig. 11.9). Examples of anti-tissue antibodies are those that react with the glomerular basement membrane and induce inflammation, a form of glomerulonephritis. Antibodies against cells include those that opsonize blood cells and target them for phagocytosis, as in autoimmune hemolytic anemia (red cell destruction) and autoimmune thrombocytopenia (destruction of platelets). Antibodies that interfere with hormones or their receptors were mentioned earlier. In most of these cases, the antibodies are autoantibodies, but less commonly, antibodies produced against a microbe may cross-react with an antigen in the tissues. For instance, in rare instances, streptococcal infection stimulates the production of antibacterial antibodies that cross-react with antigens in the heart, producing the cardiac inflammation that is characteristic of rheumatic fever.

Therapy for antibody-mediated diseases is intended mainly to limit inflammation and its injurious consequences with drugs such as corticosteroids. In severe cases, plasmapheresis is used to reduce levels of circulating antibodies. In hemolytic anemia and thrombocytopenia, splenectomy is of clinical benefit because the spleen is the major organ where opsonized blood cells are phagocytosed. Some of these diseases respond well to treatment with intravenous IgG (IVIG) pooled from healthy donors. How IVIG works is not known; it may bind to the inhibitory Fc receptor on myeloid cells and B cells and thus block activation of these cells (see Chapter 7, Fig. 7.15), or it may reduce the half-life of pathogenic antibodies by competing for binding to the neonatal Fc receptor in endothelial cells and macrophages (see Chapter 8, Fig. 8.2). Treatment of patients with an antibody specific for CD20, a surface protein of mature B cells, results in depletion of the B cells and may be useful for treating some antibody-mediated disorders. Other approaches in development for inhibiting the production of autoantibodies include treating patients with antibodies that block CD40 or its ligand and thus inhibit helper T cell–dependent B cell activation and antibodies to block cytokines that promote the survival of B cells and plasma cells. There is also interest in inducing tolerance in cases in which the autoantigens are known.

DISEASES CAUSED BY ANTIGEN-ANTIBODY COMPLEXES

Antibodies may cause disease by forming immune complexes that deposit in blood vessels (Fig. 11.7B). Many acute and chronic hypersensitivity disorders are caused by, or are associated with, immune complexes (Fig. 11.10); these are called type III hypersensitivity disorders. Immune complexes usually deposit in blood vessels, especially vessels through which plasma is filtered at high pressure (e.g., in renal glomeruli and joint synovium). Therefore, in contrast to diseases caused by tissue antigen-specific antibodies, immune complex diseases tend to be systemic and often manifest as widespread vasculitis involving sites that are particularly susceptible to immune complex deposition, such as kidneys and joints.

Immune complex disease	Antibody specificity	Clinicopathologic manifestations
Systemic lupus erythematosus	DNA, nucleoproteins, others	Nephritis, arthritis, vasculitis
Polyarteritis nodosa	In some cases, microbial antigens (e.g., hepatitis B virus surface antigen); most cases unknown	Vasculitis
Poststreptococcal glomerulonephritis	Streptococcal cell wall antigen(s)	Nephritis
Serum sickness (clinical and experimental)	Various protein antigens	Systemic vasculitis, nephritis, arthritis
Arthus reaction (experimental)	Various protein antigens	Cutaneous vasculitis

Fig. 11.10 Immune complex diseases (type III hypersensitivity). Examples of human diseases caused by the deposition of immune complexes, as well as two experimental models. In the diseases, immune complexes are detected in the blood or in the tissues that are the sites of injury. In all the disorders, injury is caused by complement-mediated and Fc receptor–mediated inflammation.

Etiology, Examples, and Therapy of Immune Complex–Mediated Diseases

Antigen-antibody complexes, which are produced during normal immune responses, cause disease only when they are formed in excessive amounts, are not efficiently removed by phagocytes, and become deposited in tissues. Complexes containing positively charged antigens are particularly pathogenic because they bind avidly to negatively charged components of the basement membranes of blood vessels and kidney glomeruli. Once deposited in the vessel walls, the Fc regions of the antibodies activate complement and bind Fc receptors on neutrophils, activating the cells to release damaging proteases and reactive oxygen species. This inflammatory response within the vessel wall, called vasculitis, may cause local hemorrhage or thrombosis leading to ischemic tissue injury. In the kidney glomerulus, the vasculitis can impair the normal filtration function, leading to renal disease.

The first immune complex disease studied was **serum sickness,** seen in subjects who received antitoxin-containing serum from immunized animals for the treatment of infections. Some of these treated individuals subsequently developed a systemic inflammatory disease. This illness could be recreated in experimental animals by systemic administration of a protein antigen, which elicits an antibody response and leads to the formation of circulating immune complexes. This can occur as a complication of any therapy involving injection of foreign proteins, such as antibodies against microbial toxins, snake venoms and T cells that are usually made in goats or rabbits, and even some humanized monoclonal antibodies that are used to treat different diseases and may differ only slightly from normal human Ig.

A localized immune complex reaction called the **Arthus reaction** was first studied in experimental animals. It is induced by subcutaneous administration of a protein antigen to a previously immunized animal; it results in the formation of immune complexes at the site of antigen injection and a local vasculitis. In a small percentage of vaccine recipients who have previously been vaccinated or already have antibodies against the vaccine antigen, a painful swelling that develops at the injection site represents a clinically relevant Arthus reaction.

In human immune complex diseases, the antibodies may be specific for self antigens or microbial antigens. In several systemic autoimmune diseases, many of the clinical manifestations are caused by vascular injury when complexes of the antibodies and self antigens deposit in vessels in different organs. For example, in systemic lupus erythematosus, immune complexes of anti-DNA antibodies and DNA can deposit in the blood vessels of almost any organ, causing vasculitis and impaired blood flow, leading to a multitude of different organ pathologies and symptoms. Several immune complex diseases are initiated by infections. For example, in response to some streptococcal infections, individuals make antistreptococcal antibodies that form complexes with the bacterial antigens. These complexes deposit in kidney glomeruli, causing an inflammatory process called poststreptococcal glomerulonephritis that can lead to renal failure. Other immune complex diseases caused by complexes of antimicrobial antibodies and microbial antigens lead to vasculitis. This may occur in patients with chronic infections with certain viruses (e.g., the hepatitis virus) or parasites (e.g., malaria).

DISEASES CAUSED BY T LYMPHOCYTES

T cells play a central role in chronic immunologic diseases in which inflammation is a prominent component. Many of the newly developed therapies that have shown efficacy in such diseases are drugs that inhibit the recruitment and activities of T cells.

Etiology of T Cell–Mediated Diseases

The major causes of T cell–mediated hypersensitivity reactions are autoimmunity and exaggerated or persistent responses to microbial or other environmental antigens. The autoimmune reactions usually are directed against cellular antigens with restricted tissue distribution. Therefore, T cell–mediated autoimmune diseases tend to be limited to a few organs and usually are not systemic. Examples of T cell–mediated hypersensitivity reactions against environmental antigens include contact sensitivity to chemicals (e.g., various therapeutic drugs and substances found in plants such as poison ivy). Tissue injury also may accompany T cell responses to microbes. For example, in tuberculosis, a T cell–mediated immune response develops against protein antigens of *Mycobacterium tuberculosis*, and the response becomes chronic because the infection is difficult to eradicate. The resultant granulomatous inflammation causes injury to normal tissues at the site of infection.

Excessive polyclonal T cell activation by certain microbial toxins produced by some bacteria and viruses can lead to production of large amounts of inflammatory cytokines, causing a syndrome similar to septic shock. These toxins are called **superantigens** because they stimulate large numbers of T cells. Superantigens bind to invariant parts of T cell receptors on many different clones of T cells, regardless of antigen specificity, thereby activating these cells.

Mechanisms of Tissue Injury

In different T cell–mediated diseases, tissue injury is caused by inflammation induced by cytokines that are produced mainly by CD4+ T cells or by killing of host cells by CD8+ cytotoxic T lymphocytes (CTLs) (Fig. 11.11). These mechanisms of tissue injury are the same as the mechanisms used by T cells to eliminate cell-associated microbes.

CD4+ T cells may react against cell or tissue antigens and secrete cytokines that induce local inflammation and activate macrophages. Different diseases may be associated with activation of Th1 and Th17 cells. Th1 cells are the source of interferon-γ (IFN-γ), the principal macrophage-activating cytokine, and Th17 cells are responsible for the recruitment of leukocytes, including neutrophils. The actual tissue injury in these diseases is caused mainly by the macrophages and neutrophils.

The typical reaction mediated by T cell cytokines is **delayed-type hypersensitivity** (DTH), so called because it occurs 24 to 48 hours after an individual previously exposed to a protein antigen is challenged with the antigen (i.e., the reaction is delayed). The delay occurs because it takes several hours for circulating effector T lymphocytes to home to the site of antigen challenge, respond to the antigen at this site, and secrete cytokines that induce a detectable reaction. DTH reactions are manifested by infiltrates of T cells and blood monocytes in the tissues (Fig. 11.12), edema and fibrin deposition caused by increased vascular permeability in response to cytokines produced by CD4+ T cells, and tissue damage induced by leukocyte products, mainly from macrophages that are activated by the T cells. DTH reactions often are used to determine if people have been previously exposed to and have responded to an antigen. For example, a DTH reaction to a mycobacterial antigen, PPD (purified protein derivative), applied to the skin, is an indicator of past or active mycobacterial infection.

CD8+ T cells specific for antigens on host cells may directly kill these cells. CD8+ T cells also produce cytokines, including IFN-γ that may induce inflammation

Fig. 11.11 Mechanisms of T cell–mediated tissue injury (type IV hypersensitivity). T cells may cause tissue injury and disease by two mechanisms. **A,** Inflammation may be triggered by cytokines produced mainly by CD4+ T cells in which tissue injury is caused by activated macrophages and inflammatory cells. **B,** Direct killing of target cells is mediated by CD8+ cytotoxic T lymphocytes (CTLs). *APC,* Antigen-presenting cell.

in some hypersensitivity diseases. In many T cell–mediated autoimmune diseases, both CD4+ T cells and CD8+ T cells specific for self antigens are present, and both contribute to tissue injury.

Clinical Syndromes and Therapy

Many organ-specific autoimmune diseases in humans are believed to be caused by T cells, based on the identification of these cells in lesions and similarities with animal models in which the diseases are known to be T cell mediated (Fig. 11.13). These disorders typically are chronic and progressive, in part because long-lived memory T cells are generated, and the inciting antigens, such as tissue antigens or proteins expressed by resident microbes, are often never cleared. Also, tissue injury causes release and alteration of self proteins, which may result in reactions against these newly encountered proteins. This phenomenon has been called epitope spreading to indicate that the initial immune response against one or a few self antigen epitopes may spread to include responses against many more self antigens.

The therapy for T cell–mediated hypersensitivity disorders is designed to reduce inflammation and to inhibit T cell responses. The mainstay of treatment of such diseases has been the potent antiinflammatory steroids, but these drugs have significant side effects. The development of more targeted therapies based on understanding of the fundamental mechanisms of these diseases has been one of the most impressive accomplishments of immunology. Antagonists of inflammatory cytokines have proved to be very effective in patients with various inflammatory and autoimmune diseases. For example, monoclonal antibodies that block TNF or IL-6 receptor, and small molecule inhibitors of the inflammatory cytokine signaling molecule Janus kinase 3 (JAK3), are now used to treat rheumatoid arthritis, and IL-17 blocking antibodies are used to treat psoriasis. Other agents developed to inhibit T cell responses include drugs that block costimulators such as B7. Clinical trials are underway to test the efficacy of transferring in vitro expanded Tregs and administering IL-2 to expand endogenous Tregs for the treatment of autoimmune diseases such as type 1 diabetes and lupus. There also is active research on methods for inducing tolerance in pathogenic T cells.

NEUROIMMUNOLOGY: INTERACTIONS BETWEEN THE IMMUNE AND NERVOUS SYSTEMS

Reflex neural circuits affect innate and adaptive immune responses and the development of inflammatory diseases. It is well known that the nervous system is the target of autoimmune reactions, as in multiple sclerosis and myasthenia gravis, and inflammation may contribute to the development of neurodegenerative disorders such as Alzheimer disease. The interesting new developments are the elucidation of molecular communications between the nervous and immune systems, often via secreted molecules. The idea that neural circuits modulate immunity and the immune system alters neural functions has fascinated biologists and clinicians for decades. Some of the earliest findings suggesting the existence of such interactions were clinical observations that psychological stresses affected the severity of allergic (Th2-dominant) and contact sensitivity (Th1-dominant) reactions. These associations were usually interpreted to reflect the actions of neuropeptides, produced during psychological alterations, on lymphocytes and other immune cells. More recently, sophisticated genetic and other tools have been used to dissect bidirectional neural-immune interactions with greater precision. Among the findings potentially relevant to the development of disease states, the following are some interesting examples.

Fig. 11.12 Delayed-type hypersensitivity reaction in the skin. **A,** Perivascular accumulation (cuffing) of mononuclear inflammatory cells (lymphocytes and macrophages), with associated dermal edema and fibrin deposition. **B,** Immunoperoxidase staining reveals a predominantly perivascular cellular infiltrate that marks positively with anti-CD4 antibodies. (**B,** Courtesy Dr. Louis Picker, Department of Pathology, Oregon Health Sciences University, Portland, OR.)

Disease	Specificity of pathogenic T cells	Clinicopathologic manifestations
Multiple sclerosis	Myelin proteins	Demyelination in the central nervous system, sensory and motor dysfunction
Rheumatoid arthritis	Unknown antigens in joint	Inflammation of synovium and erosion of cartilage and bone in joints
Type 1 diabetes	Pancreatic islet antigens	Impaired glucose metabolism, vascular disease
Crohn disease	Unknown, ? role of intestinal microbes	Inflammation of the bowel wall; abdominal pain, diarrhea, hemorrhage
Psoriasis	Unknown	Chronic skin inflammation
Contact sensitivity (e.g., poison ivy, drug reaction)	Modified skin proteins	DTH reaction in skin, rash
Chronic infections (e.g., tuberculosis)	Microbial proteins	Chronic (e.g., granulomatous) inflammation

Fig. 11.13 T cell–mediated diseases. Diseases in which T cells play a dominant role in causing tissue injury; antibodies and immune complexes may also contribute. Note that multiple sclerosis, rheumatoid arthritis, and type 1 diabetes are autoimmune disorders. Crohn disease, an inflammatory bowel disease, is likely caused by reactions against microbes in the intestine and may have a component of autoimmunity. The other diseases are caused by reactions against foreign (microbial or environmental) antigens. In most of these diseases, the role of T cells is inferred from the detection and isolation of T cells reactive with various antigens from the blood or lesions, and from the similarity with experimental models in which the involvement of T cells has been established by a variety of approaches. The specificity of pathogenic T cells has been defined in animal models and in some of the human diseases. Viral hepatitis and toxic shock syndrome are disorders in which T cells play an important pathogenic role, but these are not considered examples of hypersensitivity. *CTL*, Cytotoxic T lymphocyte; *DTH*, delayed-type hypersensitivity; *HBV*, hepatitis B virus; *HCV*, hepatitis C virus.

- Activation of the efferent vagus nerve inhibits the production of pro-inflammatory innate cytokines such as TNF, providing a novel mechanism for regulating inflammation. This has led to clinical trials of vagus nerve stimulation in patients with rheumatoid arthritis.
- Cholinergic and adrenergic signals in the spleen regulate antibody production.
- Neuropeptides produced in response to microbes and other local stimuli influence the activation of type 2 innate lymphoid cells in the airways and hence type 2 immunity, the basis of allergic diseases.
- The gut microbiome induces signals from enteric nerves that induce macrophages to develop an anti-inflammatory and tissue-protective phenotype and regulates the balance between pro-inflammatory Th17 cells and protective Treg cells. Thus, the microbiome uses neural circuits to maintain immune homeostasis in the gut, raising the possibility that

abnormalities in this circuit contribute to intestinal inflammation.

- In addition to these examples of neural signals affecting immune responses, the converse is also true, that immune reactions alter neurological and psychological functions. For instance, neuronal development is regulated by complement breakdown products and cytokines, and cytokines produced by immune cells may influence cognitive functions such as memory and social behavior.

Many other neural-immune interactions have been described, and their impact on autoimmune and allergic diseases is being explored. The hope is that elucidation of these pathways will lead to the development of new classes of therapies for these diseases.

SUMMARY

- Immune responses that cause tissue injury are called hypersensitivity reactions, and the diseases caused by these reactions are called hypersensitivity diseases.
- Hypersensitivity reactions may arise from uncontrolled or abnormal responses to foreign antigens or autoimmune responses against self antigens.
- Hypersensitivity reactions are classified according to the mechanism of tissue injury.
- Immediate hypersensitivity (type I, commonly called allergy) is caused by the activation of Th2 cells and IL-4-producing Tfh cells and production of IgE antibody against environmental antigens or drugs (allergens), sensitization of mast cells by the IgE, and degranulation of these mast cells on subsequent encounter with the allergen.
- Clinicopathologic manifestations of immediate hypersensitivity result from the actions of mediators secreted by the mast cells: amines increase vascular permeability of and dilate blood vessels, arachidonic acid metabolites cause bronchial smooth muscle contraction, and cytokines induce inflammation, the hallmark of the late-phase reaction. Treatment of allergies is designed to inhibit the production of mediators, antagonize their actions, and counteract their effects on end organs.

- Antibodies against cell and tissue antigens may cause tissue injury and disease (type II hypersensitivity). IgM and IgG antibodies activate complement, which promotes phagocytosis of cells to which they bind, induces inflammation, and causes cell lysis. IgG also promotes Fc receptor–mediated phagocytosis of cells and leukocyte recruitment. Antibodies may interfere with the functions of cells by binding to essential molecules and receptors.
- In immune complex diseases (type III hypersensitivity), antibodies may bind to circulating antigens to form immune complexes, which deposit in vessels, leading to inflammation in the vessel wall (vasculitis), which secondarily causes tissue injury due to impaired blood flow.
- T cell–mediated diseases (type IV hypersensitivity) result from inflammation caused by cytokines produced by CD4+ Th1 and Th17 cells, or killing of host cells by CD8+ CTLs.

REVIEW QUESTIONS

1. What are the major types of hypersensitivity reactions?
2. What types of antigens may induce immune responses that cause hypersensitivity reactions?
3. What is the sequence of events in a typical immediate hypersensitivity reaction? What is the late-phase reaction, and how is it caused?
4. What are some examples of immediate hypersensitivity disorders, what is their pathogenesis, and how are they treated?
5. How do antibodies cause tissue injury and disease?

6. What are some examples of diseases caused by antibodies specific for cell surface or tissue matrix antigens?
7. How do immune complexes cause disease, and how are the clinical manifestations different from most diseases caused by antibodies specific for cell surface or tissue matrix proteins?
8. What are some examples of diseases caused by T cells, what is their pathogenesis, and what are their principal clinical and pathologic manifestations?

Answers to and discussion of the Review Questions are available at Student Consult.

Congenital and Acquired Immunodeficiencies
Diseases Caused by Defective Immunity

CHAPTER OUTLINE

Defects in the development and functions of the immune system result in increased susceptibility to infections and some cancers. The infections may be newly acquired or the reactivation of latent infections such as cytomegalovirus, Epstein-Barr virus, and tuberculosis, in which the normal immune response keeps the infection in check but does not eradicate it. These consequences of defective immunity are predictable because, as emphasized throughout this book, the normal function of the immune system is to defend individuals against infections and cancers. Disorders caused by defective immunity are called **immunodeficiency diseases**. Some of these diseases may result from genetic abnormalities in components of the immune system; these are called **congenital** (or **primary**) **immunodeficiencies**. Other defects in immunity may result from infections, nutritional abnormalities, or medical treatments that cause loss or inadequate function of various components of the immune

system; these are called **acquired** (or **secondary**) **immunodeficiencies**.

In this chapter we describe the causes and pathogenesis of congenital and acquired immunodeficiencies. Among the acquired diseases, we emphasize acquired immunodeficiency syndrome (AIDS), which results from infection by human immunodeficiency virus (HIV) and is one of the most devastating health problems worldwide. We address the following questions:

- What are the mechanisms by which immunity is compromised in the most common congenital immunodeficiency diseases?
- How does HIV cause the clinical and pathologic abnormalities of AIDS?
- What approaches are being used to treat immunodeficiency diseases?

Information about the clinical features of these disorders can be found in textbooks of pediatrics and medicine.

Type of immunodeficiency	Histopathology and laboratory abnormalities	Common infectious consequences
B cell deficiencies	Often absent or reduced follicles and germinal centers in lymphoid organs Reduced serum Ig levels	Pyogenic bacterial infections, enteric bacterial and viral infections
T cell deficiencies	May be reduced T cell zones in lymphoid organs Reduced DTH reactions to common antigens Defective T cell proliferative responses to mitogens in vitro	Viral and other intracellular microbial infections (e.g., *Pneumocystis jiroveci*, other fungi, nontuberculous mycobacteria) Some cancers (e.g., EBV-associated lymphomas, skin cancers)
Innate immune deficiencies	Variable, depending on which component of innate immunity is defective	Variable; pyogenic bacterial and viral infections

Fig. 12.1 Features of immunodeficiency diseases. The figure summarizes the important diagnostic features and clinical manifestations of immunodeficiencies affecting different components of the immune system. Within each group, different diseases, and even different patients with the same disease, may show considerable variation. Reduced numbers of circulating B or T cells are often detected in some of these diseases. *DTH,* Delayed-type hypersensitivity; *EBV,* Epstein-Barr virus; *Ig,* immunoglobulin.

CONGENITAL (PRIMARY) IMMUNODEFICIENCIES

Congenital immunodeficiencies are caused by genetic defects that lead to impaired maturation or function of different components of the immune system. It is estimated that as many as 1 in 500 individuals in the United States and Europe suffer from congenital immune deficiencies of varying severity. These immunodeficiencies share several features, the most common being increased susceptibility to infections (Fig. 12.1). Congenital immunodeficiency diseases may, however, differ considerably in clinical and pathologic manifestations. Some of these disorders result in greatly increased incidence of infections that may manifest early after birth and may be fatal unless the immunologic defects are corrected. Other congenital immunodeficiencies lead to mild infections and may first be detected in adult life.

Mutations in over 300 different genes have been identified as causes of primary immunodeficiencies. Predictably, most of these genes are expressed in immune cells. Some interesting features of these mutations are worth noting. First, immune deficiency is more frequently caused by mutations in X-linked genes than in autosomal genes. Because boys have only one X chromosome,

mutations in only one gene will cause the disease in boys (and girls with the mutation will be carriers but not affected because they have two X chromosomes). Autosomal recessive diseases are seen in populations in which cosanguinous marriages are common, and these are being detected more frequently now because of the widespread use of whole genome sequencing. Second, while a complete loss-of-function mutation in a gene might lead to one disease state, a hypomorphic mutation in the same gene, which only partially compromises the function of the encoded protein, may lead to a very different disease. As an example, complete loss of function mutations in *RAG1* or *RAG2*, discussed below, lead to a disorder called severe combined immunodeficiency (SCID), whereas a hypomorphic mutation in one of these genes can lead to a very different disease (called Omenn syndrome) in which autoimmunity predominates. The third interesting feature is that mutations in certain sets of genes contribute to susceptibility to specific subsets of pathogens. For example, mutations affecting Toll-like receptor 3 (TLR3) and proteins in the TLR3 signaling pathway contribute to herpes simplex virus infection of the brain (encephalitis), while mutations in interleukin-12 (IL-12) and genes related to Th1 cell development or function result in atypical mycobacterial infections.

Disease	Functional deficiencies	Mechanisms of defect
Chronic granulomatous disease	Defective production of reactive oxygen species by phagocytes; recurrent intracellular bacterial and fungal infections	Mutations in genes of phagocyte oxidase complex; phox-91 (cytochrome b_{558} α subunit) is mutated in X-linked form
Leukocyte adhesion deficiency type 1	Defective leukocyte adhesion to endothelial cells and migration into tissues linked to decreased or absent expression of $β_2$ integrins; recurrent bacterial and fungal infections	Mutations in gene encoding the β chain (CD18) of β2 integrins
Leukocyte adhesion deficiency type 2	Defective leukocyte rolling on endothelium and migration into tissues because of decreased or absent expression of leukocyte ligands for endothelial E- and P-selectins; recurrent bacterial and fungal infections	Mutations in gene encoding GDP-fucose transporter-1, required for transport of fucose into the Golgi and its incorporation into sialyl-Lewis X
Chediak-Higashi syndrome	Defective vesicle fusion and lysosomal function in neutrophils, macrophages, dendritic cells, NK cells, cytotoxic T cells, and many other cell types; recurrent infections by pyogenic bacteria	Mutations in gene encoding LYST, a protein involved in fusion of vesicles (including lysosomes)
Toll-like receptor signaling defects	Recurrent infections caused by defects in TLR signaling	Mutations in TLR3 and MyD88 compromise NF-κB activation and type I interferon production in response to microbes

Fig. 12.2 **Congenital immunodeficiencies caused by defects in innate immunity.** The figure lists immunodeficiency diseases caused by defects in various components of the innate immune system. *NF-κB*, NF-nuclear factor κB; *NK*, natural killer, *TLR*, toll-like receptors.

Mutations in complement genes encoding proteins that form the membrane attack complex contribute to *Neisseria* infections. These restricted clinical phenotypes suggest considerable redundancy in host defense mechanisms, so defects in one pathway can be compensated by other pathways, and patients are not susceptible to a wide variety of infections. Clearly the immune system has evolved numerous pathways that are often specialized for combating subsets of pathogens.

The following discussion summarizes the pathogenesis of select immunodeficiencies, several of which were mentioned in earlier chapters to illustrate the physiologic importance of various components of the immune system. Congenital deficiencies in molecules involved in self-tolerance are manifested as autoimmune diseases, as discussed in Chapter 9.

Defects in Innate Immunity

Abnormalities in two components of innate immunity, phagocytes and the complement system, are important causes of immunodeficiency (Fig. 12.2).

- **Chronic granulomatous disease** (CGD) is caused by mutations in genes encoding subunits of the enzyme phagocyte NADPH oxidase, which catalyzes the production of microbicidal reactive oxygen species in lysosomes (see Chapter 2). Affected neutrophils and macrophages are unable to kill the microbes they phagocytose. The most common infections in CGD patients are bacteria that make the enzyme catalase, as well as *Aspergillus* and *Candida* species of fungi. Catalase-producing bacteria can degrade hydrogen peroxide, which is an alternative source of free radicals that CGD leukocytes could use to kill bacteria. The

Fig. 12.3 Congenital immunodeficiencies caused by genetic defects in lymphocyte maturation. Lymphocyte maturation pathways are described in Chapter 4. Janus kinase 3 *(JAK3)* is a kinase involved in signaling by many cytokine receptors; ARTEMIS is a protein involved in antigen receptor gene recombination; Bruton tyrosine kinase *(BTK)* is a kinase that delivers signals from the pre–B cell receptor *(BCR)* and BCR; ZAP70 is a kinase involved in TCR signaling; and TAP proteins transport peptides for presentation by class I MHC molecules. *ADA,* Adenosine deaminase; *CLP,* common lymphoid progenitor; *HSC,* hematopoietic stem cell; *PNP,* purine nucleoside phosphorylase; *RAG,* recombination-activating gene; *TCR,* T cell receptor.

immune system tries to compensate for this defective microbial killing by calling in more macrophages and by activating T cells, which stimulate recruitment and activation of phagocytes. Therefore, collections of macrophages accumulate around foci of infections to try to control the infections. These collections resemble granulomas, giving rise to the name of this disease. The most common form of CGD is X-linked, caused by mutations in a subunit of the NADPH oxidase that is encoded by a gene on the X chromosome.

- **Leukocyte adhesion deficiency** is caused by mutations in genes encoding integrins, enzymes required for the expression of ligands for selectins, or signaling molecules activated by chemokine receptors that are required to activate integrins. Integrins and selectin ligands are involved in the adhesion of leukocytes to other cells. As a result of these mutations, blood leukocytes do not bind firmly to vascular endothelium and are not recruited normally to sites of infection.
- Deficiencies of almost every complement protein, and many complement regulatory proteins, have been described (see Chapter 8). C3 deficiency results in severe infections and may be fatal. Deficiencies of C2 and C4, two components of the classical pathway of complement activation, may result in increased bacterial or viral infection or increased incidence of

systemic lupus erythematosus, presumably because of defective clearance of immune complexes. Deficiencies of complement regulatory proteins lead to various syndromes associated with excessive complement activation.

- The **Chédiak-Higashi syndrome** is an immunodeficiency disease in which the lysosomal granules of leukocytes do not function normally. The immune defect affects phagocytes and natural killer (NK) cells and manifests as increased susceptibility to bacterial infection.

Rare patients have been described with mutations affecting TLRs or signaling pathways downstream of TLRs, including molecules required for activation of the nuclear factor κB (NF-κB) transcription factor. As mentioned earlier, several of these mutations make patients susceptible to only a limited set of infections. For example, mutations affecting MyD88, an adaptor protein required for signaling by most TLRs, are associated with severe bacterial (most often pneumococcal) pneumonias, and mutations affecting TLR3 are associated with recurrent herpesvirus encephalitis but apparently not other viral infections.

Defects in Lymphocyte Maturation

Many congenital immunodeficiencies are the result of genetic abnormalities that cause blocks in the

Severe combined immunodeficiency (SCID)

Disease	Functional deficiencies	Mechanism of defect
X-linked SCID	Markedly decreased T cells; normal or increased B cells; reduced serum Ig	Cytokine receptor common γ chain gene mutations, defective T cell maturation due to lack of IL-7 signals
Autosomal recessive SCID due to ADA, PNP deficiency	Progressive decrease in T and B cells (mostly T); reduced serum Ig in ADA deficiency, normal B cells and serum Ig in PNP deficiency	ADA or PNP deficiency leads to accumulation of toxic metabolites in lymphocytes
Autosomal recessive SCID due to other causes	Decreased T and B cells; reduced serum Ig	Defective maturation of T and B cells; may be mutations in *RAG* genes and other genes involved in VDJ recombination or IL-7R signaling
DiGeorge syndrome	Decreased T cells; normal B cells; normal or decreased serum Ig	Anomalous development of 3rd and 4th branchial pouches, leading to thymic hypoplasia

B cell immunodeficiencies

Disease	Functional deficiencies	Mechanism of defect
X-linked agammaglobulinemia	Decrease in all serum Ig isotypes; reduced B cell numbers	Block in maturation beyond pre-B cells, because of mutation in Bruton tyrosine kinase (BTK)
Ig heavy chain deficiencies	IgG1, IgG2, or IgG4 absent; sometimes associated with absent IgA or IgE	Chromosomal deletion involving Ig heavy-chain locus at 14q32

Fig. 12.4 Features of congenital immunodeficiencies caused by defects in lymphocyte maturation. The figure summarizes the principal features of the most common congenital immunodeficiencies in which the genetic blocks are known. *ADA,* Adenosine deaminase; *Ig,* immunoglobulin; *IL-7R,* interleukin-7 receptor; *PNP,* purine nucleoside phosphorylase; *RAG,* recombination-activating gene.

maturation of B lymphocytes, T lymphocytes, or both (Figs. 12.3 and 12.4).

Severe Combined Immunodeficiency (SCID)

Disorders manifesting as defects in both the B cell and T cell arms of the adaptive immune system are classified as SCID. The underlying cause of SCID is a defect in T cell development or function. Several different genetic abnormalities may cause SCID.
- **X-linked SCID**, affecting only male children, accounts for about half of the cases of SCID. More than 99% of these cases are caused by mutations in the common γ

(γc) chain signaling subunit of the receptors for several cytokines, including IL-2, IL-4, IL-7, IL-9, IL-15, and IL-21. (Because the γc chain was first identified as one of the three chains of the IL-2 receptor, it is also called the IL-2Rγ chain.) When the γc chain is not functional, immature lymphocytes, especially pro-T cells, cannot proliferate in response to IL-7, which is the major growth factor for these cells. Defective responses to IL-7 result in reduced survival and maturation of lymphocyte precursors. In humans, the defect affects mainly T cell maturation (whereas in mice, B cells are also reduced). The consequence of this developmental block is a profound decrease in the numbers of mature T cells, deficient cell-mediated immunity, and defective humoral immunity because of absent T cell help (even though B cells may mature almost normally). NK cells also are deficient, because the γc chain is also part of the receptor for IL-15, the major cytokine involved in NK cell proliferation and maturation. An autosomal recessive form of SCID is caused by mutations in the gene encoding a kinase called Janus kinase 3 (JAK3) that is involved in signaling by the γc cytokine receptor chain. Such mutations result in the same abnormalities as those in X-linked SCID caused by γc mutations.

- About half the cases of **autosomal recessive SCID** are caused by mutations in an enzyme called adenosine deaminase (ADA), which is involved in the breakdown of adenosine. Deficiency of ADA leads to the accumulation of toxic purine metabolites in cells that are actively synthesizing DNA—namely, proliferating cells. Lymphocytes are particularly susceptible to injury by purine metabolites because these cells undergo tremendous proliferation during their maturation. ADA deficiency results in a block in T cell maturation more than in B cell maturation; defective humoral immunity is largely a consequence of the lack of T cell helper function. A similar phenotype is seen in individuals who have a deficiency in purine nucleotide phosphorylase (PNP).

- Other, less common, causes of autosomal recessive SCID include mutations in the *RAG1* or *RAG2* gene, which encode the recombinase that is required for immunoglobulin (Ig) and T cell receptor (TCR) gene recombination and lymphocyte maturation. In the absence of RAG1 or RAG2, B and T cells fail to develop (see Chapter 4). Mutations in the Artemis gene, which encodes an endonuclease involved in VDJ recombination, also result in failure of B and T cell development.

- **DiGeorge syndrome** (also known as 22q11 syndrome) is a defect in T cell maturation. It results from a deletion on chromosome 22, which interferes with the development of the thymus (and parathyroid glands). The condition tends to improve with age, probably because the small amount of thymic tissue that does develop is able to support some T cell maturation.

With the increasing application of newborn screening to identify congenital immunodeficiencies, many other rare causes of SCID have been discovered.

Selective B Cell Deficiency

- The most common clinical syndrome caused by a block in B cell maturation is **X-linked agammaglobulinemia** (first described as Bruton agammaglobulinemia). In this disorder, pre-B cells in the bone marrow fail to expand, resulting in a marked decrease or absence of mature B lymphocytes and serum immunoglobulins. The disease is caused by mutations in the gene encoding a kinase called Bruton tyrosine kinase (BTK), resulting in defective production or function of the enzyme. The enzyme is activated by the pre-B cell receptor expressed in pre-B cells, and it delivers signals that promote the survival, proliferation, and maturation of these cells. The *BTK* gene is located on the X chromosome. Therefore, women who carry a mutant *BTK* allele on one of their X chromosomes are carriers of the disease, but male offspring who inherit the abnormal X chromosome are affected. In about a fourth of patients with X-linked agammaglobulinemia, autoimmune diseases, notably arthritis, develop as well. A link between an immunodeficiency and autoimmunity seems paradoxical. One possible explanation for this association is that BTK contributes to B cell receptor signaling and is required for B cell tolerance, so defective BTK may result in the accumulation of autoreactive B cells.

Defects in Lymphocyte Activation and Function

Numerous immunodeficiency diseases are caused by mutations affecting molecules involved in lymphocyte activation (Fig. 12.5).

Defects in B Cell Responses

Defective antibody production may result from abnormalities in B cells or in helper T cells.

- The **X-linked hyper-IgM syndrome** is characterized by defective B cell heavy-chain isotype (class) switching, so immunoglobulin M (IgM) is the major serum antibody, and by deficient cell-mediated immunity against intracellular microbes. The disease is caused by mutations in the X chromosome gene encoding CD40 ligand (CD40L), the helper T cell protein that binds to CD40 on B cells, dendritic cells, and macrophages and thus mediates T cell–dependent activation of these cells (see Chapters 6 and 7). Failure to express functional CD40L leads to defective germinal center reactions in T cell–dependent B cell responses, so there is poor humoral immunity with little Ig isotype

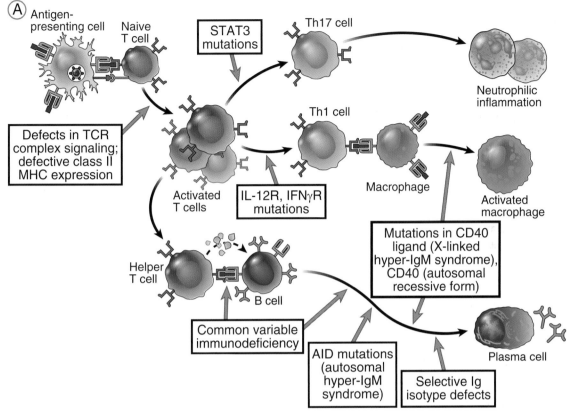

Fig. 12.5 Congenital immunodeficiencies associated with defects in lymphocyte activation and effector functions. Congenital immunodeficiencies may be caused by genetic defects in the expression of molecules required for antigen presentation to T cells, T or B lymphocyte antigen receptor signaling, helper T cell activation of B cells and macrophages, and differentiation of antibody-producing B cells. A, Examples showing the sites at which immune responses may be blocked.

switching and no affinity maturation. In addition, there is defective T cell–dependent macrophage activation in cell-mediated immunity. Boys with this disease are especially susceptible to infection by *Pneumocystis jiroveci*, a fungus that survives within phagocytes in the absence of T cell help. An autosomal recessive form of hyper-IgM syndrome with a similar phenotype to that seen in the X-linked disease is observed in individuals with mutations in CD40. Another autosomal recessive form of hyper-IgM syndrome in which there are humoral abnormalities but no defect in cellular immunity is seen in individuals with mutations affecting the enzyme activation-induced deaminase (AID), which is involved in B cell isotype switching and affinity maturation (see Chapter 7).
- Genetic deficiencies in the production of selected Ig isotypes are quite common. **IgA deficiency** is believed

to affect as many as 1 in 700 people but causes no clinical problems in most patients and sinus, lung, and intestinal infections in a minority. The defect causing these deficiencies is not known in a majority of cases; rarely, the deficiencies may be caused by mutations of Ig heavy-chain constant (C) region genes.
- **Common variable immunodeficiency** (CVID) is a heterogeneous group of disorders that are characterized by poor antibody responses to infections and reduced serum levels of IgG, IgA, and sometimes IgM. The underlying causes of CVID include defects in various genes involved in B cell maturation and activation or in T-B cell collaboration. Some patients have mutations in genes encoding receptors for B cell growth factors or costimulators that play a role in T cell–B cell interactions. Patients have recurrent infections, autoimmune disease, and lymphomas.

B

Disease	Functional deficiencies	Mechanisms of defect
X-linked hyper-IgM syndrome	Defects in helper T cell–dependent B cell and macrophage activation	Mutations in CD40 ligand
Selective Ig deficiency	Reduced or no production of selective Ig isotypes; susceptibility to infections or no clinical problem	Mutations in Ig genes or unknown mutations
Common variable immunodeficiency	Reduced immunoglobulins; susceptibility to bacterial infections	Mutations in receptors for B cell growth factors, costimulators
Defective class II MHC expression: The bare lymphocyte syndrome	Lack of class II MHC expression and impaired CD4+ T cell activation; defective cell–mediated immunity and T cell–dependent humoral immunity	Mutations in genes encoding transcription factors required for class II MHC gene expression
Defects in T cell receptor complex expression or signaling	Decreased T cells or abnormal ratios of CD4+ and CD8+ subsets; decreased cell–mediated immunity	Mutations or deletions in genes encoding CD3 proteins, ZAP-70
Defects in Th1 differentiation	Decreased T cell–mediated macrophage activation; susceptibility to infection by atypical mycobacteria and other intracellular pathogens	Mutations in genes encoding IL-12, the receptors for IL-12 or interferon-γ, STAT1
Defects in Th17 differentiation	Decreased T cell–mediated inflammatory responses; mucocutaneous candidiasis, bacterial skin abscesses	Mutations in genes encoding STAT3, IL-17, IL-17R
X-linked lymphoproliferative syndrome	Uncontrolled EBV-induced B cell proliferation and CTL activation; defective NK cell and CTL function and antibody responses	Mutations in gene encoding SAP (an adaptor protein involved in signaling in lymphocytes)

Fig. 12.5, cont'd B, This figure summarizes the features of select congenital immunodeficiency disorders. Note that abnormalities in class II MHC expression and TCR complex signaling can cause defective T cell maturation (see Fig. 12.2), as well as defective activation of the cells that do mature, as shown here. *AID,* Activation-induced deaminase; *CTL,* cytotoxic T lymphocyte; *EBV,* Epstein-Barr virus; *IFNγR,* IFN-γ receptor; *Ig,* immunoglobulin; *IL-12R,* IL-12 receptor; *MHC,* major histocompatibility complex; *NK,* natural killer; *SAP,* SLAM-associated protein; *ZAP-70,* ζ chain–associated protein of 70 kD.

Defective Activation of T Lymphocytes

A variety of inherited abnormalities may interfere with T cell activation.

- The **bare lymphocyte syndrome** is a disease caused by a failure to express class II major histocompatibility complex (MHC) molecules, as a result of mutations in the transcription factors that normally induce class II MHC expression. Recall that class II MHC molecules display peptide antigens for recognition by CD4+ T cells and this recognition is critical for maturation and activation of the T cells. The disease is manifested by a profound decrease in CD4+ T cells because of defective maturation of these cells in the thymus and poor activation of the cells in peripheral lymphoid organs.

- Rare cases of selective T cell deficiency are caused by mutations affecting various signaling pathways or cytokines and receptors involved in differentiation of naive T cells into effector cells. Depending on the mutation and the extent of the defect, affected patients show severe T cell deficiency or deficiency in particular arms of T cell–mediated immunity, such as in Th1 responses (associated with nontuberculous mycobacterial infections) and Th17 responses (associated with fungal and bacterial infections). These defects have revealed the importance of various pathways of T cell activation, but these are rare disorders.
- **Hemophagocytic lymphohistiocytosis** (HLH) syndromes are characterized by systemic, sometimes life-threatening, activation of immune cells including macrophages, usually in response to infections. Many cases of HLH occur as a manifestation of genetic disorders in which cytotoxic CD8⁺ T cells and NK cells are unable to kill virus-infected target cells. These include patients with mutations in the gene encoding perforin as well as mutations in genes that encode proteins involved in granule exocytosis. These mutations result in persistent infections, usually viral, and excessive production of IFNγ by T cells and NK cells, which in turn causes excessive macrophage activation. Some of these highly activated macrophages ingest red blood cells, giving the syndrome its name.

Lymphocyte Abnormalities Associated With Other Diseases

Some systemic diseases that involve multiple organ systems, and whose major manifestations are not immunologic, may have a component of immunodeficiency.

- **Wiskott-Aldrich syndrome** is characterized by eczema, reduced blood platelets, and immunodeficiency. This X-linked disease is caused by a mutation in a gene that encodes a protein that binds to various adaptor molecules and cytoskeletal components in hematopoietic cells. Because of the absence of this protein, platelets and leukocytes do not develop normally, are small, and fail to migrate normally.
- **Ataxia-telangiectasia** is characterized by gait abnormalities (ataxia), vascular malformations (telangiectasia), and immunodeficiency. The disease is caused by mutations in a gene whose product is involved in DNA repair. Defects in this protein lead to abnormal DNA repair (e.g., during recombination of antigen receptor gene segments), resulting in defective lymphocyte maturation.

Therapy of Congenital Immunodeficiencies

Treatment of primary immunodeficiencies varies with the disease. SCID is fatal in early life unless the patient's immune system is reconstituted. The most widely used treatment is hematopoietic stem cell transplantation, with careful matching of donor and recipient to avoid potentially serious graft-versus-host disease. For selective B cell defects, patients may be given intravenous injections of pooled immunoglobulin (IVIG) from healthy donors to provide passive immunity. IVIG replacement therapy has provided enormous benefit in patients with X-linked agammaglobulinemia. Although the ideal treatment for all congenital immunodeficiencies is to replace the defective gene, this remains a distant goal for most diseases. Successful gene therapy has been reported in patients with X-linked SCID; a normal γc gene was introduced into their bone marrow stem cells, which were then transplanted back into the patients. In all patients with these diseases, infections are treated with antibiotics as needed.

ACQUIRED (SECONDARY) IMMUNODEFICIENCIES

Deficiencies of the immune system often develop because of abnormalities that are not genetic but are acquired during life (Fig. 12.6). The most serious of these abnormalities worldwide is HIV infection, as described later. The most frequent causes of secondary immunodeficiencies in developed countries are cancers involving the bone marrow (leukemias) and immunosuppressive therapies. Cancer treatment with chemotherapeutic drugs and irradiation may damage proliferating cells, including precursors of leukocytes in the bone marrow and mature lymphocytes, resulting in immunodeficiency. Immunosuppressive drugs used to prevent graft rejection or treat inflammatory diseases, including some of the newer therapies (e.g., cytokine antagonists, leukocyte adhesion molecule blockers), are designed to blunt immune responses. Therefore, immunodeficiency is a complication of such therapies. Protein-calorie malnutrition results in deficiencies of virtually all components of the immune system and is a common cause of immunodeficiency in countries with widespread poverty or famines.

ACQUIRED IMMUNODEFICIENCY SYNDROME

Although AIDS was first recognized as a distinct entity in the 1980s, it has become one of the most devastating

Cause	Mechanism
Human immunodeficiency virus infection	Depletion of CD4+ helper T cells
Irradiation and chemotherapy treatments for cancer	Decreased bone marrow precursors for all leukocytes
Immunosuppression for graft rejection and inflammatory diseases	Depletion or functional impairment of lymphocytes
Involvement of bone marrow by cancers (metastases, leukemias)	Reduced site of leukocyte development
Protein-calorie malnutrition	Metabolic derangements inhibit lymphocyte maturation and function
Removal of spleen	Decreased phagocytosis of microbes

Fig. 12.6 Acquired (secondary) immunodeficiency. The figure lists the most common causes of acquired immunodeficiency diseases and how they lead to defects in immune responses.

afflictions in history. AIDS is caused by infection with HIV. Of the estimated 37 million HIV-infected people worldwide, about 70% are in Africa and 20% in Asia. More than 35 million deaths are attributable to HIV/AIDS, with over 1 million deaths annually. Effective antiretroviral drugs have been developed, but the infection continues to spread in parts of the world where these therapies are not widely available, and in some African countries, more than 30% of the population has HIV infection. This section describes the important features of HIV, how it infects humans, and the disease it causes, ending with a brief discussion of the current status of therapy and vaccine development.

Human Immunodeficiency Virus

HIV is a retrovirus that infects cells of the immune system, mainly CD4+ T lymphocytes, and causes progressive destruction of these cells. An infectious HIV particle consists of two RNA strands within a protein core, surrounded by a lipid envelope derived from infected host cells but containing viral proteins (Fig. 12.7). The viral RNA encodes structural proteins, various enzymes, and proteins that regulate transcription of viral genes and the viral life cycle.

The life cycle of HIV consists of the following sequential steps: infection of cells, production of a DNA copy of viral RNA and its integration into the host genome, expression of viral genes, and production of viral particles (Fig. 12.8). HIV infects cells by virtue of its major envelope glycoprotein, called gp120 (for 120-kD glycoprotein), which binds to CD4 and to particular chemokine receptors on human cells (mainly CXCR4 and CCR5). The major cell types that express these surface molecules and thus may be infected by HIV are CD4+ T lymphocytes; additionally, macrophages and dendritic cells may acquire the virus mainly by phagocytosis. After binding to cellular receptors, the viral membrane fuses with the host cell membrane, and the virus enters the cell's cytoplasm. Here the virus is uncoated by viral protease, and its RNA is released. A DNA copy of the viral RNA is synthesized by the viral reverse transcriptase enzyme (a process characteristic of all retroviruses), and the DNA integrates into the host cell's DNA by the action of the integrase enzyme. The integrated viral DNA is called a provirus. If the infected T cell is activated by some extrinsic stimulus, such as another infectious microbe or cytokines, the cell responds by turning on the transcription of many of its own genes and often by producing cytokines itself. A negative consequence

Fig. 12.7 Structure and genes of the human immunodeficiency virus (HIV). **A,** An HIV-1 virion is shown next to a T cell surface. HIV-1 consists of two identical strands of RNA (the viral genome) and associated enzymes, including reverse transcriptase, integrase, and protease, packaged in a cone-shaped core composed of the p24 capsid protein with a surrounding p17 protein matrix, all surrounded by a phospholipid membrane envelope derived from the host cell. Virally encoded envelope proteins (gp41 and gp120) bind to CD4 and chemokine receptors on the host cell surface. **B,** The HIV-1 genome consists of genes whose positions are indicated here as different-colored blocks. Some genes contain sequences that overlap with sequences of other genes, as shown by overlapping blocks, but are read differently by host cell RNA polymerase. Similarly shaded blocks separated by lines (*tat, rev*) indicate genes whose coding sequences are separated in the genome and require RNA splicing to produce functional messenger RNA. The major functions of the proteins encoded by different viral genes are listed. *MHC*, Major histocompatibility complex. (**A,** Modified from front cover, The new face of AIDS. *Science* 272:1841–2102, 1996. Copyright Terese Winslow. **B,** Modified from Greene WC: *AIDS and the immune system.* Copyright 1993 by Scientific American, Inc. All rights reserved.)

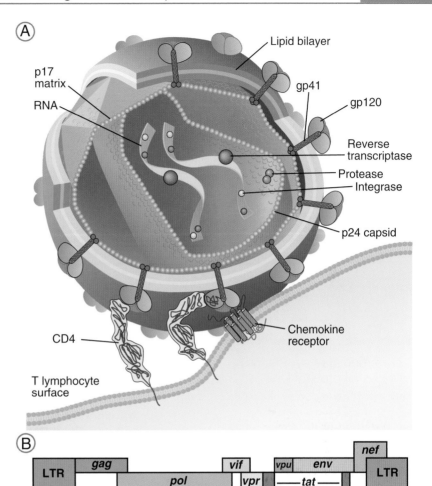

LTR Long terminal repeat: Integration of viral DNA into host genome; binding site for transcription factors

gag Pr55gag: Nuclear import of viral DNA

pol Polymerase: Encodes a variety of viral enzymes

vif Viral infectivity factor (p23): Overcomes inhibitory effects of host cell factors

vpr Viral protein R (p15): Promotes infection of macrophages by regulating nuclear import of HIV preintegration complex

tat Transcriptional activator (p14): Promotes cell cycle arrest and enhances integrated viral DNA transcription

rev Regulator of viral gene expression (p19): Inhibits viral RNA splicing and promotes export of incompletely spliced viral RNA

vpu Viral protein U: Promotes CD4 degradation and influences virion release

env Envelope protein gp160: Cleaved into gp120, which mediates CD4 and chemokine receptor binding, and gp41, which mediates fusion

nef Negative effector: Promotes downregulation of surface CD4 and class I MHC expression; blocks apoptosis; enhances virion infectivity

Fig. 12.8 Life cycle of human immunodeficiency virus (HIV). The sequential steps in HIV reproduction are shown, from initial infection of a host cell to release of new virus particles (virions).

of this normal protective response is that the cytokines, and the process of cellular activation, may activate the provirus, leading to production of viral RNAs and then proteins. The virus is then able to form a core structure, which migrates to the cell membrane, acquires a lipid envelope from the host, and is shed as an infectious viral particle, ready to infect another cell. The integrated HIV DNA provirus may remain latent within infected cells for months or years, hidden from the patient's immune system (and even from antiviral therapies, discussed later).

It is believed that macrophages and follicular helper T cells are important reservoirs for the virus.

Most cases of AIDS are caused by HIV-1 (i.e., HIV type 1). A related virus, HIV-2, causes some cases of the disease.

Pathogenesis of AIDS

AIDS develops over many years as latent HIV becomes activated and destroys cells of the immune system. Virus production leads to death of infected cells, as well as to death of uninfected lymphocytes, subsequent

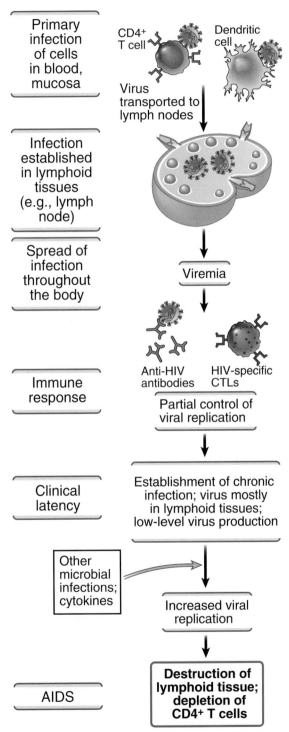

Fig. 12.9 Pathogenesis of disease caused by human immunodeficiency virus (HIV). The development of HIV disease is associated with the spread of HIV from the initial site of infection to lymphoid tissues throughout the body. The immune response of the host temporarily controls acute infection but does not prevent establishment of chronic infection of cells in lymphoid tissues. Cytokines produced in response to HIV and other microbes serve to enhance HIV production and progression to acquired immunodeficiency syndrome (AIDS). *CTLs*, Cytotoxic T lymphocytes.

immune deficiencies, and clinical AIDS (Fig. 12.9). HIV infection is acquired by sexual intercourse, sharing contaminated needles used by intravenous drug users, transplacental transfer, or transfusion of infected blood or blood products. After infection there may be a brief acute viremia, when the virus is detected in the blood, and the host may respond as in any mild viral infection and present with nonspecific symptoms such as fever, body aches, and malaise. The virus primarily infects CD4$^+$ T cells at sites of entry through mucosal epithelia, in lymphoid organs such as lymph nodes, and in the circulation. In mucosal tissues at the sites of entry, there may be considerable destruction of infected T cells. Because a large fraction of the body's lymphocytes, and especially memory T cells, reside in these tissues, the result of the local destruction may be a significant functional deficit that is not reflected in the presence of infected cells in the blood or the depletion of circulating T cells. Dendritic cells may capture the virus as it enters through mucosal epithelia and transport it to peripheral lymphoid organs, where it infects T cells. The integrated provirus may be activated in infected cells, as described previously, leading to production of viral particles and spread of the infection. During the course of HIV infection, the major source of infectious viral particles is activated CD4$^+$ T cells. As mentioned earlier, follicular helper T cells and macrophages may become reservoirs of infection, wherein the virus may lie dormant and be reactivated months or years later.

The depletion of CD4$^+$ T cells after HIV infection is caused by a cytopathic effect of the virus resulting from production of viral particles in infected cells, as well as death of uninfected cells. Active viral gene expression and protein production may interfere with the synthetic machinery of the infected T cells. Therefore, T cells in which the virus is replicating are killed during this process. The number of T cells lost during the progression to AIDS appears to be greater than the number of infected cells. The mechanism of this T cell loss remains poorly defined.

Other infected cells, such as dendritic cells and macrophages, may also die, resulting in destruction of the architecture of lymphoid organs. Many studies have suggested that immune deficiency results not only from depletion of T cells but also from various functional abnormalities in T lymphocytes and other immune cells (dendritic cells and macrophages). The significance of these functional defects has not been established, however, and loss of T cells (followed by a fall in the blood

CD4$^+$ T cell count) remains the most reliable indicator of disease progression.

Clinical Features of HIV Infection and AIDS

The clinical course of HIV infection is characterized by several phases, culminating in immune deficiency (Fig. 12.10A).

- **Acute HIV syndrome.** Early after HIV infection, patients may experience a mild acute illness with fever and malaise, correlating with the initial viremia. This illness subsides within a few days, and the disease enters a period of clinical latency.
- **Latency.** During latency, there may be few clinical problems, but there usually is a progressive loss of CD4$^+$ T cells in lymphoid tissues and destruction of the architecture of these tissues. Eventually, the blood CD4$^+$ T cell count begins to decline, and when the count falls below 200 cells/mm^3 (normal level about 1500 cells/mm^3), patients become susceptible to infections and are diagnosed as having AIDS.
- **Clinical AIDS. AIDS ultimately causes increased susceptibility to infections and some cancers, as a consequence of immune deficiency.** Patients not given antiretroviral drugs often are infected by intracellular microbes, such as viruses, the fungal pathogen *Pneumocystis jiroveci*, and nontuberculous mycobacteria, all of which normally are combated by T cell–mediated immunity. Many of these microbes are present in the environment, but they do not infect healthy persons with intact immune systems. Because these infections are seen in immunodeficient persons, in whom the microbes have an opportunity to establish infection, these types of infections are said to be opportunistic. Reactivation of latent viruses, such as cytomegalovirus and Epstein-Barr virus (EBV), may also occur because patients with AIDS show defective cytotoxic T lymphocyte (CTL) responses to viruses. Even though HIV does not infect CD8$^+$ T cells, the CTL responses are defective probably because CD4$^+$ helper T cells (the main targets of HIV) are required for full CD8$^+$ CTL responses against many viruses (see Chapters 5 and 6). Latent viruses, which are normally kept in check by CTL responses, become reactivated in AIDS patients and cause severe disease. AIDS patients are at increased risk for infections by extracellular bacteria, probably because of impaired helper T cell–dependent antibody responses to bacterial antigens. Patients also become susceptible to cancers caused by

Fig. 12.10 Clinical course of human immunodeficiency virus (HIV) disease. **A,** Blood-borne virus (plasma viremia) is detected early after infection and may be accompanied by systemic symptoms typical of acute HIV syndrome. The virus spreads to lymphoid organs, but plasma viremia falls to very low levels (detectable only by sensitive reverse transcriptase–polymerase chain reaction assays) and stays this way for many years. CD4+ T cell counts steadily decline during this clinical latency period because of active viral replication and T cell destruction in lymphoid tissues. As the level of CD4+ T cells falls, there is increasing risk of infection and other clinical components of acquired immunodeficiency syndrome. **B,** Magnitude and kinetics of immune responses, shown in arbitrary relative units. *CTLs,* Cytotoxic T lymphocytes. (Reproduced with permission from Pantaleo G, Graziosi C, Fauci AS: The immunopathogenesis of human immunodeficiency virus infection, *New England Journal of Medicine* 328:327–335, 1993.)

oncogenic viruses. The two most common types of cancers are B cell lymphomas, caused by EBV, and a tumor of small blood vessels called Kaposi sarcoma, caused by a herpesvirus. Patients with advanced AIDS often have a wasting syndrome with significant loss of body mass, caused by altered metabolism and reduced caloric intake. The dementia that develops in some patients with AIDS is likely caused by infection of macrophages (microglial cells) in the brain.

The clinical course of HIV infection has been dramatically changed by effective antiretroviral drug therapy. With appropriate treatment, patients exhibit much slower progression of the disease, fewer opportunistic infections, and greatly reduced incidence of cancers and dementia.

The immune response to HIV is ineffective in controlling spread of the virus and its pathologic effects. Infected patients produce antibodies and CTLs against viral antigens, and the responses help limit the early, acute HIV syndrome (see Fig. 12.10B). But these immune responses usually do not prevent progression of the disease. Antibodies against envelope glycoproteins, such as gp120, may be ineffective because the virus rapidly mutates the region of gp120 that is the target of

most antibodies. CTLs often are ineffective in killing infected cells because the virus inhibits the expression of class I MHC molecules by the infected cells. Immune responses to HIV may paradoxically promote spread of the infection. Antibody-coated viral particles may bind to Fc receptors on macrophages and follicular dendritic cells in lymphoid organs, thus increasing virus entry into these cells and creating additional reservoirs of infection. If CTLs are able to kill infected cells, the dead cells may be cleared by macrophages, which can migrate to other tissues and spread the infection. By infecting and thus interfering with the function of immune cells, the virus is able to prevent its own eradication.

A small fraction of patients control HIV infection without therapy; these individuals are often referred to as elite controllers or long-term nonprogressors. There has been great interest in defining the genes that may protect these individuals, because elucidation of these genes may suggest therapeutic approaches. The presence of certain HLA alleles, such as HLA-B57 and HLA-B27, seems to be protective, perhaps because these HLA molecules are particularly efficient at presenting HIV peptides to CD8+ T cells. In addition, a 32 base pair deletion in the CCR5 gene is a known polymorphism, especially in Northern Europeans. Rare individuals with a homozygous form of this polymorphism lack functional CCR5, rendering these individuals completely resistant to HIV infection.

Therapy and Vaccination Strategies

The current treatment for AIDS is aimed at controlling replication of HIV and the infectious complications of the disease. Combinations of drugs that block the activity of the viral reverse transcriptase, protease, and integrase enzymes are now being administered early in the course of the infection. This therapeutic approach is called combination antiretroviral therapy (ART). In societies with widely available ART therapy, opportunistic infections (e.g., by Pneumocystis) and some tumors (e.g., Kaposi sarcoma, EBV-induced lymphoma), which were devastating complications in the past, are now rarely seen in AIDS patients. In fact, treated patients are living quite long life spans and are dying of cardiovascular and other diseases that also afflict individuals who age without HIV (although they may be accelerated as a consequence of HIV infection, for unknown reasons). Even these highly effective drugs do not completely eradicate HIV infection. The virus is capable of mutating its genes, which may render it resistant to the drugs used, and reservoirs of latent virus (e.g., in lymphoid tissues) may be inaccessible to these drugs. For patients resistant to the older antiviral drugs, agents that inhibit virus entry and fusion have been developed.

The development of effective vaccines will likely be necessary for control of HIV infection worldwide. A successful vaccine probably needs to induce high titers of broadly neutralizing antibodies that can recognize a wide range of virus isolates and a strong T cell response, as well as mucosal immunity. It has proved difficult to achieve all these goals with current vaccination strategies. The tremendous mutability of the virus allows it to mutate away from most neutralizing antibodies; the goal of current vaccination attempts is to create immunogens that can elicit broadly neutralizing antibodies. This goal has not as yet been met and so far, vaccine trials for HIV have proved disappointing.

◼ SUMMARY

- Immunodeficiency diseases are caused by defects in various components of the immune system that result in increased susceptibility to infections and some cancers. Congenital (primary) immunodeficiency diseases are caused by genetic abnormalities. Acquired (secondary) immunodeficiencies are the result of infections, cancers, malnutrition, or treatments for other conditions that adversely affect the cells of the immune system.

- SCID results from blocks in lymphocyte maturation. It may be caused by mutations in the cytokine receptor γc chain that reduce the IL-7–driven proliferation of immature lymphocytes, by mutations in enzymes involved in purine metabolism, or by other defects in lymphocyte maturation.

- Selective B cell maturation defects are seen in X-linked agammaglobulinemia, caused by abnormalities in an enzyme involved in B cell maturation (BTK), and selective T cell maturation defects are seen in the DiGeorge syndrome, in which the thymus does not develop normally.

- Some immunodeficiency diseases are caused by defects in lymphocyte activation. The X-linked hyper-IgM syndrome is caused by mutations in the gene encoding CD40 ligand, resulting in defective helper T cell–dependent B cell responses (e.g., Ig heavy chain class switching) and T cell–dependent macrophage activation. The bare lymphocyte syndrome is caused by reduced expression of class II MHC proteins, resulting in impaired maturation and activation of CD4+ T cells.

- AIDS is caused by the retrovirus HIV, which infects CD4+ T cells, macrophages, and dendritic cells by using an envelope protein (gp120) to bind to CD4 and chemokine receptors. The viral RNA is reverse transcribed, and the resulting DNA integrates into the host genome, where it may be activated to produce infectious virus. Infected cells die during this process of virus replication, and death of cells of the immune system is the principal mechanism by which the virus causes immune deficiency.

- The clinical course of HIV infection typically consists of acute viremia, clinical latency with progressive destruction of CD4+ T cells and dissolution of lymphoid tissues, and ultimately AIDS, with severe immunodeficiency resulting in opportunistic infections, some cancers, weight loss, and occasionally dementia. Treatment of HIV infection is designed to interfere with the life cycle of the virus. Vaccine development is ongoing.

REVIEW QUESTIONS

1. What are the most common clinicopathologic manifestations of immunodeficiency diseases?
2. What are some of the proteins affected by mutations that may block the maturation of T and B lymphocytes in human immunodeficiency diseases?
3. What are some of the mutations that may block activation or effector functions of both mature CD4+ T cells and B cells, and what are the clinicopathologic consequences of these mutations?
4. How does HIV infect cells and replicate inside infected cells?
5. What are the principal clinical manifestations of advanced HIV infection, and what is the pathogenesis of these manifestations?

Answers to and discussion of the Review Questions are available at Student Consult.

SELECTED READINGS

The references listed below are a guide for students interested in learning about particular areas of immunology in depth. The reference list is not intended to be comprehensive or complete in terms of topics and authors.

CHAPTER 1

General Introduction and Foundations of Immunology

Burnet FM: A modification of Jerne's theory of antibody production using the concept of clonal selection, *Australian Journal of Science* 20:67–69, 1957.

Jerne NK: The natural-selection theory of antibody formation, *Proceedings of the National Academy of Sciences of the United States of America* 41:849–857, 1955.

Silverstein AM: *Paul Ehrlich's receptor immunology: the magnificent obsession*, New York, 2001, Academic Press.

Lymphocytes: Life History and Functions

Roederer M, Quaye L, Mangino M, et al.: The genetic architecture of the human immune system: a bioresource for autoimmunity and disease pathogenesis, *Cell* 161:387–403, 2015.

Surh CD, Sprent J: Homeostasis of naive and memory T cells, *Immunity* 29:848–862, 2008.

Cells and Tissues of the Immune System

Boehm T: Thymus development and function, *Current Opinion in Immunology* 20:178–184, 2008.

Bronte V, Pittet MJ: The spleen in local and systemic regulation of immunity, *Immunity* 39:806–818, 2013.

Lymphocyte Migration

Masopust D, Schenkel JM: The integration of T cell migration, differentiation and function, *Nature Reviews Immunology* 13:309–320, 2013.

CHAPTER 2

Pattern Recognition Receptors and Their Ligands

Blasius AL, Beutler B: Intracellular toll-like receptors, *Immunity* 32:305–315, 2010.

Broz P, Dixit V: Inflammasomes: mechanisms of assembly, regulation and signaling, *Nature Reviews Immunology* 16:407–420, 2016.

Brubaker SW, Bonham KS, Zanoni I, Kagan JC: Innate immune pattern recognition: a cell biological perspective, *Annual Review of Immunology* 33:257–290, 2015.

Chen G, Shaw MH, Kim YG, Nuñez G: Nod-like receptors: role in innate immunity and inflammatory disease, *Annual Review of Pathology* 4:365–398, 2009.

Chen Q, Sun L, Chen ZJ: Regulation and function of the cGAS-STING pathway of cytosolic DNA sensing, *Nature Immunology* 17:1142–1149, 2016.

Pandey S, Kawai T, Akira S: Microbial sensing by Toll-like receptors and intracellular nucleic acid sensors, *Cold Spring Harbor Perspectives in Biology* 7, 2014:a016246.

Yin Q, Fu T-M, Li J, Wu H: Structural biology of innate immunity, *Annual Review of Immunology* 33:393–416, 2015.

Cells of the Innate Immune System

Colonna M: Innate Lymphoid cells: diversity, plasticity, and unique functions in immunity, *Immunity* 48:1104–1117, 2018.

Flannagan RS, Jaumouille V, Grinstein S: The cell biology of phagocytosis, *Annual Review of Pathology: Mechanisms of Disease* 7:61–98, 2012.

Ginhoux F, Guilliams M: Tissue-resident macrophage ontogeny and homeostasis, *Immunity* 44:439–449, 2016.

Gordon S: Phagocytosis: an immunobiologic process, *Immunity* 44:463–475, 2016.

Klose CSN, Artis D: Innate lymphoid cells as regulators of immunity, inflammation and tissue homeostasis, *Nature Immunology* 17:765–774, 2016.

Lanier LL: NK cell recognition, *Annual Review of Immunology* 23:225–274, 2005.

Nicolas-Avila JA, Adrover JM, Hidalgo A: Neutrophils in homeostasis, immunity and cancer, *Immunity* 46:15–28, 2017.

Selsted ME, Ouellette AJ: Mammalian defensins in the anti-microbial immune response, *Nature Immunology* 6:551–557, 2005.

Varol C, Mildner A, Jung S: Macrophages: development and tissue specialization, *Annual Review of Immunology* 33:643–675, 2015.

Vivier E, Artis D, Colonna M, et al.: Innate lymphoid cells: 10 years on. *Cell* 174:1054–1066, 2018.

Vivier E, Tomasello E, Baratin M, et al.: Functions of natural killer cells, *Nature Immunology* 9:503–510, 2008.

Acute Inflammation

Ley K, Laudanna C, Cybulsky MI, et al.: Getting to the site of inflammation: the leukocyte adhesion cascade updated, *Nature Reviews Immunology* 7:678–689, 2007.

Rock KL, Latz E, Ontiveros F, et al.: The sterile inflammatory response, *Annual Review of Immunology* 28:321–342, 2010.

Sokol CL, Luster AD: The chemokine system in innate immunity, *Cold Spring Harbor Perspectives in Biology* 7:1–18, 2015.

Zlotnik A, Yoshie O: The chemokine superfamily revisited, *Immunity* 36:705–716, 2012.

Antiviral Innate Immunity

Klotman ME, Chang TL: Defensins in innate antiviral immunity, *Nature Reviews Immunology* 6:447–456, 2006.

Pichlmair A, Reis e Sousa C: Innate recognition of viruses, *Immunity* 27:370–383, 2007.

Other Functions of Innate Immunity

Iwasaki A, Medzhitov R: Control of adaptive immunity by the innate immune system, *Nature Immunology* 16:343–353, 2015.

Diseases of Innate Immunity

Angus DC, van der Poll T: Severe sepsis and septic shock, *New England Journal of Medicine* 369:840–851, 2013.

Manthiram K, Zhou Q, Aksentijevich I, Kastner DL: The monogenic autoinflammatory diseases define new pathways in human innate immunity and inflammation, *Nature Immunology* 18:832–842, 2017.

CHAPTER 3

Dendritic Cells in Antigen Capture and Presentation

Anderson DA, Murphy KM, Briseneo CG: Development, diversity, and function of dendritic cells in mouse and human, *Cold Spring Harbor Perspectives in Biology Sept* 27:a028613, 2017.

Bousso P: T-cell activation by dendritic cells in the lymph node: lessons from the movies, *Nature Reviews Immunology* 8:675–684, 2008.

Collin M, McGovern N, Haniffa M: Human dendritic cell subsets, *Immunology* 140:22–30, 2013.

Merad M, Sathe P, Helft J, et al.: The dendritic cell lineage: ontogeny and function of dendritic cells and their subsets in the steady state and inflamed setting, *Annual Review of Immunology* 31:563–604, 2013.

Mildner A, Jung S: Development and function of dendritic cell subsets, *Immunity* 40:642–645, 2014.

Murphy TL, Grajales-Reyes GE, Wu X, et al.: Transcriptional control of dendritic cell development, *Annual Review Immunology* 34:93–119, 2016.

Shortman K, Sathe P, Vremec D, et al.: Plasmacytoid dendritic cell development, *Advances in Immunology* 120:105–126, 2013.

Structure of MHC Genes, MHC Molecules, and Peptide-MHC Complexes

Bjorkman PJ, Saper MA, Samraoui B, et al.: Structure of the human class I histocompatibility antigen HLA-A2, *Nature* 329:506–512, 1987.

Horton R, Wilming L, Rand V, et al.: Gene map of the extended human MHC, *Nature Reviews Genetics* 5:889–899, 2004.

Kaufman J: Unfinished business: evolution of the MHC and the adaptive immune system of jawed vertebrates, *Annual Review of Immunology* 36:383–409, 2018.

Protein Antigen Processing and MHC-Associated Presentation of Peptide Antigens

Basler M, Kirk CJ, Groettrup M: The immunoproteasome in antigen processing and other immunological functions, *Current Opinion in Immunology* 25:74–80, 2013.

Blum JS, Wearsch PA, Cresswell P: Pathways of antigen processing, *Annual Review of Immunology* 31:443–473, 2013.

Roche PA, Furuta K: The ins and outs of MHC class II–mediated antigen processing and presentation, *Nature Reviews Immunology* 15:203–216, 2015.

van de Weijer ML, Luteijn RD, Wiertz EJ: Viral immune evasion: lessons in MHC class I antigen presentation, *Seminars in Immunology* 27:125–137, 2015.

Cross-Presentation

Blander JM: Regulation of the cell biology of antigen cross-presentation, *Annual Review of Immunology* 36:717–753, 2018.

Cruz FM, Colbert JD, Merino E, et al.: The biology and underlying mechanisms of cross-presentation of exogenous antigens on MHC-I molecules, *Annual Review of Immunology* 35:149–176, 2017.

Schuette V, Burgdorf S: The ins-and-outs of endosomal antigens for cross-presentation, *Current Opinion in Immunology* 26:63–68, 2014.

Non-Classical Antigen Presentation

Adams EJ, Luoma AM: The adaptable major histocompatibility complex (MHC) fold: structure and function of non-classical and MHC class I–like molecules, *Annual Review of Immunology* 31:529–561, 2013.

Cohen NR, Garg S, Brenner MB: Antigen presentation by CD1: lipids, T cells, and NKT cells in microbial immunity, *Advances in Immunology* 102:1–94, 2009.

CHAPTER 4

Structure and Function of Antibodies

Corti D, Lanzavecchia A: Broadly neutralizing antiviral antibodies, *Annual Review of Immunology* 31:705–742, 2013.

Fagarasan S: Evolution, development, mechanism and function of IgA in the gut, *Current Opinion in Immunology* 20:170–177, 2008.

Law M, Hengartner L: Antibodies against viruses: passive and active immunization, *Current Opinion in Immunology* 20:486–492, 2008.

Structure and Function of the T Cell Receptor for Antigen

Klein L, Hinterberger M, Wirnsberger G, et al.: Antigen presentation in the thymus for positive selection and central tolerance induction, *Nature Reviews Immunology* 9:833–844, 2009.

Kuhns MS, Davis MM, Garcia KC: Deconstructing the form and function of the TCR/CD3 complex, *Immunity* 24:133–139, 2006.

Rossjohn J, Gras S, Miles JJ, et al.: T cell antigen receptor recognition of antigen-presenting molecules, *Annual Review of Immunology* 33:169–200, 2015.

Rudolph MG, Stanfield RL, Wilson IA: How TCRs bind MHCs, peptides, and coreceptors, *Annual Review of Immunology* 24:419–466, 2006.

B and T Lymphocyte Development

Boehm T, Swann JB: Origin and evolution of adaptive immunity, *Annual Review of Animal Bioscience* 2:259–283, 2014.

Klein L, Kyewski B, Allen PM, et al.: Positive and negative selection of the T cell repertoire: what thymocytes see (and don't see), *Nature Reviews Immunology* 14:377–391, 2014.

Lo WL, Allen PM: Self-peptides in TCR repertoire selection and peripheral T cell function, *Current Topics in Microbiology and Immunology* 373:49–67, 2014.

Reth M, Nielsen P: Signaling circuits in early B-cell development, *Advances in Immunology* 122:129–175, 2014.

Stritesky GL, Jameson SC, Hogquist K: Selection of self-reactive T cells in the thymus, *Annual Review of Immunology* 30:95–114, 2012.

Taniuchi I, Ellmeier W: Transcriptional and epigenetic regulation of CD4/CD8 lineage choice, *Advances in Immunology* 110:71–110, 2011.

CHAPTER 5

T Cell Antigen Recognition and Costimulation

Chen L, Flies DB: Molecular mechanisms of T cell co-stimulation and co-inhibition, *Nature Reviews Immunology* 13:227–242, 2013.

Esensten JH, Helou YA, Chopra G, Weiss A, Bluestone JA: CD28 costimulation: from mechanism to therapy, *Immunity* 44:973–988, 2016.

Fooksman DR, Vardhana S, Vasiliver-Shamis G, et al.: Functional anatomy of T cell activation and synapse formation, *Annual Review of Immunology* 28:79–105, 2010.

Huppa JB, Davis MM: The interdisciplinary science of T-cell recognition, *Advances in Immunology* 119:1–50, 2013.

Malissen B, Bongrand P: Early T cell activation: integrating biochemical, structural, and biophysical cues, *Annual Review of Immunology* 33:539–561, 2015.

Biochemical Signals in T Cell Activation

Chakraborty A, Weiss A: Insights into the initiation of TCR signaling, *Nature Immunology* 15:798–807, 2014.

Gallo EM, Cante-Barrett K, Crabtree GR: Lymphocyte calcium signaling from membrane to nucleus, *Nature Immunology* 7:25–32, 2006.

Malissen B, Gregoire C, Malissen M, et al.: Integrative biology of T cell activation, *Nature Immunology* 15:790–797, 2014.

Functional Responses to T Cell Activation

Boyman O, Sprent J: The role of interleukin-2 during homeostasis and activation of the immune system, *Nature Reviews Immunology* 12:180–190, 2012.

Kumar BV, Connore TJ, Farber DL: Human T cell development, localization, and function throughout life, *Immunity* 48:202–213, 2018.

Zhu J, Yamane H, Paul WE: Differentiation of effector CD4 T cell populations, *Annual Review of Immunology* 28:445–489, 2010.

Memory T Cells

Farber DL, Netea MG, Radbruch A, Rajewsky K, Zinkernagel RM: Immunological memory: lessons from the past and a look to the future, *Nature Reviews Immunology* 16:124–128, 2016.

Mueller SN, Mackay LK: Tissue-resident memory T cells: local specialists in immune defence, *Nature Reviews Immunology* 16:79–89, 2016.

Pepper M, Jenkins MK: Origin of CD4+ effector and central memory T cells, *Nature Immunology* 12:467–471, 2011.

Sallusto F, Lanzavecchia A: Heterogeneity of CD4+ memory T cells: functional modules for tailored immunity, *European Journal of Immunology* 39:2076–2082, 2009.

Sprent J, Surh CD: Normal T cell homeostasis: the conversion of naive cells into memory-phenotype cells, *Nature Immunology* 12:478–484, 2011.

T Cell Migration

Bajénoff M, Egen JG, Qi H, et al.: Highways, byways and breadcrumbs: directing lymphocyte traffic in the lymph node, *Trends in Immunology* 28:346–352, 2007.

Bromley SK, Mempel TR, Luster AD: Orchestrating the orchestrators: chemokines in control of T cell traffic, *Nature Immunology* 9:970–980, 2008.

Masopust D, Schenkel JM: The integration of T cell migration, differentiation and function, *Nature Reviews Immunology* 13:309–320, 2013.

CHAPTER 6

CD4⁺ Helper T Cell Subsets

Annunziato F, Romagnani S: Heterogeneity of human effector CD4+ T cells, *Arthritis Research and Therapy* 11:257–264, 2009.

Gordon S, Martinez FO: Alternative activation of macrophages: mechanisms and functions, *Immunity* 32:593–604, 2010.

Kanno Y, Golnaz V, Hirahara K, et al.: Transcriptional and epigenetic control of T helper cell specification: molecular mechanisms underlying commitment and plasticity, *Annual Review of Immunology* 30:707–731, 2012.

Korn T, Bettelli E, Oukka M, et al.: IL-17 and TH17 cells, *Annual Review of Immunology* 27:485–517, 2009.

Murphy KM, Stockinger B: Effector T cell plasticity: flexibility in the face of changing circumstances, *Nature Immunology* 11:674–680, 2010.

O'Shea JJ, Paul WE: Mechanisms underlying lineage commitment and plasticity of helper CD4+ T cells, *Science* 327:1098–1102, 2010.

Pulendran B, Artis D: New paradigms in type 2 immunity, *Science* 337:431–435, 2012.

Stockinger B, Omenetti S: The dichotomous nature of T helper 17 cells, *Nature Reviews Immunology* 17:535–544, 2017.

Van Dyken SJ, Locksley RM: Interleukin-4- and interleukin-13-mediated alternatively activated macrophages: roles in homeostasi and disease, *Annual Review of Immunology* 31:317–343, 2013.

Walker JA, McKenzie ANJ: Th2 cell development and function, *Nature Reviews Immunology* 18:121–133, 2018.

Zhu J, Yamane H, Paul WE: Differentiation of effector CD4 T cell populations, *Annual Review of Immunology* 28:445–489, 2010.

CD8⁺ Cytotoxic T Lymphocytes

Kaech SM, Cui W: Transcriptional control of effector and memory CD8+ T cell differentiation, *Nature Reviews Immunology* 12:749–761, 2012.

Williams MA, Bevan MJ: Effector and memory CTL differentiation, *Annual Review of Immunology* 25:171–192, 2007.

Zhang N, Bevan MJ: CD8(+) T cells: foot soldiers of the immune system, *Immunity* 35:161–168, 2011.

CHAPTER 7

Helper T Cell–Dependent Antibody Responses

Gonzalez SF, Degn SE, Pitcher LA, et al.: Trafficking of B cell antigen in lymph nodes, *Annual Review of Immunology* 29:215–233, 2011.

Goodnow CC, Vinuesa CG, Randall KL, et al.: Control systems and decision making for antibody production, *Nature Immunology* 11:681–688, 2010.

Heesters BA, Myers RC, Carroll MC: Follicular dendritic cells: dynamic antigen libraries, *Nature Reviews Immunology* 14:495–504, 2014.

McHeyzer-Williams M, Okitsu S, Wang N, et al.: Molecular programming of B cell memory, *Nature Reviews Immunology* 12:24–34, 2012.

Mesin L, Ersching J, Victora GD: Germinal center B cell dynamics, *Immunity* 45:471–482, 2016.

Nutt SL, Hodgkin PD, Tarlinton DM, et al.: The generation of antibody-secreting plasma cells, *Nature Reviews Immunology* 15:160–171, 2015.

Peled JU, Kuang FL, Iglesias-Ussel MD, et al.: The biochemistry of somatic hypermutation, *Annual Review of Immunology* 26:481–511, 2008.

Stavnezer J, Schrader CE: IgH chain class switch recombination: mechanism and regulation, *Journal of Immunology* 193:5370–5378, 2014.

Takemori T, Kaji T, Takahashi Y, et al.: Generation of memory B cells inside and outside germinal centers, *European Journal of Immunology* 44:1258–1264, 2014.

Ueno H, Banchereau J, Vinuesa CG: Pathophysiology of T follicular helper cells in humans and mice, *Nature Immunology* 16:142–152, 2015.

Vinuesa CG, Linterman MA, Yu D, MacLennan ICM: Follicular helper T cells, *Annual Review of Immunology* 34:335–368, 2016.

Weisel F, Shlomchik M: Memory B cells of mice and humans, *Annual Review of Immunology* 35:255–284, 2017.

T-Independent B Cell Responses

Cerutti A, Cols M, Puga I: Marginal zone B cells: virtues of innate-like antibody-producing lymphocytes, *Nature Reviews Immunology* 13:118–132, 2013.

CHAPTER 8

Antibody Effector Functions and Fc Receptors

Nimmerjahn F, Ravetch JV: FcγRs in health and disease, *Current Topics in Microbiology and Immunology* 350:105–125, 2011.

Schwab I, Nimmerjahn F: Intravenous immunoglobulin therapy: how does IgG modulate the immune system? *Nature Reviews Immunology* 13:176–189, 2013.

Vidarsson l, Dekkers G, Rispens T: IgG subclasses and allotypes: from structure to effector functions, *Frontiers in Immunology* 5:520, 2014.

Ward ES: Acquiring maternal immunoglobulin: different receptors, similar functions, *Immunity* 20:507–508, 2004.

Complement

Carroll MV, Sim RB: Complement in health and disease, *Advances in Drug Delivery Reviews* 63:965–975, 2011.

Hajishengallis G, et al.: Novel mechanisms and functions of complement, *Nature Immunology* 18:1288–1298, 2017.

Holers VM: Complement and its receptors: new insights into human disease, *Annual Review of Immunology* 32:433–459, 2015.

Liszewski M, Atkinson JP: Complement regulators in human disease: lessons from modern genetics, *Journal of Internal Medicine* 277:294–305, 2015.

Ricklin D, Lambris JD: Complement in immune and inflammatory disorders, *Journal of Immunology* 190:3831–3847, 2013.

CHAPTER 9

Immunological Tolerance: General Mechanisms

Baxter AG: Hodgkin PD: Activation rules: the two-signal theories of immune activation, *Nature Reviews Immunology* 2:439–446, 2002.

Goodnow CC, Sprent J, Fazekas de St Groth B, et al.: Cellular and genetic mechanisms of self tolerance and autoimmunity, *Nature* 435:590–597, 2005.

Mueller DL: Mechanisms maintaining peripheral tolerance, *Nature Immunology* 11:21–27, 2010.

Redmond WL, Sherman LA: Peripheral tolerance of CD8 T lymphocytes, *Immunity* 22:275–284, 2005.

Schwartz RH: Historical overview of immunological tolerance, *Cold Spring Harbor Perspectives in Biology* 4(a006908), 2012.

Shlomchik MJ: Sites and stages of autoreactive B cell activation and regulation, *Immunity* 28:18–28, 2008.

Central Tolerance

Anderson MS, Su MA: AIRE expands: new roles in immune tolerance and beyond, *Nature Reviews Immunology* 16:247–258, 2016.

Cheng M, Anderson MS: Thymic tolerance as a key brake on autoimmunity, *Nature Immunology* 19:659–664, 2018.

Klein L, Kyewski B, Allen PM, Hogquist KA: Positive and negative selection of the T cell repertoire: what thymocytes see (and don't see), *Nature Reviews Immunology* 14:377–391, 2014.

Nemazee D: Mechanisms of central tolerance for B cells, *Nature Reviews Immunology* 17:281–294, 2017.

Anergy; Inhibitory Receptors

Okazaki T, Chikuma S, Iwai Y, et al.: A rheostat for immune responses: the unique properties of PD-1 and their advantages for clinical applications, *Nature Immunology* 14:1212–1218, 2013.

Schildberg FA, Klein SR, Freeman GJ, Sharpe AH: Coinhibitory pathways in the B7-CD28 ligand-receptor family, *Immunity* 44:955–972, 2016.

Walker LS, Sansom DM: Confusing signals: recent progress in CTLA-4 biology, *Trends in Immunology* 36:63–70, 2015.

Wells AD: New insights into the molecular basis of T cell anergy: anergy factors, avoidance sensors, and epigenetic imprinting, *Journal of Immunology* 182:7331–7341, 2009.

Apoptosis

Arakaki R, Yamada A, Kudo Y, et al.: Mechanism of activation-induced cell death of T cells and regulation of FasL expression, *Critical Reviews of Immunology* 34:301–314, 2014.

Bidere N, Su HC, Lenado MJ: Genetic disorders of programmed cell death in the immune system, *Annual Review of Immunology* 24:321–352, 2006.

Griffith TS, Ferguson TA: Cell death in the maintenance and abrogation of tolerance: the five Ws of dying cells, *Immunity* 35:456–466, 2011.

Regulatory T Cells

Dominguez-Villar M, Hafler DA: Regulatory T cells in autoimmune disease, *Nature Immunology* 19:665–673, 2018 .

Josefowicz SZ, Lu L-F, Rudensky Y: Regulatory T cells: mechanisms of differentiation and function, *Annual Review of Immunology* 30:531–564, 2012.

Kitagawa Y, Sakaguchi S: Molecular control of regulatory T cell development and function, *Current Opinion in Immunology* 49:64–70, 2017.

Panduro M, Benoist C, Mathis D: Tissue Tregs, *Annual Review of Immunology* 34:609–633, 2016.

Rosenblum MD, Way SS, Abbas AK: Regulatory T cell memory, *Nature Reviews Immunology* 16:90–101, 2016.

Mechanisms of Autoimmunity: Genetics and Environment

Bach J-F: The hygiene hypothesis in autoimmunity: the role of pathogens and commensals, *Nature Reviews Immunology* 18:105–120, 2018.

Bluestone JA, Bour-Jordan H, Cheng M, Anderson M: T cells in the control of organ-specific autoimmunity, *Journal of Clinical Investigation* 125:2250–2260, 2015.

Cheng MH, Anderson MS: Monogenic autoimmunity, *Annual Review of Immunology* 30:393–427, 2012.

Dendrou CA, Petersen J, Rossjohn J, Fugger L: HLA variation and disease, *Nature Reviews Immunology* 18:325–339, 2018.

Fourneau JM, Bach JM, van Endert PM, et al.: The elusive case for a role of mimicry in autoimmune diseases, *Molecular Immunology* 40:1095–1102, 2004.

Inshaw JRJ, Cutler AJ, Burren OS, Stefana MI, Todd JA: Approaches and advances in the genetic causes of autoimmunity and their implications, *Nature Immunology* 19:674–684, 2018.

Lenardo M, Lo B, Lucas CL: Genomics of immune diseases and new therapies, *Annual Review of Immunology* 34:121–149, 2016.

Marson A, Housley WJ, Hafler DA: Genetic basis of autoimmunity, *Journal of Clinical Investigation* 125:2234–2241, 2015.

Suurmond J, Diamond B: Autoantibodies in systemic autoimmune diseases: specificity and pathogenicity, *Journal of Clinical Investigation* 125:2194–2202, 2015.

Theofilopoulos A, Kono DH, Baccala R: The multiple pathways to autoimmunity, *Nature Immunology* 18:716–724, 2017.

Zenewicz L, Abraham C, Flavell RA, et al.: Unraveling the genetics of autoimmunity, *Cell* 140:791–797, 2010.

CHAPTER 10

Immune Responses to Tumors

Burnet FM: The concept of immunological surveillance, *Progress in Experimental Tumor Research* 13:1–27, 1970.

Coussens LM, Zitvogel L, Palucka AK: Neutralizing tumor-promoting chronic inflammation: a magic bullet? *Science* 339:286–291, 2013.

Gajewski TF, Schreiber H, Fu YX: Innate and adaptive immune cells in the tumor microenvironment, *Nature Immunology* 14:1014–1022, 2013.

Grivennikov SI, Greten FR, Karin M: Immunity, inflammation, and cancer, *Cell* 140:883–899, 2010.

Mantovani A, Allavena P, Sica A, et al.: Cancer-related inflammation, *Nature* 454:436–444, 2008.

Schreiber RD, Old LJ, Smyth MJ: Cancer immunoediting: integrating immunity's roles in cancer suppression and promotion, *Science* 331:1565–1570, 2011.

Ward JP, Gubin MM, Schreiber RD: The role of neoantigens in naturally occurring and therapeutically induced immune responses to cancer, *Advances in Immunology* 130:25–74, 2016.

Tumor Immunotherapy

Callahan MK, Postow MA, Wolchok JD: Targeting T cell co-receptors for cancer therapy, *Immunity* 44:1069–1078, 2016.

June CH, O'Connor RS, Kawalekar OU, Ghassemi S, Milone MC: CAR T cell immunotherapy for human cancer, *Science* 359:1361–1365, 2018.

Mellman I, Coukos G, Dranoff G: Cancer immunotherapy comes of age, *Nature* 480:480–489, 2012.

Palucka K, Banchereau J: Dendritic cell-based therapeutic cancer vaccines, *Immunity* 39:38–48, 2013.

Patel SA, Minn AJ: Combination cancer therapy with immune checkpoint blockade: mechanisms and strategies, *Immunity* 48:417–433, 2018.

Rosenberg SA, Restifo NP: Adoptive cell transfer as personalized immunotherapy for human cancer, *Science* 348:62–68, 2015.

Schumacher TN, Schreiber RD: Neoantigens in cancer immunotherapy, *Science* 348:69–74, 2015.

Sharma P, Allison JP: Immune checkpoint targeting in cancer therapy: toward combination strategies with curative potential, *Cell* 161:205–214, 2015.

Topalian SL, Drake CG, Pardoll DM: Immune checkpoint blockade: a common denominator approach to cancer therapy, *Cancer Cell* 27:450–461, 2015.

Recognition and Rejection of Allogeneic Transplants

Abrahimi P, Liu R, Pober JS: Blood vessels in allotransplantation, *American Journal of Transplantation* 15, 2015. 1748-54.

Gras S, Kjer-Nielsen L, Chen Z, et al.: The structural bases of direct T-cell allorecognition: implications for T-cell-mediated transplant rejection, *Immunology and Cell Biology* 89:388–395, 2011.

Lakkis FG, Lechler RI: Origin and biology of the allogeneic response, *Cold Spring Harbor Perspectives in Medicine* 3:1–10, 2013.

Li XC, Rothstein DM, Sayegh MH: Costimulatory pathways in transplantation: challenges and new developments, *Immunological Reviews* 229:271–293, 2009.

Nagy ZA: Alloreactivity: an old puzzle revisited, *Scandinavian Journal of Immunology* 75:463–470, 2012.

Nankivell BJ, Alexander SI: Rejection of the kidney allograft, *New England Journal of Medicine* 363:1451–1462, 2010.

Valenzuela NM, Reed EF: Antibody-mediated rejection across solid organ transplants: manifestations, mechanisms, and therapies, *Journal of Clinical Investigation* 127:2492–2504, 2017.

Wood KJ, Goto R: Mechanisms of rejection: current perspectives, *Transplantation* 93:1–10, 2012.

Clinical Transplantation

Blazar BR, Murphy WJ, Abedi M: Advances in graft-versus-host disease biology and therapy, *Nature Reviews Immunology* 12:443–458, 2012.

Li HW, Sykes M: Emerging concepts in haematopoietic cell transplantation, *Nature Reviews Immunology* 12:403–416, 2012.

Immunosuppression and Tolerance Induction to Allografts

Chidgey AP, Layton D, Trounson A, et al.: Tolerance strategies for stem-cell-based therapies, *Nature* 453:330–377, 2008.

Halloran PF: Immunosuppressive drugs for kidney transplantation, *New England Journal of Medicine* 351:2715–2729, 2004.

Kinnear G, Jones ND, Wood KJ: Costimulation blockade: current perspectives and implications for therapy, *Transplantation* 95:527–535, 2013.

McDonald-Hyman C, Turka LA, Blazar BR: Advances and challenges in immunotherapy for solid organ and hematopoietic stem cell transplantation, *Science Translational Medicine* 7(280r), 2015.

CHAPTER 11

Immediate Hypersensitivity

Abraham SN: St John AL: Mast cell-orchestrated immunity to pathogens, *Nature Reviews Immunology* 10:440–452, 2010.

Galli SJ, Tsai M: IgE and mast cells in allergic disease, *Nature Medicine* 18:693–704, 2012.

Gurish MF, Austen KF: Developmental origin and functional specialization of mast cell subsets, *Immunity* 37:25–33, 2012.

Holgate ST: Innate and adaptive immune responses in asthma, *Nature Medicine* 18:673–683, 2012.

Lambrecht BN, Hammad H: The immunology of asthma, *Nature Immunology* 16:45–56, 2015.

Licona-Limon P, Kim LK, Flavell RA: TH2, allergy and group 2 innate lymphoid cells, *Nature Immunology* 14:536–542, 2013.

Rothenberg ME, Hogan SP: The eosinophil, *Annual Review of Immunology* 24:147–174, 2006.

Stone KD, Prussin C, Metcalfe DD: IgE, mast cells, basophils, and eosinophils, *Journal of Allergy and Clinical Immunology* 125:S73–S80, 2010.

Voehringer D: Protective and pathological roles of mast cells and basophils, *Nature Reviews Immunology* 13:362–375, 2013.

Wu LC, Zarrin AA: The production and regulation of IgE by the immune system, *Nature Reviews Immunology* 14:247–259, 2014.

Wynn TA: Type 2 cytokines: mechanisms and therapeutic strategies, *Nature Reviews Immunology* 15:271–282, 2015.

Diseases Caused by T Lymphocytes

Chavan SS, Pavlov VA, Tracey KJ: Mechanisms and therapeutic relevance of neuro-immune communication, *Immunity* 46:927–942, 2016.

Weaver CT, Elson CO, Fouser LA, Kolls JK: The Th17 pathway and inflammatory diseases of the intestines, lungs, and skin, *Annual Review of Pathology* 8:477–512, 2013.

CHAPTER 12

Congenital (Primary) Immunodeficiencies

Casanova JL, Abel L: Human genetics of infectious diseases: unique insights into immunological redundancy, *Seminars in Immunology* 36:1–12, 2018.

Conley ME, Dobbs AK, Farmer DM, et al.: Primary B cell immunodeficiencies: comparisons and contrasts, *Annual Review of Immunology* 27:199–227, 2009.

Durandy A, Kracker S, Fischer A: Primary antibody deficiencies, *Nature Reviews Immunology* 13:519–533, 2013.

Fischer A, Notarangelo LD, Neven B, Cavazzana M, Puck JM: Severe combined immunodeficiencies and related disorders, *Nature Reviews Disease Primers* 1:15061, 2015.

Milner JD, Holland SM: The cup runneth over: lessons from the ever-expanding pool of primary immunodeficiency diseases, *Nature Reviews Immunology* 13:635–668, 2013.

Notarangelo LD, Fleisher TA: Targeted strategies directed at the molecular defect: toward precision medicine for select primary immunodeficiency disorders, *Journal of Allergy and Clinical Immunology* 139:715–723, 2017.

Parvaneh N, Casanova JL, Notarangelo LD, et al.: Primary immunodeficiencies: a rapidly evolving story, *Journal of Allergy and Clinical Immunology* 131:314–323, 2013.

Pieper K, Grimbacher B, Eibel H: B-cell biology and development, *Journal of Allergy and Clinical Immunology* 131:959–971, 2013.

HIV and AIDS

Barouch DH: Challenges in the development of an HIV-1 vaccine, *Nature* 455:613–619, 2008.

Burton DR, Mascola JR: Antibody responses to envelope glycoproteins in HIV-1 infection, *Nature Immunology* 16:571–576, 2015.

Haynes BF, Shaw GM, Korber B, et al.: HIV-host interactions: implications for vaccine design, *Cell Host Microbe* 19:292–303, 2016.

McLaren PJ, Carrington M: The impact of host genetic variation on infection with HIV-1, *Nature Immunology* 16:577–583, 2015.

Migueles SA, Connors M: Success and failure of the cellular immune response against HIV-1, *Nature Immunology* 16:563–570, 2015.

Moir S, Chun TW, Fauci AS: Pathogenic mechanisms of HIV disease, *Annual Review of Pathology: Mechanisms of Disease* 6:223–248, 2011.

Piot P, Abdool Karim SS, Hecht R: UNAIDS–Lancet Commission. Defeating AIDS—advancing global health, *Lancet* 386:171–218, 2015.

Walker BD, Yu XG: Unraveling the mechanisms of durable control of HIV-1, *Nature Reviews Immunology* 13:487–498, 2013.

Zhang Q, Frange P, Blanche S, Casanova JL: Pathogenesis of infections in HIV-infected individuals: insights from primary immunodeficiencies, *Current Opinion in Immunology* 48:122–133, 2017.

GLOSSARY

A

αβ T cell receptor (αβ TCR) The most common form of TCR, expressed on both CD4$^+$ and CD8$^+$ T cells. The αβ TCR recognizes peptide antigen bound to an MHC molecule. Both α and β chains contain highly variable (V) regions that together form the antigen-binding site as well as constant (C) regions. TCR V and C regions are structurally homologous to the V and C regions of Ig molecules.

ABO blood group antigens Carbohydrate antigens attached mainly to cell surface proteins or lipids that are present on many cell types, including red blood cells. These antigens differ among individuals, depending on inherited alleles encoding the enzymes required for synthesis of the carbohydrate. The ABO antigens act as alloantigens that are responsible for blood transfusion reactions and hyperacute rejection of allografts.

Acquired immunodeficiency A deficiency in the immune system that is acquired after birth, usually because of infection (e.g., AIDS), and that is not related to a genetic defect. Synonymous with secondary immunodeficiency.

Acquired immunodeficiency syndrome (AIDS) A disease caused by human immunodeficiency virus (HIV) infection that is characterized by depletion of CD4$^+$ T cells, leading to a profound defect in cell-mediated immunity. Clinically, AIDS includes opportunistic infections, malignant tumors, wasting, and encephalopathy.

Activation-induced cell death (AICD) Apoptosis of activated lymphocytes, generally used for T cells.

Activation-induced (cytidine) deaminase (AID) An enzyme expressed in B cells that catalyzes the conversion of cytosine into uracil in DNA, which is a step required for somatic hypermutation and affinity maturation of antibodies and for Ig class switching.

Activation protein 1 (AP-1) A family of DNA-binding transcription factors composed of dimers of two proteins that bind to one another through a shared structural motif called a leucine zipper.

The best-characterized AP-1 factor is composed of the proteins Fos and Jun. AP-1 is involved in transcriptional regulation of many different genes that are important in the immune system, such as cytokine genes.

Active immunity The form of adaptive immunity that is induced by exposure to a foreign antigen and activation of lymphocytes and in which the immunized individual plays an active role in responding to the antigen. This type contrasts with passive immunity, in which an individual receives antibodies or lymphocytes from another individual who was previously actively immunized.

Acute-phase proteins Proteins, mostly synthesized in the liver in response to inflammatory cytokines such as IL-1, IL-6, and TNF, whose plasma concentrations increase shortly after infection as part of the acute phase response. Examples include C-reactive protein, complement proteins, fibrinogen, and serum amyloid A protein. The acute-phase reactants play various roles in the innate immune response to microbes. Also called acute phase reactants.

Acute-phase response The increase in plasma concentrations of several proteins, called acute-phase reactants, that occurs as part of the early innate immune response to infections.

Acute rejection A form of graft rejection involving vascular and parenchymal injury mediated by T cells, macrophages, and antibodies that usually occurs days or weeks after transplantation but may occur later if pharmacologic immunosuppression becomes inadequate.

Adaptive immunity The form of immunity that is mediated by lymphocytes and stimulated by exposure to foreign antigens. In contrast to innate immunity, adaptive immunity is characterized by exquisite specificity for distinct molecules and by long-term memory, which is the ability to respond more vigorously to repeated exposure to the same microbe. Adaptive immunity is also called specific immunity or acquired immunity.

Adaptor protein A protein involved in intracellular signal transduction pathways

by serving as a bridge molecule or scaffold for the recruitment of other signaling molecules. During lymphocyte antigen receptor or cytokine receptor signaling, adaptor molecules may be phosphorylated on tyrosine residues to enable them to bind other proteins containing Src homology 2 (SH2) domains. Adaptor molecules involved in T cell activation include LAT, SLP-76, and Grb-2.

Addressin An adhesion molecule expressed on endothelial cells in different anatomic sites that directs organ-specific lymphocyte homing. Mucosal addressin cell adhesion molecule 1 (MadCAM-1) is an example of an addressin expressed in Peyer patches in the intestinal wall that binds to the integrin α4β7 on gut-homing T cells.

Adhesion molecule A cell surface molecule whose function is to promote adhesive interactions with other cells or the extracellular matrix. Leukocytes express various types of adhesion molecules, such as selectins, integrins, and members of the Ig superfamily, and these molecules play crucial roles in cell migration and cellular activation in innate and adaptive immune responses.

Adjuvant A substance, distinct from antigen, that enhances T and B cell activation mainly by promoting innate immune responses, which enhance the accumulation and activation of antigen-presenting cells (APCs) at the site of antigen exposure. Adjuvants stimulate expression of T cell-activating costimulators and cytokines by APCs and may also prolong the expression of peptide-MHC complexes on the surface of APCs.

Adoptive transfer The process of transferring cells from one individual into another or back into the same individual after in vitro expansion and activation. Adoptive transfer is used in research to define the role of a particular cell population (e.g., T cells) in an immune response. Clinically, adoptive transfer of tumor-specific T lymphocytes and tumor antigen-presenting dendritic cells is used in cancer therapy, and transfer of regulatory T cells is being developed for autoimmune diseases and graft rejection.

Affinity The strength of the binding between a single binding site of a molecule (e.g., an antibody) and a ligand (e.g., an antigen). The affinity of a molecule X for a ligand Y is represented by the dissociation constant (K_d), which is the concentration of Y that is required to occupy the combining sites of half the X molecules present in a solution. A smaller K_d indicates a stronger or higher affinity interaction, and a lower concentration of ligand is needed to occupy the sites.

Affinity maturation The process that leads to increased affinity of antibodies for a particular antigen as a T cell-dependent antibody response progresses. Affinity maturation takes place in germinal centers of lymphoid tissues and is the result of somatic mutation of immunoglobulin genes, followed by selective survival of the B cells producing the highest affinity antibodies.

Allele One of different forms of the same gene in different individuals present at a particular chromosomal locus. An individual who is heterozygous at a locus has two different alleles, each on a different member of a pair of chromosomes, one inherited from the mother and one from the father. If a particular gene in a population has different alleles, the gene or locus is said to be polymorphic. MHC genes have many alleles (i.e., they are highly polymorphic).

Allelic exclusion The exclusive expression of only one of two inherited alleles encoding Ig heavy and light chains and TCR β chains. Allelic exclusion occurs when the protein product of one productively recombined antigen receptor locus on one chromosome blocks rearrangement and expression of the corresponding locus on the other chromosome. This property ensures that each lymphocyte will express a single antigen receptor and that all antigen receptors expressed by one clone of lymphocytes will have the identical specificity. Because the TCR α chain locus does not show allelic exclusion, some T cells do express two different TCRs.

Allergen An antigen that elicits an immediate hypersensitivity (allergic) reaction. Allergens are proteins or chemicals bound to proteins that induce IgE antibody responses in atopic individuals.

Allergy A disorder caused by an immediate hypersensitivity reaction, often named according to the type of antigen (allergen) that elicits the disease, such as food allergy, bee sting allergy, and penicillin allergy. All of these conditions are the result of IgE production stimulated by IL-4–producing helper T cells, followed by allergen and IgE-dependent mast cell activation.

Alloantibody An antibody specific for an alloantigen (i.e., specific for an antigen present in some individuals of a species but not in others).

Alloantigen A cell or tissue antigen that is present in some individuals of a species but not in others and that is recognized as foreign on an allograft. Alloantigens are usually products of polymorphic genes.

Alloantiserum The alloantibody-containing serum of an individual who has previously been exposed to one or more alloantigens.

Allogeneic graft An organ or tissue graft from a donor who is of the same species but genetically nonidentical to the recipient (also called an allograft).

Alloreactive Reactive to alloantigens; describes T cells or antibodies from one individual that will recognize antigens on cells or tissues of another genetically nonidentical individual.

Allotype The property of a group of antibody molecules defined by their sharing of a particular antigenic determinant found on the antibodies of some individuals but not others. Such determinants are called **allotopes**. Antibodies that share a particular allotope belong to the same allotype. *Allotype* is also often used synonymously with *allotope*.

Alternative macrophage activation Macrophage activation by IL-4 and IL-13 leading to an antiinflammatory and tissue-reparative phenotype, in contrast to classical macrophage activation by interferon-γ and TLR ligands.

Alternative pathway of complement activation An antibody-independent pathway of activation of the complement system that occurs when the C3b fragment of the C3 protein binds to microbial cell surfaces. The alternative pathway is a component of the innate immune system and mediates inflammatory responses to infection as well as direct lysis of microbes. The alternative pathway, as well as the classical and lectin pathways, terminate with formation of the membrane attack complex.

Anaphylatoxins The C5a, C4a, and C3a complement fragments that are generated during complement activation. The anaphylatoxins bind specific cell surface receptors and promote acute inflammation by stimulating neutrophil chemotaxis and activating mast cells.

Anaphylaxis A severe form of immediate hypersensitivity in which there is systemic mast cell or basophil activation, and the released mediators cause bronchial constriction, tissue edema, and cardiovascular collapse.

Anchor residues The amino acid residues of a peptide whose side chains fit into pockets in the peptide-binding cleft of an MHC molecule. The side chains bind to complementary amino acids in the MHC molecule and therefore serve to anchor the peptide in the cleft of the MHC molecule.

Anergy A state of unresponsiveness to antigenic stimulation. Lymphocyte anergy (also called clonal anergy) is the failure of clones of T or B cells to react to antigen and is a mechanism of maintaining immunologic tolerance to self. Clinically, anergy describes the lack of T cell–dependent cutaneous delayed-type hypersensitivity reactions to common antigens.

Angiogenesis New blood vessel formation regulated by a variety of protein factors elaborated by cells of the innate and adaptive immune systems and often accompanying chronic inflammation and tumor growth.

Antibody A type of glycoprotein molecule, also called immunoglobulin (Ig), produced by B lymphocytes that binds antigens, often with a high degree of specificity and affinity. The basic structural unit of an antibody is composed of two identical heavy chains and two identical light chains. The N-terminal variable regions of the heavy and light chains form the antigen-binding sites, whereas the C-terminal constant regions of the heavy chains functionally interact with other molecules in the immune system. Every individual has millions of different antibodies, each with a unique antigen-binding site. Secreted antibodies perform various effector functions, including neutralizing antigens, activating complement, and promoting leukocyte-dependent destruction of microbes.

Antibody-dependent cell-mediated cytotoxicity (ADCC)   A process by which NK cells are targeted to IgG-coated cells, resulting in lysis of the antibody-coated cells. A specific receptor for the constant region of IgG, called FcγRIII (CD16), is expressed on the NK cell membrane and mediates binding to the IgG.

Antibody feedback   The downregulation of antibody production by secreted IgG antibodies that occurs when antigen-antibody complexes simultaneously engage B cell membrane Ig and one type of Fcγ receptor (FcγRIIb). Under these conditions, the cytoplasmic tail of FcγRIIb transduces inhibitory signals inside the B cell.

Antibody repertoire   The collection of different antibody specificities expressed in an individual.

Antibody-secreting cell   A B lymphocyte that has undergone differentiation and produces the secretory form of Ig. Antibody-secreting cells are generated from naive B cells in response to antigen and reside in the spleen and lymph nodes as well as in the bone marrow. Often used synonymously with plasma cells.

Antigen   A molecule that binds to an antibody or a TCR. Antigens that bind to antibodies include all classes of molecules. Most TCRs bind only peptide fragments of proteins complexed with MHC molecules; both the peptide ligand and the native protein from which it is derived are called **T cell antigens**.

Antigen presentation   The display of antigens on the surface of cells for recognition by lymphocytes, most often referring to display of peptides bound by MHC molecules on the surface of an APC that permits specific recognition by TCRs and activation of T cells.

Antigen-presenting cell (APC)   A cell that displays peptide fragments of protein antigens, in association with MHC molecules, on its surface and activates antigen-specific T cells. In addition to displaying peptide-MHC complexes, APCs also express costimulatory molecules to optimally activate T lymphocytes.

Antigen processing   The intracellular conversion of protein antigens derived from the extracellular space or the cytosol into peptides and loading of these peptides onto MHC molecules for display to T lymphocytes.

Antigenic variation   The process by which antigens expressed by microbes may change by various genetic mechanisms, and therefore allow the microbe to evade immune responses. One example of antigenic variation is the change in influenza virus surface proteins hemagglutinin and neuraminidase, which necessitates the use of new vaccines each year.

Antiretroviral therapy (ART)   Combination chemotherapy for HIV infection, usually consisting of two nucleoside reverse transcriptase inhibitors and either one viral protease inhibitor or one nonnucleoside reverse transcriptase inhibitor. ART can reduce plasma virus titers to below detectable levels for more than 1 year and slow the progression of HIV disease. Also called highly active antiretroviral therapy (HAART).

Antiserum   Serum from an individual previously immunized with an antigen that contains antibody specific for that antigen.

Apoptosis   A process of cell death characterized by activation of intracellular caspases, DNA cleavage, nuclear condensation and fragmentation, and plasma membrane blebbing that leads to phagocytosis of cell fragments without inducing an inflammatory response. This type of cell death is important in development of lymphocytes, return to homeostasis after an immune response to an infection, maintenance of tolerance to self antigens, and killing of infected cells by cytotoxic T lymphocytes and natural killer cells.

Arthus reaction   A localized form of experimental immune complex–mediated vasculitis induced by injection of an antigen subcutaneously into a previously immunized animal or into an animal that has been given intravenous antibody specific for the antigen. Circulating antibodies bind to the injected antigen and form immune complexes that are deposited in the walls of small arteries at the injection site and give rise to a local cutaneous vasculitis with necrosis.

Asthma   An inflammatory disease usually caused by repeated immediate hypersensitivity reactions in the lung that leads to intermittent and reversible airway obstruction, chronic bronchial inflammation with eosinophils, and bronchial smooth muscle cell hypertrophy and hyperreactivity.

Atopy   The propensity of an individual to produce IgE antibodies in response to various environmental antigens and to develop strong immediate hypersensitivity (allergic) responses. People who have allergies to environmental antigens, such as pollen or house dust, are said to be atopic.

Autoantibody   An antibody produced in an individual that is specific for a self antigen. Autoantibodies can cause damage to cells and tissues and are produced in excess in autoimmune diseases, such as systemic lupus erythematosus and myasthenia gravis.

Autocrine factor   A molecule that acts on the same cell that produces the factor. For example, IL-2 is an autocrine T cell growth factor that stimulates mitotic activity of the T cell that produces it.

Autoimmune disease   A disease caused by a breakdown of self tolerance such that the adaptive immune system responds to self-antigens and mediates cell and tissue damage. Autoimmune diseases can be caused by immune attack against one organ or tissue (e.g., multiple sclerosis, thyroiditis, or type 1 diabetes) or against multiple and systemically distributed antigens (e.g., systemic lupus erythematosus).

Autoimmune polyendocrine syndrome type 1 (APS-1)   Also known as autoimmune polyendocrinopathy-candidiasis–ectodermal dystrophy/dysplasia (APECED). A rare autoimmune disease caused by genetic deficiency of the autoimmune regulator protein (AIRE) required for central T cell tolerance to many different tissue antigens. APS-1 patients suffer from immune injury to multiple endocrine organs.

Autoimmune regulator (AIRE)   A protein that functions to stimulate expression of peripheral tissue protein antigens in thymic medullary epithelial cells. Mutations in the *AIRE* gene in humans and mice lead to an autoimmune disease (autoimmune polyendocrine syndrome type 1) affecting multiple organs because of defective expression of tissue antigens in the thymus and failure to delete T cells or generate some regulatory T cells specific for these antigens.

Autoimmunity   The state of adaptive immune system responsiveness to self antigens that occurs when mechanisms of self tolerance fail.

Autologous graft   A tissue or organ graft in which the donor and recipient are the same individual. Autologous bone marrow and skin grafts are performed in clinical medicine.

Autophagy   The normal process by which a cell degrades its own components by lysosomal catabolism. Autophagy plays a role in innate immune defense against infections, and polymorphisms of genes that regulate autophagy are linked to risk for some autoimmune diseases.

Avidity   The overall strength of interaction between two molecules, such as an antibody and antigen. Avidity depends on both the affinity and the valency of interactions.

Therefore, the avidity of a pentameric IgM antibody, with 10 antigen-binding sites, for a multivalent antigen is much greater than the affinity of a single antibody combining site specific for the same antigen. Avidity can be used to describe the strength of cell-cell interactions, which are mediated by many binding interactions between cell surface molecules.

B

B lymphocyte The only cell type capable of producing antibody molecules and therefore the mediator of humoral immune responses. B lymphocytes, or B cells, develop in the bone marrow, and mature B cells are found mainly in lymphoid follicles in secondary lymphoid tissues, in bone marrow, and in the circulation.

B-1 lymphocytes A subset of B lymphocytes that develop earlier during ontogeny than do conventional (follicular) B cells, express a limited repertoire of V genes with little junctional diversity, and secrete IgM antibodies that bind T-independent antigens. Many B-1 cells express the CD5 molecule.

Bare lymphocyte syndrome An immunodeficiency disease characterized by a lack of class II MHC molecule expression that leads to defects in maturation and activation of CD4$^+$ T cells and cell-mediated immunity. The disease is caused by mutations in genes encoding factors that regulate class II MHC gene transcription.

Basophil A type of bone marrow–derived circulating granulocyte with structural and functional similarities to mast cells that has granules containing many of the same inflammatory mediators as mast cells and expresses a high-affinity Fc receptor for IgE. Basophils that are recruited into tissue sites where antigen is present may contribute to immediate hypersensitivity reactions.

Bcl-6 A transcriptional repressor that is required for germinal center B cell development and for Tfh development.

Bcl-2 family proteins A family of structurally homologous cytoplasmic and mitochondrial membrane proteins that regulate apoptosis by influencing mitochondrial outer membrane permeability. Members of this family can be pro-apoptotic (such as Bax, Bad, and Bak) or anti-apoptotic (such as Bcl-2 and Bcl-X$_L$).

B cell receptor (BCR) The cell surface antigen receptor on B lymphocytes, which is a membrane-bound immunoglobulin molecule.

B cell receptor complex (BCR complex) A multiprotein complex expressed on the surface of B lymphocytes that recognizes antigen and transduces activating signals into the cell. The BCR complex includes membrane Ig, which is responsible for binding antigen, and Igα and Igβ proteins, which initiate signaling events.

BLIMP-1 A transcriptional repressor that is required for plasma cell generation.

Bone marrow The tissue within the central cavity of bone that is the site of generation of all circulating blood cells in adults, including immature lymphocytes, and the site of B cell maturation.

Bone marrow transplantation See **hematopoietic stem cell transplantation**.

Bruton tyrosine kinase (Btk) A Tec family tyrosine kinase that is essential for B cell maturation. Mutations in the gene encoding Btk cause X-linked agammaglobulinemia, a disease characterized by failure of B cells to mature beyond the pre-B cell stage.

Burkitt lymphoma A malignant B cell tumor that is diagnosed by histologic features but almost always carries a reciprocal chromosomal translocation involving *Ig* gene loci and the cellular *MYC* gene on chromosome 8. Many cases of Burkitt lymphoma in Africa are associated with Epstein-Barr virus infection.

C

C (constant region) gene segments The DNA sequences in the *Ig* and *TCR* gene loci that encode the nonvariable portions of Ig heavy and light chains and TCR α, β, γ, and δ chains.

C1 A serum complement system protein composed of several polypeptide chains that initiates the classical pathway of complement activation by attaching to the Fc portions of IgG or IgM antibody that has bound antigen.

C1 inhibitor (C1 INH) A plasma protein inhibitor of the classical pathway of complement activation as well as proteases in fibrinolytic, coagulation, and kinin pathways. C1 INH is a serine protease

inhibitor (serpin) that mimics the normal substrates of the C1r and C1s components of C1. A genetic deficiency in C1 INH causes the disease hereditary angioedema.

C2 A classical complement pathway protein that is proteolytically cleaved by activated C1 to generate C2a, which forms part of the classical pathway C3 convertase.

C3 The central and most abundant complement system protein; it is involved in both the classical and alternative pathway cascades. C3 is proteolytically cleaved during complement activation to generate a C3b fragment, which covalently attaches to cell or microbial surfaces, and a C3a fragment, which has various proinflammatory activities.

C3 convertase A multiprotein enzyme complex generated by the early steps of classical, lectin, and alternative pathways of complement activation. C3 convertase cleaves C3, which gives rise to two proteolytic products called C3a and C3b.

C4 A classical complement pathway protein that is proteolytically cleaved by activated C1 to generate C4b, which forms part of the classical pathway C3 convertase.

C5 A protein that is cleaved by C5 convertases in all complement pathways, generating a C5b fragment, which initiates formation of the membrane attack complex, and a released C5a fragment, which has various proinflammatory activities.

C5 convertase A multiprotein enzyme complex generated by C3b binding to C3 convertase. C5 convertase cleaves C5 and initiates the late steps of complement activation leading to formation of the membrane attack complex and lysis of cells.

Calcineurin A cytoplasmic serine/threonine phosphatase that dephosphorylates the transcription factor NFAT, thereby allowing NFAT to enter the nucleus. Calcineurin is activated by calcium signals generated through TCR signaling in response to antigen recognition, and the immunosuppressive drugs cyclosporine and tacrolimus work by blocking calcineurin activity.

Carcinoembryonic antigen (CEA, CD66) A highly glycosylated membrane protein; increased expression of CEA in many carcinomas of the colon, pancreas, stomach, and breast results in a rise in serum levels. The level of serum CEA is used to monitor the persistence or recurrence of metastatic carcinoma after treatment.

Caspases Intracellular proteases with cysteines in their active sites that cleave substrates at the C-terminal sides of aspartic acid residues. Most are components of enzymatic cascades that cause apoptotic death of cells, but caspase-1, which is part of the inflammasome, drives inflammation by processing inactive precursor forms of the cytokines IL-1 and IL-18 into their active forms.

Cathelicidins Polypeptides produced by neutrophils and various barrier epithelia that serve various functions in innate immunity, including direct toxicity to microorganisms, activation of leukocytes, and neutralization of lipopolysaccharide.

Cathepsins Thiol and aspartyl proteases with broad substrate specificities, which are abundant in the endosomes in APCs, and play an important role in generating peptide fragments from exogenous protein antigens that bind to class II MHC molecules.

CD molecules Cell surface molecules expressed on various cell types in the immune system that are designated by the "cluster of differentiation" or CD number. See Appendix I for a list of CD molecules.

Cell-mediated immunity (CMI) The form of adaptive immunity that is mediated by T lymphocytes and serves as the defense mechanism against various types of microbes that are taken up by phagocytes or infect nonphagocytic cells. Cell-mediated immune responses include CD4+ T cell–mediated activation of phagocytes and CD8+ CTL–mediated killing of infected cells.

Central tolerance A form of self tolerance induced in generative (central) lymphoid organs as a consequence of immature self-reactive lymphocytes recognizing self antigens and subsequently leading to their death or inactivation. Central tolerance prevents the emergence of lymphocytes with high-affinity receptors for the self antigens that are expressed in the bone marrow or thymus.

Centroblasts Rapidly proliferating B cells in the dark zone of germinal centers

of secondary lymphoid tissues, which give rise to thousands of progeny, express activation-induced deaminase (AID), and undergo somatic mutation of their *V* genes. Centroblasts become the centrocytes of the light zone of germinal centers.

Centrocytes B cells in the light zone of germinal centers of secondary lymphoid organs, which are the progeny of proliferating centroblasts of the dark zone. Centrocytes that express high-affinity Ig are positively selected to survive and undergo isotype switching and further differentiation into long-lived plasma cells and memory B cells.

Checkpoint blockade A form of cancer immunotherapy in which blocking antibodies specific for T cell inhibitory molecules, including PD-1, PD-L1, and CTLA-4, are administered to cancer patients to boost antitumor T cell responses; also called immune checkpoint blockade. This approach has been successful in effectively treating several kinds of widely metastatic cancers that are unresponsive to other therapies.

Chédiak-Higashi syndrome A rare autosomal recessive immunodeficiency disease caused by a defect in the cytoplasmic granules of various cell types that affects the lysosomes of neutrophils and macrophages as well as the granules of CTLs and NK cells. Patients show reduced resistance to infection with pyogenic bacteria.

Chemokine receptors Cell surface receptors for chemokines that transduce signals stimulating the migration of leukocytes. There are at least 19 different mammalian chemokine receptors, each of which binds a different set of chemokines; all are members of the seven-transmembrane α-helical, G protein–coupled receptor family.

Chemokines A large family of structurally homologous low–molecular-weight cytokines that stimulate leukocyte chemotaxis, regulate the migration of leukocytes from the blood to tissues by activating leukocyte integrins, and maintain the spatial organization of different subsets of lymphocytes and antigen-presenting cells within lymphoid organs.

Chemotaxis Movement of a cell directed by a chemical concentration gradient. The

movement of leukocytes within various tissues is often directed by gradients of low–molecular-weight cytokines called chemokines.

Chimeric antigen receptor (CAR) Genetically engineered receptors with tumor antigen–specific binding sites encoded by recombinant Ig-variable genes and cytoplasmic tails containing signaling domains of both the TCR and costimulatory receptors. When T cells are engineered to express chimeric antigen receptors these cells can recognize and kill cells that the extracellular domain recognizes. Adoptive transfer of CAR-expressing T cells has been used successfully for the treatment of some types of hematologic cancers.

Chromosomal translocation A chromosomal abnormality in which a segment of one chromosome is transferred to another. Many malignant diseases of lymphocytes are associated with chromosomal translocations involving an Ig or TCR locus and a chromosomal segment containing a cellular oncogene.

Chronic granulomatous disease A rare inherited immunodeficiency disease caused by mutations in genes encoding components of the phagocyte oxidase enzyme complex that is needed for microbial killing by polymorphonuclear leukocytes and macrophages. The disease is characterized by recurrent intracellular bacterial and fungal infections, often accompanied by chronic cell-mediated immune responses and the formation of granulomas.

Chronic rejection A form of allograft rejection characterized by fibrosis with loss of normal organ structures occurring during a prolonged period. In many cases, the major pathologic event in chronic rejection is graft arterial occlusion caused by proliferation of intimal smooth muscle cells, which is called graft arteriosclerosis.

c-Kit ligand (stem cell factor) A protein required for hematopoiesis, early steps in T cell development in the thymus, and mast cell development. c-Kit ligand is produced in membrane-bound and secreted forms by stromal cells in the bone marrow and thymus, and it binds to the c-Kit tyrosine kinase membrane receptor on pluripotent stem cells.

Class I major histocompatibility complex (MHC) molecule One of two forms of polymorphic heterodimeric membrane proteins that bind and display peptide fragments of protein antigens on the surface of APCs for recognition by T lymphocytes. Class I MHC molecules usually display peptides derived from proteins that are proteolytically processed by proteasomes in the cytosol of the cell, for recognition by CD8+ T cells.

Class II-associated invariant chain peptide (CLIP) A peptide remnant of the invariant chain that sits in the class II MHC peptide-binding cleft and is removed by action of the HLA-DM molecule before the cleft becomes accessible to peptides produced from extracellular protein antigens that are internalized into vesicles.

Class II major histocompatibility complex (MHC) molecule One of two major classes of polymorphic heterodimeric membrane proteins that bind and display peptide fragments of protein antigens on the surface of APCs for recognition by T lymphocytes. Class II MHC molecules usually display peptides derived from extracellular proteins that are internalized into phagocytic or endocytic vesicles, for recognition by CD4+ T cells.

Classical macrophage activation Macrophage activation by interferon-γ, Th1 cells, and TLR ligands, leading to a proinflammatory and microbicidal phenotype. "Classically activated" macrophages are also called M1 macrophages.

Classical pathway of complement activation The complement pathway that is an effector arm of humoral immunity, generating inflammatory mediators, opsonins for phagocytosis of antigens, and lytic complexes that destroy cells. The classical pathway is initiated by binding of antigen-antibody complexes to the C1 molecule, leading to proteolytic cleavage of C4 and C2 proteins to generate the classical pathway C3 convertase. The classical pathway, as well as the alternative and lectin pathways, terminate with formation of the membrane attack complex.

Clonal anergy A state of antigen unresponsiveness of a clone of T lymphocytes experimentally induced by recognition of antigen in the absence of additional signals (costimulatory signals) required for functional activation. Clonal anergy is considered a model for one mechanism of tolerance to self antigens and may be applicable to B lymphocytes as well.

Clonal deletion A mechanism of lymphocyte tolerance in which an immature T cell in the thymus or an immature B cell in the bone marrow undergoes apoptotic death as a consequence of recognizing a self antigen.

Clonal expansion The approximately 1000- to 100,000-fold increase in the number of lymphocytes specific for an antigen that results from antigen stimulation and proliferation of naive T and B cells. Clonal expansion occurs in lymphoid tissues and is required to generate enough antigen-specific effector T lymphocytes and plasma cells from rare naive precursors to eradicate infections.

Clonal ignorance A form of lymphocyte unresponsiveness in which self antigens are ignored by the immune system even though lymphocytes specific for those antigens remain viable and functional.

Clonal selection A fundamental tenet of the immune system meaning that every individual possesses numerous clonally derived lymphocytes, each clone having arisen from a single precursor, expresses one antigen receptor, and is capable of recognizing and responding to a distinct antigenic determinant. When an antigen enters, it selects a specific preexisting clone and activates it.

Clone A group of cells, all derived from a single common precursor, which maintain many of the genotypic and phenotypic features shared by the cell of origin. In adaptive immunity, all members of a clone of lymphocytes share the same clonally unique recombined *Ig* or *TCR* genes. The rearranged *Ig V* genes of different cells within a clone of B cells may change in sequence due to somatic hypermutation that occurs after activation of mature B cells.

Coinhibitor A cell surface protein expressed by antigen-presenting cells or tissue cells that binds to coinhibitory receptors on effector T cells, inducing signals that block T cell activation by antigen and costimulators. An example is PD-L1, a coinhibitor expressed on various cell types, which binds to PD-1 on effector T cells. The PD-L1/PD-1 pathway is being therapeutically targeted to enhance antitumor T cell responses.

Collectins A family of proteins, including mannose-binding lectin, that is characterized by a collagen-like domain and a lectin (i.e., carbohydrate-binding) domain. Collectins play a role in the innate immune system by acting as microbial pattern recognition receptors, and they may activate the complement system by binding to C1q.

Colony-stimulating factors (CSFs) Cytokines that promote the expansion and differentiation of bone marrow progenitor cells. CSFs are essential for the maturation of red blood cells, granulocytes, monocytes, and lymphocytes. Examples of CSFs include granulocyte-monocyte colony-stimulating factor (GM-CSF), granulocyte colony-stimulating factor (G-CSF), and IL-3.

Combinatorial diversity The diversity of Ig and TCR specificities generated by the use of many different combinations of different variable, diversity, and joining segments during somatic recombination of DNA in the Ig and TCR loci in developing B and T cells. Combinatorial diversity is one mechanism, which works together with junctional diversity, for the generation of large numbers of different antigen receptor genes from a limited number of DNA gene segments.

Complement A system of serum and cell surface proteins that interact with one another and with other molecules of the immune system to generate important effectors of innate and adaptive immune responses. The classical, alternative, and lectin pathways of the complement system are activated by antigen-antibody complexes, microbial surfaces, and plasma lectins binding to microbes, respectively, and consist of a cascade of proteolytic enzymes that generate inflammatory mediators and opsonins. All three pathways lead to the formation of a common terminal cell lytic complex that is inserted in cell membranes.

Complement receptor type 1 (CR1) A receptor for the C3b and C4b fragments of complement. Phagocytes use CR1 to mediate internalization of C3b- or C4b-coated particles. CR1 on erythrocytes serves in the clearance of immune complexes from the circulation. CR1 is also a regulator of complement activation.

Complement receptor type 2 (CR2) A receptor expressed on B cells and follicular dendritic cells that binds proteolytic fragments of the C3 complement protein, including C3d, C3dg, and iC3b. CR2 (also called CD21) functions to stimulate humoral immune responses by enhancing B cell activation by antigen and by promoting the trapping of antigen-antibody complexes in germinal centers. CR2 is also the receptor for Epstein-Barr virus.

Complementarity-determining region (CDR) Short segments of Ig and TCR proteins that contain most of the sequence differences between antibodies or TCRs expressed by different clones of B cells and T cells and make contact with antigen; also called **hypervariable regions.** Three CDRs are present in the variable domain of each antigen receptor polypeptide chain, and six CDRs are present in an intact Ig or TCR molecule. These hypervariable segments assume loop structures that together form a surface complementary to the three-dimensional structure of the bound antigen.

Congenic mouse strains Inbred mouse strains that are identical to one another at every genetic locus except the one for which they are selected to differ; such strains are created by repetitive back cross breeding and selection for a particular trait. Congenic strains that differ from one another only at a particular MHC allele have been useful in defining the function of MHC molecules.

Congenital immunodeficiency A genetic defect in which an inherited deficiency in some aspect of the innate or adaptive immune system leads to an increased susceptibility to infections. Congenital immunodeficiency is frequently manifested early in infancy and childhood but is sometimes clinically detected later in life. Synonymous with **primary immunodeficiency.**

Constant (C) region The portion of Ig or TCR polypeptide chains that does not vary in sequence among different clones and is not involved in antigen binding.

Contact sensitivity A state of immune responsiveness to certain chemical agents leading to T cell–mediated delayed-type hypersensitivity reactions upon skin contact. Substances that elicit contact sensitivity, including nickel ions, urushiols in poison ivy, and many therapeutic drugs,

bind to and modify self proteins on the surfaces of APCs, which are then recognized by CD4+ or CD8+ T cells.

Coreceptor A lymphocyte surface receptor that binds to an antigen at the same time that membrane Ig or TCR binds the antigen and delivers signals required for optimal lymphocyte activation. CD4 and CD8 are T cell coreceptors that bind nonpolymorphic parts of an MHC molecule concurrently with the TCR binding to polymorphic MHC residues and the displayed peptide. CR2 is a coreceptor on B cells that binds to complement-coated antigens at the same time that membrane Ig binds another part of the antigen.

Costimulator A molecule expressed on the surface of APCs in response to innate immune stimuli, which provides a stimulus (the "second signal"), in addition to antigen (the "first signal"), required for the activation of naive T cells. The best defined costimulators are the B7 molecules (CD80 and CD86) on APCs that bind to the CD28 receptor on T cells.

CpG nucleotides Unmethylated cytidine-guanine sequences found mainly in microbial DNA that stimulate innate immune responses. Strings of repeated CpG nucleotides are recognized by Toll-like receptor 9, and thereby activate innate immune responses.

C-reactive protein (CRP) A member of the pentraxin family of plasma proteins involved in innate immune responses to bacterial infections. CRP is an acute-phase reactant, and it binds to the capsule of pneumococcal bacteria. CRP also binds to C1q and may thereby activate complement or act as an opsonin by interacting with phagocyte C1q receptors. Increased serum CRP is a marker of inflammation.

Cross-matching A screening test performed to minimize the chance of adverse transfusion reactions or graft rejection, in which a patient in need of a blood transfusion or organ allograft is tested for the presence of preformed antibodies against donor cell surface antigens (usually blood group antigens or MHC antigens). The test involves mixing the recipient serum with leukocytes or red blood cells from potential donors and analyzing for agglutination or complement-dependent lysis of the cells.

Cross-presentation A mechanism by which a dendritic cell activates (or

primes) a naive CD8+ CTL specific for the antigens of a third cell (e.g., a virus-infected or tumor cell). Cross-presentation occurs, for example, when protein antigens from an infected cell are ingested by a dendritic cell and the microbial antigens are processed and presented in association with class I MHC molecules, unlike the general rule for phagocytosed antigens, which are presented in association with class II MHC molecules. The dendritic cell also provides costimulation for the T cells. Also called **cross-priming.**

CTLA-4 An Ig superfamily protein expressed on the surface of activated effector T cells and Treg, which binds B7-1 and B7-2 with high affinity and plays an essential role in inhibiting T cell responses. CTLA-4 (also called CD152) is essential for Treg function and T cell tolerance to self antigens.

C-type lectin A member of a large family of calcium-dependent carbohydrate-binding proteins, many of which play important roles in innate and adaptive immunity. For example, soluble C-type lectins bind to microbial carbohydrate structures and mediate phagocytosis or complement activation (e.g., mannose-binding lectin, dectins, collectins, ficolins).

Cutaneous immune system The components of the innate and adaptive immune systems found in the skin that function together in a specialized way to detect and respond to pathogens on or in the skin and to maintain homeostasis with commensal microbes. Components of the cutaneous immune system include keratinocytes, Langerhans cells, dermal dendritic cells, intraepithelial lymphocytes, and dermal lymphocytes.

Cyclic GMP-AMP synthase A cytosolic DNA sensor that generates cyclic GMP-AMP as a second messenger which interacts with the STING adaptor to induce type I interferon synthesis.

Cyclosporine A calcineurin inhibitor widely used as an immunosuppressive drug to prevent allograft rejection by blocking T cell activation. Cyclosporine (also called cyclosporin A) binds to a cytosolic protein called cyclophilin, and cyclosporine-cyclophilin complexes bind to and inhibit calcineurin, thereby inhibiting activation and nuclear translocation of the transcription factor NFAT.

Cytokines Proteins that are produced and secreted by many different cell types, and mediate inflammatory and immune reactions. Cytokines are principal mediators of communication between cells of the immune system (see Appendix II).

Cytosolic DNA sensors (CDSs) Molecules that detect microbial double-stranded DNA in the cytosol and activate signaling pathways that initiate antimicrobial responses, including type 1 interferon production and autophagy.

Cytotoxic (or cytolytic) T lymphocyte (CTL) A type of T lymphocyte whose major effector function is to recognize and kill host cells infected with viruses or other intracellular microbes as well as tumor cells. CTLs usually express CD8 and recognize peptides derived from cytosolic microbial and tumor antigens displayed by class I MHC molecules. CTL killing of infected and tumor cells involves delivery of the contents of cytoplasmic granules into the cytosol of the cells, leading to apoptotic death.

D

Damage-associated molecular patterns (DAMPs) Endogenous molecules that are produced by or released from damaged and dying cells that bind to pattern recognition receptors and stimulate innate immune responses. Examples include high-mobility group box 1 (HMGB1) protein, extracellular ATP, and uric acid.

Death receptors Plasma membrane receptors expressed on various cell types that, upon ligand binding, transduce signals that lead to recruitment of the Fas-associated protein with death domain (FADD) adaptor protein, which activates caspase-8, leading to apoptotic cell death. All death receptors, including FAS, TRAIL, and TNFR, belong to the TNF receptor superfamily.

Dectins Pattern recognition receptors expressed on dendritic cells that recognize fungal cell wall carbohydrates and induce signaling events that promote inflammation and activate the dendritic cells.

Defensins Cysteine-rich peptides produced by epithelial barrier cells in the skin, gut, lung, and other tissues and in neutrophil granules that act as broad-spectrum antibiotics to kill a wide variety of bacteria and fungi. The synthesis of defensins is increased in response to stimulation of innate immune system receptors such as Toll-like receptors and inflammatory cytokines such as IL-1 and TNF.

Delayed-type hypersensitivity (DTH) An immune reaction in which T cell-dependent macrophage activation and inflammation cause tissue injury. A DTH reaction to the subcutaneous injection of antigen is often used as an assay for cell-mediated immunity (e.g., the purified protein derivative skin screening test for immunity to *Mycobacterium tuberculosis*).

Dendritic cells Bone marrow–derived cells found in epithelial and lymphoid tissues that are morphologically characterized by thin membranous projections. Many subsets of dendritic cells exist with diverse functions. Classical (conventional) dendritic cells function as innate sentinel cells and APCs for naive T lymphocytes, and they are important for initiation of adaptive immune responses to protein antigen. Immature (resting) classical dendritic cells are important for induction of tolerance to self antigens. Plasmacytoid dendritic cells produce type 1 interferons in response to exposure to viruses.

Desensitization A method of treating immediate hypersensitivity disease (allergies) that involves repetitive administration of low doses of an antigen to which individuals are allergic. This process often prevents severe allergic reactions on subsequent environmental exposure to the allergen, but the mechanisms are not well understood.

Determinant The specific portion of a macromolecular antigen to which an antibody or T cell receptor binds. In the case of a protein antigen recognized by a T cell, the determinant is the peptide portion that binds to an MHC molecule for recognition by the TCR. Synonymous with **epitope**.

Diacylglycerol (DAG) A signaling molecule generated by phospholipase C (PLCγ1)-mediated hydrolysis of the plasma membrane phospholipid phosphatidylinositol 4,5-bisphosphate (PIP$_2$) during antigen activation of lymphocytes. The main function of DAG is to activate an enzyme called protein kinase C that participates in the generation of active transcription factors.

DiGeorge syndrome A selective T cell deficiency caused by a congenital malformation that results in defective development of the thymus, parathyroid glands, and other structures that arise from the third and fourth pharyngeal pouches.

Direct antigen presentation (direct allorecognition) Presentation of cell surface allogeneic MHC molecules by graft APCs to a graft recipient's T cells that leads to activation of the alloreactive T cells. In direct recognition of allogeneic MHC molecules, a TCR that was selected to recognize a self MHC molecule plus foreign peptide cross-reacts with the allogeneic MHC molecule plus peptide. Direct presentation is partly responsible for strong T cell responses to allografts.

Diversity The existence of a large number of lymphocytes with different antigenic specificities in any individual. Diversity is a fundamental property of the adaptive immune system and is the result of variability in the structures of the antigen-binding sites of lymphocyte receptors for antigens (antibodies and TCRs).

Diversity (D) segments Short coding sequences between the variable (V) and constant (C) gene segments in the Ig heavy chain and TCR β and γ loci that together with J segments are somatically recombined with V segments during lymphocyte development. The resulting recombined VDJ DNA codes for the carboxyl-terminal ends of the antigen receptor V regions, including the third hypervariable (CDR) regions. Random use of D segments contributes to the diversity of the antigen receptor repertoire.

DNA vaccine A vaccine composed of a bacterial plasmid containing a complementary DNA encoding a protein antigen. DNA vaccines presumably work because professional APCs are transfected in vivo by the plasmid and express immunogenic peptides that elicit specific responses. Furthermore, the plasmid DNA contains CpG nucleotides that act as potent adjuvants.

Double-negative thymocyte A subset of developing T cells in the thymus (thymocytes) that express neither CD4 nor CD8. Most double-negative thymocytes are at an early developmental stage and do not express antigen receptors. They will later express both CD4 and CD8 during the intermediate double-positive stage before further maturation to single-positive T cells expressing only CD4 or CD8.

Double-positive thymocyte A subset of developing T cells in the thymus (thymocytes) that express both CD4 and CD8 and are at an intermediate developmental stage. Double-positive thymocytes also express TCRs and are subject to selection processes, and they mature to single-positive T cells expressing only CD4 or CD8.

E

Ectoparasites Parasites that live on the surface of an animal, such as ticks and mites. Both the innate and adaptive immune systems may play a role in protection against ectoparasites, often by destroying the larval stages of these organisms.

Effector cells The cells that perform effector functions during an immune response, such as secreting cytokines (e.g., helper T cells), killing microbes (e.g., macrophages), killing microbe-infected host cells (e.g., CTLs), or secreting antibodies (e.g., differentiated B cells).

Effector phase The phase of an immune response in which a foreign antigen is destroyed or inactivated. For example, in a humoral immune response, the effector phase may be characterized by antibody-dependent complement activation and phagocytosis of antibody- and complement-opsonized bacteria.

Endosome An intracellular membrane-bound vesicle into which extracellular proteins are internalized during antigen processing. Endosomes have an acidic pH and contain proteolytic enzymes that degrade proteins into peptides that bind to class II MHC molecules. A subset of class II MHC-rich endosomes, called MIIC, play a special role in antigen processing and presentation by the class II pathway. (Endosomes are found in all cells and participate in internalization events that are not linked to antigen presentation.)

Endotoxin A component of the cell wall of gram-negative bacteria, also called **lipopolysaccharide** (LPS), that is released from dying bacteria and stimulates innate immune inflammatory responses by binding to TLR4 on many different cell types, including phagocytes, endothelial cells, dendritic cells, and barrier epithelial cells. Endotoxin contains both lipid components and carbohydrate (polysaccharide) moieties.

Enhancer A regulatory nucleotide sequence in a gene that is located either upstream or downstream of the promoter, binds transcription factors, and increases the activity of the promoter. In cells of the immune system, enhancers are responsible for integrating cell surface signals that lead to induced transcription of genes encoding many of the effector proteins of an immune response, such as cytokines.

Envelope glycoprotein (Env) A membrane glycoprotein encoded by a retrovirus that is expressed on the plasma membrane of infected cells and on the host cell-derived membrane coat of viral particles. Env proteins are often required for viral infectivity. The Env proteins of HIV include gp41 and gp120, which bind to CD4 and chemokine receptors, respectively, on human T cells and mediate fusion of the viral and T cell membranes.

Enzyme-linked immunosorbent assay (ELISA) A method of quantifying an antigen immobilized on a solid surface by use of a specific antibody with a covalently coupled enzyme. The amount of antibody that binds the antigen is proportional to the amount of antigen present and is determined by spectrophotometrically measuring the conversion of a clear substrate to a colored product by the coupled enzyme.

Eosinophil A bone marrow–derived granulocyte that is abundant in the inflammatory infiltrates of immediate hypersensitivity late-phase reactions and contributes to many of the pathologic processes in allergic diseases. Eosinophils are important in defense against extracellular parasites, including helminths.

Epitope The specific portion of a macromolecular antigen to which an antibody or T cell receptor binds. In the case of a protein antigen recognized by a T cell, an epitope is the peptide portion that binds to an MHC molecule for recognition by the TCR. Synonymous with **determinant**.

Epitope spreading In autoimmunity, the development of immune responses to multiple epitopes as an autoimmune disease originally targeting one epitope progresses, likely caused by further breakdown in tolerance and release of additional tissue antigens due to the inflammatory process stimulated by the initial response.

Epstein-Barr virus (EBV) A double-stranded DNA virus of the herpesvirus family that is the etiologic agent of infectious mononucleosis and is associated with some B cell malignant tumors and nasopharyngeal carcinoma. EBV infects B lymphocytes and some epithelial cells by specifically binding to CR2 (CD21).

Experimental autoimmune encephalomyelitis (EAE) An animal model of multiple sclerosis, an autoimmune demyelinating disease of the central nervous system. EAE is induced in rodents by immunization with components of the myelin sheath (e.g., myelin basic protein) of nerves, mixed with an adjuvant. The disease is mediated in large part by cytokine-secreting CD4$^+$ T cells specific for the myelin sheath proteins.

F

Fab (fragment, antigen-binding) A part of an antibody, first produced by proteolysis of IgG, that includes one complete light chain paired with one heavy chain fragment containing the variable domain and only the first constant domain. Fab fragments, which can be generated from all antibodies, retain the ability to monovalently bind an antigen but cannot interact with IgG Fc receptors on cells or with complement. Therefore Fab preparations are used in research and therapeutic applications when antigen binding is desired without activation of effector functions. (The Fab′ fragment retains the hinge region of the heavy chain.)

F(ab′)2 A part of an Ig molecule (first produced by proteolysis of IgG) that includes two complete light chains but only the variable domain, first constant domain, and hinge region of the two heavy chains. F(ab′)$_2$ fragments retain the entire bivalent antigen-binding region of an intact Ig molecule but cannot bind complement or Fc receptors. They are used in research and therapeutic applications when antigen binding is desired without antibody effector functions.

Fas (CD95) A death receptor of the TNF receptor family that is expressed on the surface of T cells and many other cell types and initiates a signaling cascade leading to apoptotic death of the cell. The death pathway is initiated when Fas binds to Fas ligand expressed on activated T cells. Fas-mediated killing of lymphocytes is important for the maintenance of self tolerance. Mutations in the *FAS* gene cause systemic autoimmune disease (see also **death receptors**).

Fas ligand (CD95 ligand) A membrane protein that is a member of the TNF family of proteins expressed on activated T cells. Fas ligand binds to the death receptor Fas, thereby stimulating a signaling pathway leading to apoptotic death of the Fas-expressing cell. Mutations in the Fas ligand gene cause systemic autoimmune disease in mice.

Fc (fragment, crystalline) A region of an antibody molecule that can be isolated by proteolysis of IgG that contains only the disulfide-linked carboxyl-terminal regions of the two heavy chains. The Fc region of Ig molecules mediates effector functions by binding to cell surface receptors or the C1q complement protein. (Fc fragments are so named because they tend to crystallize out of solution.)

Fc receptor A cell surface receptor specific for the carboxyl-terminal constant region of an Ig molecule. Fc receptors are typically multichain protein complexes that include signaling components and Ig-binding components. Several types of Fc receptors exist, including those specific for different IgG isotypes, IgE, and IgA. Fc receptors mediate many of the cell-dependent effector functions of antibodies, including phagocytosis of antibody-bound antigens, antigen-induced activation of mast cells, and targeting and activation of NK cells.

FcεRI A high-affinity receptor for the carboxyl-terminal constant region of IgE molecules that is expressed on mast cells, basophils, and eosinophils. FcεRI molecules on mast cells are usually occupied by IgE, and antigen-induced cross-linking of these IgE-FcεRI complexes activates the mast cell and initiates immediate hypersensitivity reactions.

Fcγ receptor (FcγR) A cell surface receptor specific for the carboxyl-terminal constant region of IgG molecules. There are several different types of Fcγ receptors, including a high-affinity FcγRI that mediates phagocytosis by macrophages and neutrophils, a low-affinity FcγRIIB that transduces inhibitory signals in B cells and myeloid cells, and a low-affinity FcγRIIIA that mediates recognition of opsonized cells by and activation of NK cells.

Ficolins Hexameric innate immune system plasma proteins, containing collagen-like domains and fibrinogen-like carbohydrate-recognizing domains, which bind to cell wall components of gram-positive bacteria, opsonizing them and activating complement.

First-set rejection Allograft rejection in an individual who has not previously received a graft or otherwise been exposed to tissue alloantigens from the same donor. First-set rejection usually takes approximately 7 to 14 days.

Flow cytometry A method of analysis of the phenotype of cell populations requiring a specialized instrument (flow cytometer) that can detect fluorescence on individual cells in a suspension and thereby determine the number of cells expressing the molecule to which a fluorescent probe binds, as well as the relative amount of the molecule expressed. Suspensions of cells are incubated with fluorescently labeled antibodies or other probes, and the amount of probe bound by each cell in the population is measured by passing the cells one at a time through a fluorimeter with a laser-generated incident beam.

Fluorescence-activated cell sorter (FACS) An adaptation of the flow cytometer that is used for the purification of cells from a mixed population according to which and how much fluorescent probe the cells bind. Cells are first stained with fluorescently labeled probe, such as an antibody specific for a surface antigen of a cell population. The cells are then passed one at a time through a fluorimeter with a laser-generated incident beam and are deflected into different collection tubes by electromagnetic fields whose strength and direction are varied according to the measured intensity of the fluorescence signal.

Follicle See **lymphoid follicle**.

Follicular dendritic cells (FDCs) Cells in lymphoid follicles of secondary lymphoid organs that express complement receptors and Fc receptors, and have long cytoplasmic processes that form a meshwork integral to the architecture of the follicles. Follicular dendritic cells display antigens on their surface for B cell recognition and are involved in the activation and selection of B cells expressing high-affinity membrane Ig during the process of affinity maturation. They are nonhematopoietic cells (not of bone marrow origin).

Follicular helper T cell (Tfh cell) See **T follicular helper (Tfh) cells**.

N-Formylmethionine An amino acid that initiates all bacterial proteins (except those synthesized within mitochondria) and serves as a signal to the innate immune system of infection. Specific receptors for N-formyl-methionine–containing peptides are expressed on neutrophils and mediate activation of the neutrophils.

FoxP3 A forkhead family transcription factor expressed by and required for the development and function of CD4+ regulatory T cells. Mutations in *FoxP3* in mice and humans result in an absence of CD25+ regulatory T cells and multisystem autoimmune disease.

G

γδ T cell receptor (γδ TCR) A form of TCR that is distinct from the more common αβ TCR and is expressed on a subset of T cells found mostly in epithelial barrier tissues. Although the γδ TCR is structurally similar to the αβ TCR, the forms of antigen recognized by γδ TCRs are poorly understood; they do not recognize peptide complexes bound to polymorphic MHC molecules.

G protein–coupled receptor family A diverse family of receptors for hormones, lipid inflammatory mediators, and chemokines that use associated trimeric G proteins for intracellular signaling.

G proteins Proteins that bind guanyl nucleotides and act as exchange molecules by catalyzing the replacement of bound guanosine diphosphate (GDP) by guanosine triphosphate (GTP). G proteins with bound GTP can activate a variety of cellular enzymes in different signaling cascades. Trimeric GTP-binding proteins are associated with the cytoplasmic portions of many cell surface receptors, such as chemokine receptors. Other small soluble G proteins, such as Ras and Rac, are recruited into signaling pathways by adaptor proteins.

GATA-3 A transcription factor that promotes the differentiation of Th2 cells from naive T cells.

Generative lymphoid organ An organ in which lymphocytes develop from immature precursors. The bone marrow and thymus are the major generative lymphoid organs in which B cells and T cells develop, respectively.

Germinal centers Specialized structures in peripheral (secondary) lymphoid organs generated during T-dependent humoral immune responses, where extensive B cell proliferation, isotype switching, somatic mutation, affinity maturation, memory B cell generation, and induction of long-lived plasma cells take place. Germinal centers appear as lightly staining regions within a lymphoid follicle in spleen, lymph node, and mucosal lymphoid tissue.

Germline organization The inherited arrangement of variable, diversity, joining, and constant region gene segments of the antigen receptor loci in nonlymphoid cells or in immature lymphocytes. In developing B or T lymphocytes, the germline organization is modified by somatic recombination to form functional *Ig* or *TCR* genes.

Glomerulonephritis Inflammation of the renal glomeruli, often initiated by immunopathologic mechanisms such as deposition of circulating antigen-antibody complexes in the glomerular basement membrane or binding of antibodies to antigens expressed in the glomerulus. The antibodies can activate complement and phagocytes, and the resulting inflammatory response can lead to renal failure.

Graft A tissue or organ that is removed from one site and placed in another site, usually in a different individual.

Graft arteriosclerosis Occlusion of graft arteries caused by proliferation of intimal smooth muscle cells. This process may develop within 6 months to a year after transplantation and is responsible for chronic rejection of vascularized organ grafts. The mechanism is likely to be a chronic immune response to vessel wall alloantigens. Graft arteriosclerosis is also called accelerated arteriosclerosis.

Graft rejection A specific immune response to an organ or tissue graft that leads to inflammation, graft damage, and possibly graft failure.

Graft-versus-host disease A disease occurring in hematopoietic stem cell (HSC) transplant recipients that is caused by mature T cells present in the HSC inoculum reacting with alloantigens on host cells. The disease most often affects the skin, liver, and intestines.

Granulocyte colony-stimulating factor (G-CSF) A cytokine made by activated T cells, macrophages, and endothelial cells at sites of infection that acts on bone marrow to increase the production of and mobilize neutrophils to replace those consumed in inflammatory reactions.

Granulocyte-monocyte colony-stimulating factor (GM-CSF) A cytokine made by activated T cells, macrophages, endothelial cells, and stromal fibroblasts that acts on bone marrow to increase the production of neutrophils and monocytes. GM-CSF is also a macrophage-activating factor and promotes the maturation of dendritic cells.

Granuloma A nodule of inflammatory tissue composed of clusters of activated macrophages, usually with associated fibrosis. Granulomatous inflammation is a form of chronic delayed-type hypersensitivity, often in response to persistent microbes, such as *Mycobacterium tuberculosis* and some fungi, or in response to particulate antigens that are not readily phagocytosed.

Granulysin A protein present in the granules of CTLs and NK cells that is released upon activation of these cells and disrupts the membranes of microbes and infected host cells. Granulysin plays a role in tissue damage in certain CTL-mediated reactions to drugs.

Granzyme B A serine protease found in the granules of CTLs and NK cells that is released by exocytosis, enters target cells, and proteolytically cleaves and activates caspases, which in turn cleave several substrates and induce target cell apoptosis.

Gut-associated lymphoid tissue (GALT) Collections of lymphocytes and APCs within the mucosa of the gastrointestinal tract where adaptive immune responses to intestinal microbial flora and ingested antigens are initiated (see also **mucosa-associated lymphoid tissues**).

H

H-2 molecule An MHC molecule in the mouse. The mouse MHC was originally called the H-2 locus.

Haplotype The set of tightly linked MHC alleles inherited together from one parent and present on one chromosome.

Hapten A small chemical that can bind to an antibody but must be attached to a macromolecule (carrier) to stimulate an adaptive immune response specific for that chemical. For example, immunization with dinitrophenol (DNP) alone will not stimulate an anti-DNP antibody response, but immunization with a protein with covalently attached DNP hapten will.

Heavy-chain isotype (class) switching The process by which a B lymphocyte changes the isotype, or class, of the antibodies that it produces, from IgM to IgG, IgE, or IgA, without changing the antigen specificity of the antibody. Heavy-chain isotype switching is stimulated by cytokines and CD40 ligand expressed by helper T cells and involves recombination of B cell VDJ segments with downstream heavy-chain gene segments.

Helminth A parasitic worm. Helminthic infections often elicit Th2-dependent immune responses characterized by eosinophil-rich inflammatory infiltrates and IgE production.

Helper T cells The class of T lymphocytes whose main functions are to activate macrophages and to promote inflammation in cell-mediated immune responses and to promote B cell antibody production in humoral immune responses. These functions are mediated by secreted cytokines and by T cell CD40 ligand binding to macrophage or B cell CD40. Most helper T cells recognize peptide-class II MHC complexes and express the CD4 molecule.

Hematopoiesis The development of mature blood cells, including erythrocytes, leukocytes, and platelets, from pluripotent stem cells in the bone marrow and fetal liver. Hematopoiesis is regulated by several different colony-stimulating factors produced by bone marrow stromal cells, T cells, and other cell types.

Hematopoietic stem cell An undifferentiated bone marrow cell that divides continuously and gives rise to additional stem cells and cells of multiple different lineages. A hematopoietic stem cell in the bone marrow will give rise to cells of the lymphoid, myeloid, and erythrocytic lineage.

Hematopoietic stem cell transplantation The transplantation of hematopoietic stem cells taken from the blood or bone marrow; it is performed clinically to treat inherited defects in and cancers of blood cells and is also used in various immunologic experiments in animals.

High endothelial venules (HEVs) Specialized venules that are the sites of lymphocyte migration from the blood into the stroma of secondary lymphoid tissues. HEVs are lined by plump endothelial cells that protrude into the vessel lumen and express unique adhesion molecules involved in binding naive (and central memory) B and T cells.

Hinge region The region of Ig heavy chains between the first two constant domains that can assume multiple conformations, thereby imparting flexibility in the orientation of the two antigen-binding sites. Because of the hinge region, an antibody molecule can simultaneously bind two epitopes that are separated by some distance from one another.

Histamine A vasoactive amine stored in the granules of mast cells that is one of the important mediators of immediate hypersensitivity. Histamine binds to specific receptors in various tissues and causes increased vascular permeability and contraction of bronchial and intestinal smooth muscle.

HLA See **human leukocyte antigens**.

HLA-DM A peptide exchange molecule that plays a critical role in the class II MHC pathway of antigen presentation. HLA-DM is found in the endosomes involved in class II–associated antigen presentation, where it facilitates removal of the invariant chain–derived CLIP peptide and the binding of other peptides to class II MHC molecules. HLA-DM is encoded by a gene in the MHC and is structurally similar to class II MHC molecules, but it is not polymorphic.

Homeostasis In the adaptive immune system, the maintenance of a constant number and diverse repertoire of lymphocytes, despite the emergence of new lymphocytes and tremendous expansion of individual clones that may occur during responses to immunogenic antigens. Homeostasis is achieved mainly by the death of lymphocytes that are no longer needed, such as those that have eliminated the antigen that initiated the response.

Homing receptor Adhesion molecules expressed on the surface of lymphocytes that are responsible for the different pathways of lymphocyte recirculation and tissue homing. Homing receptors bind to ligands (addressins) expressed on endothelial cells in particular vascular beds.

Human immunodeficiency virus (HIV) The etiologic agent of AIDS. HIV is a retrovirus that infects a variety of cell types, including CD4$^+$ helper T cells, macrophages, and dendritic cells, and causes chronic progressive destruction of the immune system.

Human leukocyte antigens (HLA) MHC molecules expressed on the surface of human cells. Human MHC molecules were first identified as alloantigens on the surface of white blood cells (leukocytes) that bound serum antibodies from individuals previously exposed to other individuals' cells (e.g., mothers or transfusion recipients) (see also **major histocompatibility complex [MHC] molecule**).

Humanized antibody A monoclonal antibody encoded by a recombinant hybrid gene and composed of the antigen-binding sites from a murine monoclonal antibody and the constant region of a human antibody. Humanized antibodies are less likely than mouse monoclonal antibodies to induce an anti-antibody response in humans. They are used clinically in the treatment of inflammatory diseases, tumors, and transplant rejection.

Humoral immunity The type of adaptive immune response mediated by antibodies produced by B lymphocytes. Humoral immunity is the principal defense mechanism against extracellular microbes and their toxins.

Hybridoma A cell line derived by fusion, or somatic cell hybridization, between a normal lymphocyte and an immortalized lymphocyte tumor line. B cell hybridomas created by fusion of normal B cells of defined antigen specificity with a myeloma cell line are used to produce monoclonal antibodies. T cell hybridomas created by fusion of a normal T cell of defined specificity with a T cell tumor line are commonly used in research.

Hyper-IgM syndrome Primary immune deficiency disorders caused by defective CD40-dependent functions in B cells, with impaired class switch recombination (CSR) and somatic hypermutation, leading to poor antibody-mediated immunity against extracellular pathogens and compromised defense against intracellular infections due to impaired CD40-dependent macrophage activation. The most common cause is mutations of the CD40 ligand gene on the X chromosome, but mutations in CD40 and downstream signaling molecules cause similar disorders. Mutations in the genes encoding activation-induced cytidine deaminase or uracil-DNA glycosylase result in the B cell defects seen in CD40 ligand deficiency but do not affect macrophages and characterized by failure of B cell heavy-chain isotype switching and cell-mediated immunity. Patients suffer from both pyogenic bacterial and protozoal infections.

Hyperacute rejection A form of allograft or xenograft rejection that begins within minutes to hours after transplantation and that is characterized by thrombotic occlusion of the graft vessels. Hyperacute rejection is mediated by preexisting antibodies in the host circulation that bind to donor endothelial alloantigens, such as blood group antigens or MHC molecules, and activate the complement system.

Hypersensitivity diseases Disorders caused by immune responses. Hypersensitivity diseases include autoimmune diseases, in which immune responses are directed against self antigens, and diseases that result from uncontrolled or excessive responses against foreign antigens, such as microbes and allergens. The tissue damage that occurs in hypersensitivity diseases is due to the same effector mechanisms used by the immune system to protect against microbes.

Hypervariable region Short segments of approximately 10 amino acid residues within the variable regions of antibody or TCR proteins that form loop structures that contact antigen. Three hypervariable loops are present in each antibody heavy chain and light chain and in each TCR chain. Most of the variability between different antibodies or TCRs is located within these loops (also called **complementarity determining region [CDR]**).

I

Idiotype The shared structural features of a group of antibodies or TCRs of the same specificity. The idiotype reflects the unique variable region sequences that are present in antibodies or TCRs produced by one clone of lymphocyte.

Igα and Igβ Proteins that are required for surface expression and signaling functions of membrane Ig on B cells. Igα and Igβ pairs are disulfide-linked to one another, noncovalently associated with the cytoplasmic tail of membrane Ig, and form the BCR complex. The cytoplasmic domains of Igα and Igβ contain ITAMs that are involved in early signaling events during antigen-induced B cell activation.

IL-1 receptor antagonist (IL-1RA) A natural inhibitor of IL-1 produced by macrophages and other cells that is structurally homologous to IL-1 and binds to the same receptors but is biologically inactive. IL-1RA is used as a drug to treat autoinflammatory syndromes caused by excessive IL-1 production as well as rheumatoid arthritis.

Immature B lymphocyte A membrane IgM+, IgD− B cell, recently derived from marrow precursors, that does not proliferate or differentiate in response to antigens but rather may undergo apoptotic death or become functionally unresponsive. This property is important for the negative selection of B cells that are specific for self antigens present in the bone marrow.

Immediate hypersensitivity The type of immune reaction responsible for allergic diseases, which is dependent on antigen-mediated activation of IgE-coated tissue mast cells. The mast cells release mediators that cause increased vascular permeability, vasodilation, bronchial and visceral smooth muscle contraction, and local inflammation.

Immune complex A multimolecular complex of antibody molecules with bound antigen. Because each antibody molecule has 2 to 10 antigen-binding sites and many antigens are multivalent, immune complexes can vary greatly in size. Immune complexes activate effector mechanisms of humoral immunity, such as the classical complement pathway and Fc receptor–mediated phagocytosis. Deposition of circulating immune complexes in blood vessel walls or renal glomeruli can lead to inflammation and disease.

Immune complex disease An inflammatory disease caused by the deposition of antigen-antibody complexes in blood vessel walls, resulting in local complement activation and inflammation. Immune complexes may form because of overproduction of antibodies against microbial antigens or as a result of autoantibody production in the setting of an autoimmune disease such as systemic lupus erythematosus. Immune complex deposition in the specialized capillary basement membranes of renal glomeruli can cause glomerulonephritis and impair renal function. Deposition of immune complexes in joints can cause arthritis, and deposition in arterial walls can cause vasculitis with thrombosis and ischemic damage to various organs.

Immune deviation The conversion of a T cell response associated with one set of cytokines, such as Th1 cytokines that stimulate inflammatory functions of macrophages, to a response associated with other cytokines, such as Th2 cytokines that activate eosinophils and anti-inflammatory functions of macrophages.

Immune inflammation Inflammation that is a result of an adaptive immune response to antigen. The cellular infiltrate at the inflammatory site may include cells of the innate immune system, such as neutrophils and macrophages, which are recruited as a result of the actions of T cell cytokines.

Immune response A collective and coordinated response to the introduction of foreign substances in an individual mediated by the cells and molecules of the immune system.

Immune response (Ir) genes Originally defined as genes in inbred strains of rodents that were inherited in a dominant Mendelian manner and that controlled the ability of the animals to make antibodies against simple synthetic polypeptides. We now know that *Ir* genes are the polymorphic genes that encode class II MHC molecules, which display peptides to T lymphocytes and are therefore required for T cell activation and helper T cell–dependent B cell (antibody) responses to protein antigens.

Immune surveillance The concept that a physiologic function of the immune system is to recognize and destroy clones of transformed cells before they grow into tumors and to kill tumors after they are formed. The term *immune surveillance* is sometimes used in a general sense to describe the function of T lymphocytes to detect and destroy any cell, not necessarily a tumor cell, that is expressing foreign (e.g., microbial) antigens.

Immune system The molecules, cells, tissues, and organs that collectively function to provide immunity, or protection, against foreign pathogens and cancers.

Immunity Protection against disease, usually infectious disease, mediated by the cells and tissues that are collectively called the immune system. In a broader sense, immunity refers to the ability to respond to foreign substances, including microbes and noninfectious molecules.

Immunoblot An analytical technique in which antibodies are used to detect the presence of an antigen bound to (i.e., blotted on) a solid matrix such as filter paper (also known as a Western blot).

Immunodeficiency See **acquired immunodeficiency** and **congenital immunodeficiency**.

Immunodominant epitope The epitope of a protein antigen that elicits most of the response in an individual immunized with the native protein. Immunodominant epitopes correspond to the peptides of the protein that are proteolytically generated within APCs, bind most avidly to MHC molecules, and are most likely to stimulate T cells.

Immunodysregulation polyendocrinopathy enteropathy X-linked syndrome (IPEX) A rare autoimmune disease, caused by mutations of the FOXP3 transcription factor, resulting in a failure to produce regulatory T cells. IPEX patients suffer from immune-mediated destruction of multiple endocrine organs, as well as allergies and skin and gastrointestinal inflammation.

Immunofluorescence A technique in which a molecule is detected by use of an antibody labeled with a fluorescent probe. For example, in immunofluorescence microscopy, cells that express a particular surface antigen can be stained with a fluorescein-conjugated antibody specific for the antigen and then visualized with a fluorescent microscope.

Immunogen An antigen that induces an immune response. Not all antigens are immunogens. For example, low–molecular-weight compounds (haptens) can bind to antibodies, and are therefore antigens, but will not stimulate an immune response unless they are linked to macromolecules (carriers), and thus are not immunogens.

Immunoglobulin (Ig) Synonymous with antibody (see **antibody**).

Immunoglobulin domain A three-dimensional globular structural motif (also called an Ig fold) found in many proteins in the immune system, including Igs, TCRs, and MHC molecules. Ig domains are approximately 110 amino acid residues in length, include an internal disulfide bond, and contain two layers of β-pleated sheets, each layer composed of three to five strands of antiparallel polypeptide chain.

Immunoglobulin heavy chain One of two types of polypeptide chains in an antibody molecule. The basic structural unit of an antibody includes two identical disulfide-linked heavy chains and two identical light chains. Each heavy chain is composed of a variable (V) Ig domain and three or four constant (C) Ig domains. The different antibody isotypes, including IgM, IgD, IgG, IgA, and IgE, are distinguished by structural differences in their heavy chain constant regions. The heavy chain constant regions mediate effector functions, such as complement activation and engagement of phagocytes.

Immunoglobulin light chain One of two types of polypeptide chains in an antibody molecule. The basic structural unit of an antibody includes two identical light chains, each disulfide linked to one of two identical heavy chains. Each light chain is composed of one variable (V) Ig domain and one constant (C) Ig domain. There are two light chain isotypes, called κ and λ, both functionally identical. Approximately 60% of human antibodies have κ light chains, and 40% have λ light chains.

Immunoglobulin superfamily A large family of proteins that contain a globular structural motif called an Ig domain, or Ig fold, originally described in antibodies. Many proteins of importance in the immune system, including antibodies, TCRs, MHC molecules, CD4, and CD8, are members of this superfamily.

Immunohistochemistry A technique to detect the presence of an antigen in histologic tissue sections by use of an enzyme-coupled antibody that is specific for the antigen. The enzyme converts a colorless substrate to a colored insoluble substance that precipitates at the site where the antibody and thus the antigen are localized. The position of the colored precipitate, and therefore the antigen, in the tissue section is observed by light microscopy. Immunohistochemistry is commonly used in diagnostic pathology and various fields of research.

Immunologic synapse The collection of membrane proteins that become organized at the point of juxtaposition between a T cell and an antigen-presenting cell, including the TCR complex, CD4 or CD8, costimulatory receptors, and integrins on the T cell, which bind to peptide-MHC complexes, costimulators, and integrin ligands, respectively, on the antigen presenting cell. The immune synapse is required for bidirectional functional responses between the T cell and APC, and enhances specific delivery of secreted products from the T cell to the antigen-presenting cell, such as granule contents from a CTL to its target cell.

Immunologic tolerance See **tolerance**.

Immunologically privileged site A site in the body that is inaccessible to or actively suppresses immune responses. The anterior chamber of the eye, the testes, and the brain are examples of immunologically privileged sites.

Immunoperoxidase technique A common immunohistochemical technique in which a horseradish peroxidase–coupled antibody is used to identify the presence of an antigen in a tissue section. The peroxidase enzyme converts a colorless substrate to an insoluble brown product that is observable by light microscopy.

Immunoprecipitation A technique for the isolation of a molecule from a solution by binding it to an antibody and then rendering the antigen-antibody complex insoluble, either by precipitation with a second antibody or by coupling the first antibody to an insoluble particle or bead.

Immunoreceptor tyrosine-based activation motif (ITAM) A conserved protein motif composed of two copies of the sequence tyrosine-x-x-leucine (where x is an unspecified amino acid) found in the cytoplasmic tails of various membrane proteins in the immune system that are involved in signal transduction. ITAMs are present in the ζ and CD3 proteins of the TCR complex, in Igα and Igβ proteins in the BCR complex, in receptors for costimulators, and in several Ig Fc receptors. When these receptors bind their ligands, the tyrosine residues of the ITAMs become phosphorylated and form docking sites for other molecules involved in propagating cell-activating signal transduction pathways.

Immunoreceptor tyrosine-based inhibition motif (ITIM) A six-amino-acid (isoleucine-x-tyrosine-x-x-leucine) motif found in the cytoplasmic tails of various inhibitory receptors in the immune system, including FcγRIIB on B cells, killer cell Ig-like receptors (KIRs) on NK cells, and some coinhibitory receptors of T cells. When these receptors bind their ligands, the ITIMs become phosphorylated on their tyrosine residues and form a docking site for protein tyrosine phosphatases, which in turn function to inhibit other signal transduction pathways.

Immunosuppression Inhibition of one or more components of the adaptive or innate immune system as a result of an underlying disease or intentionally induced by drugs for the purpose of preventing or treating graft rejection or autoimmune disease. A commonly used immunosuppressive drug is cyclosporine, which blocks T cell cytokine production.

Immunotherapy The treatment of a disease with therapeutic agents that promote or inhibit immune responses. For example, cancer immunotherapy involves promotion of active immune responses to tumor antigens or administration of antitumor antibodies or T cells to establish passive immunity.

Immunotoxins Reagents that may be used in the treatment of cancer and consist of covalent conjugates of a potent cellular toxin, such as ricin or diphtheria toxin, with antibodies specific for antigens expressed on the surface of tumor cells. It is hoped that such reagents can specifically target and kill tumor cells without damaging normal cells.

Inbred mouse strain A strain of mice created by repetitive mating of siblings that is characterized by homozygosity at every genetic locus. Every mouse of an inbred strain is genetically identical (syngeneic) to every other mouse of the same strain.

Indirect antigen presentation (indirect allorecognition) In transplantation immunology, a pathway of presentation of donor (allogeneic) MHC molecules by recipient APCs that involves the same mechanisms used to present microbial proteins. The allogeneic MHC proteins are processed by recipient dendritic cells, and peptides derived from the allogeneic MHC molecules are presented, in association with recipient (self) MHC molecules, to host T cells. In contrast to indirect antigen presentation, direct antigen presentation involves recipient T cell recognition of unprocessed allogeneic MHC molecules on the surface of graft cells.

Inflammasome A multiprotein complex in the cytosol of mononuclear phagocytes, dendritic cells, and other cell types that proteolytically generates the active form of IL-1β from the inactive pro-IL-1β precursor. The formation of the inflammasome complex, one variety of which includes NLRP3 (a NOD-like pattern recognition receptor), the ASC (apoptosis associated speck like protein containing a CARD domain) adaptor and procaspase-1, is stimulated by a variety of microbial products, cell damage–associated molecules, and crystals.

Inflammation A complex reaction of vascularized tissue to infection or cell injury that involves extravascular accumulation of plasma proteins and leukocytes. Acute inflammation is a common result of innate immune responses, and local adaptive immune responses can also promote inflammation. Although inflammation serves a protective function in controlling infections and promoting tissue repair, it can also cause tissue damage and disease.

Inflammatory bowel disease (IBD) A group of disorders, including ulcerative colitis and Crohn disease, characterized by chronic inflammation in the gastrointestinal tract. The etiology of IBD is not known, but some evidence indicates that it is caused by inadequate regulation of T cell responses, possibly against intestinal commensal bacteria. IBD develops in gene knockout mice lacking IL-2, IL-10, or the TCR α chain.

Innate immunity Protection against infection that relies on mechanisms that exist before infection, are capable of a rapid response to microbes, and react in essentially the same way to repeated infections. The innate immune system includes epithelial barriers, phagocytic cells (neutrophils, macrophages), NK cells, the complement system, and cytokines, largely made by dendritic cells and mononuclear phagocytes. Innate immune reactions also eliminate damaged and necrotic host tissues.

Innate lymphoid cells (ILCs) Cells that arise from the common lymphoid progenitor in the bone marrow, which have a lymphocyte morphology and perform effector functions similar to T cells, but do not express TCRs. Three groups of innate lymphoid cells, called ILC1, ILC2, and ILC3, produce cytokines and express different transcription factors analogous to the Th1, Th2, and Th17 subsets of CD4+ effector T lymphocytes, respectively. Natural killer cells are related to ILC1's.

Integrins Heterodimeric cell surface proteins whose major functions are to mediate the adhesion of cells to other cells or to extracellular matrix. Integrins are important for T cell interactions with APCs and for migration of leukocytes from blood into tissues. The ligand-binding activity of leukocyte integrins depends on signals induced by chemokines binding to chemokine receptors. Two integrins important in the immune system are VLA-4 (very late antigen 4), and LFA-1 (leukocyte function-associated antigen 1).

Interferon regulatory factors (IRFs) A family of transcription factors that are activated by TLR signals and stimulate production of type I interferons, which are cytokines that inhibit viral replication.

Interferons A group of cytokines originally named for their ability to interfere with viral infections but that have other important immunomodulatory functions. Type I interferons include interferon-α and interferon-β, whose main function is to prevent viral replication in cells; type II interferon, usually called interferon-γ, activates macrophages and various other cell types (see Appendix II).

Interleukins Molecularly defined cytokines that are named with a numerical suffix roughly sequentially in order of discovery or molecular characterization (e.g., interleukin-1, interleukin-2). Some cytokines were originally named for their biologic activities and do not have an interleukin designation (see Appendix II).

Intracellular bacterium A bacterium that survives or replicates within cells. The principal defense against intracellular bacteria, such as *Mycobacterium tuberculosis*, is T cell–mediated immunity.

Intraepithelial lymphocytes T lymphocytes present in the epidermis of the skin and in mucosal epithelia that typically express a limited diversity of antigen receptors. Some of these lymphocytes, called invariant NKT cells, may recognize microbial products, such as glycolipids, associated with nonpolymorphic class I MHC-like molecules. Others, called γδ T cells, recognize various nonpeptide antigens, not presented by MHC molecules. Intraepithelial T lymphocytes may be effector cells of innate immunity.

Invariant chain (Iᵢ) A nonpolymorphic protein that binds to newly synthesized class II MHC molecules in the endoplasmic reticulum. The invariant chain prevents loading of the class II MHC peptide-binding cleft with peptides present in the endoplasmic reticulum, so such peptides are left to associate with class I molecules. The invariant chain also promotes folding and assembly of class II molecules and directs newly formed class II molecules to the endosomal compartment where peptide loading takes place.

Isotype One of five types of antibodies, determined by which of five different forms of heavy chain is present. Antibody isotypes include IgM, IgD, IgG, IgA, and IgE, and each isotype performs a different set of effector functions. Additional structural variations characterize distinct subtypes of IgG and IgA.

J

J (joining) chain A small polypeptide that is disulfide linked to the tail pieces of IgM and IgA antibodies that joins the antibody molecules to form pentamers of IgM and dimers of IgA. The J chain also contributes to the transepithelial transport of these immunoglobulins.

JAK-STAT signaling pathway A signaling pathway initiated by cytokine binding to type I and type II cytokine receptors. This pathway sequentially involves activation of receptor-associated Janus kinase (JAK) tyrosine kinases, JAK-mediated tyrosine phosphorylation of the cytoplasmic tails of cytokine receptors, docking of signal transducers and activators of transcription (STATs) to the phosphorylated receptor chains, JAK-mediated tyrosine phosphorylation of the associated STATs, dimerization and nuclear translocation of the STATs, and STAT binding to regulatory regions of target genes causing transcriptional activation of those genes.

Janus kinases (JAKs) A family of tyrosine kinases that associate with the cytoplasmic tails of several different cytokine receptors, including the receptors for IL-2, IL-3, IL-4, IFN-γ, IL-12, and others. In response to cytokine binding and receptor dimerization, JAKs phosphorylate the cytokine receptors to permit the binding of STATs, and then the JAKs phosphorylate and thereby activate the STATs. Different JAK kinases associate with different cytokine receptors.

Joining (J) segments Short coding sequences between the variable (V) and constant (C) gene segments in all Ig and TCR loci, which together with D segments are somatically recombined with V segments during lymphocyte development. The resulting recombined VDJ DNA codes for the carboxyl-terminal ends of the antigen receptor V regions, including the third hypervariable regions (CDR3). Random use of different J segments contributes to the diversity of the antigen receptor repertoire.

Junctional diversity The diversity in antibody and TCR repertoires that is created by the random addition or removal of nucleotide sequences at junctions between V, D, and J gene segments.

K

Kaposi sarcoma A tumor of vascular cells that frequently arises in patients with AIDS. Kaposi sarcoma is associated with infection by the Kaposi sarcoma–associated herpesvirus (human herpesvirus 8).

Killer cell Ig-like receptors (KIRs) Ig superfamily receptors expressed by NK cells that recognize different alleles of HLA-A, HLA-B, and HLA-C molecules. Some KIRs have signaling components with ITIMs in their cytoplasmic tails, and these deliver inhibitory signals to inactivate the NK cells. Some members of the KIR family have short cytoplasmic tails without ITIMs but associate with other ITAM-containing polypeptides and function as activating receptors.

Knockout mouse A mouse with a targeted disruption of one or more genes that is created by homologous recombination techniques. Knockout mice lacking functional genes encoding cytokines, cell surface receptors, signaling molecules, and transcription factors have provided valuable information about the roles of these molecules in the immune system.

L

Lamina propria A layer of loose connective tissue underlying epithelium in mucosal tissues such as the intestines and airways, where dendritic cells, mast cells, lymphocytes, and macrophages mediate immune responses to invading pathogens.

Langerhans cells Immature dendritic cells found as a meshwork in the epidermal layer of the skin whose major function is to trap microbes and antigens that enter through the skin and transport the antigens to draining lymph nodes. During their migration to the lymph nodes, Langerhans cells differentiate into mature dendritic cells, which can efficiently present antigen to and activate naive T cells.

Large granular lymphocyte Another name for an NK cell based on the morphologic appearance of this cell type in the blood.

Late-phase reaction A component of the immediate hypersensitivity reaction that ensues 2 to 4 hours after mast cell degranulation and that is characterized by an inflammatory infiltrate of eosinophils, basophils, neutrophils, and lymphocytes. Repeated bouts of this late-phase inflammatory reaction can cause tissue damage.

Lck A Src family nonreceptor tyrosine kinase that noncovalently associates with the cytoplasmic tails of CD4 and CD8 molecules in T cells and is involved in the early signaling events of antigen-induced T cell activation. Lck mediates tyrosine phosphorylation of the cytoplasmic tails of CD3 and ζ proteins of the TCR complex.

Lectin pathway of complement activation A pathway of complement activation triggered by the binding of microbial polysaccharides to circulating lectins such as MBL. MBL is structurally similar to C1q and activates the C1r-C1s enzyme complex (like C1q) or activates another serine esterase, called mannose-binding protein-associated serine esterase. The remaining steps of the lectin pathway, beginning with cleavage of C4, are the same as the classical pathway.

Leishmania An obligate intracellular protozoan parasite that infects macrophages and can cause a chronic inflammatory disease involving many tissues. *Leishmania* infection in mice has served as a model system for study of the effector functions of several cytokines and the helper T cell subsets that produce them. Th1 responses to *Leishmania major* and associated IFN-γ production control infection, whereas Th2 responses with IL-4 production lead to disseminated lethal disease.

Lethal hit A term used to describe the events that result in irreversible damage to a target cell when a CTL binds to it. The lethal hit includes CTL granule exocytosis and perforin-dependent delivery of apoptosis-inducing enzymes (granzymes) into the target cell cytoplasm.

Leukemia A malignant disease of bone marrow precursors of blood cells in which large numbers of neoplastic cells usually occupy the bone marrow and often circulate in the blood stream. Lymphocytic leukemias are derived from B or T cell precursors, myelogenous leukemias are derived from granulocyte or monocyte precursors, and erythroid leukemias are derived from red blood cell precursors.

Leukocyte adhesion deficiency (LAD) One of a rare group of congenital (primary) immunodeficiency diseases with infectious complications that is caused by defective expression of leukocyte adhesion molecules required for tissue recruitment of phagocytes and lymphocytes. LAD-1 is due to mutations in the gene encoding the CD18 protein, which is part of β2 integrins. LAD-2 is caused by mutations in a gene that encodes a fucose transporter involved in the synthesis of leukocyte ligands for endothelial selectins.

Leukotrienes A class of arachidonic acid–derived lipid inflammatory mediators produced by the lipoxygenase pathway in many cell types. Mast cells make abundant leukotriene C_4 (LTC$_4$) and its degradation products LTD$_4$ and LTE$_4$, which bind to specific receptors on smooth muscle cells and cause prolonged bronchoconstriction. Leukotrienes contribute to pathology of asthma. Collectively, LTC$_4$, LTD$_4$, and LTE$_4$ constitute what was once called slow-reacting substance of anaphylaxis.

Lipopolysaccharide Synonymous with **endotoxin**.

Live virus vaccine A vaccine composed of a live but nonpathogenic (attenuated) form of a virus. Attenuated viruses carry mutations that interfere with the viral life cycle or virulence. Because live virus vaccines actually infect the recipient cells, they can effectively stimulate immune responses that are optimal for protecting against wild-type viral infection. A commonly used live virus vaccine is the Sabin oral poliovirus vaccine.

Lymph node Small nodular, encapsulated lymphocyte-rich organs situated along lymphatic channels throughout the body where adaptive immune responses to lymph-borne antigens are initiated. Lymph nodes, which are secondary or peripheral lymphoid organs, have a specialized anatomic architecture that regulates the interactions of B cells, T cells, dendritic cells, macrophages, and antigens to maximize the induction of protective immune responses. Lymph nodes also perform a filtering function, trapping microorganism and other potentially harmful constituents in tissue fluids and preventing them from draining via the lymph into the blood.

Lymphatic system A system of vessels throughout the body that collects tissue fluid called lymph, originally derived from the blood, and returns it, through the thoracic duct, to the circulation. Lymph nodes are interspersed along these vessels and trap and retain antigens present in the lymph.

Lymphocyte homing The directed migration of subsets of circulating lymphocytes into particular tissue sites. Lymphocyte homing is regulated by the selective expression of endothelial adhesion molecules and chemokines in different tissues. For example, some lymphocytes preferentially home to the intestinal mucosa, which is regulated by the chemokine CCL25 and the endothelial adhesion molecule MadCAM, both expressed in the gut, which bind respectively to the CCR9 chemokine receptor and the α4β1 integrin on gut-homing lymphocytes.

Lymphocyte maturation The process by which pluripotent hematopoietic stem cells develop into mature, antigen receptor–expressing naive B or T lymphocytes that populate peripheral lymphoid tissues. This process takes place in the specialized environments of the bone marrow (for B cells) and the thymus (for T cells). Synonymous with **lymphocyte development**.

Lymphocyte migration The movement of lymphocytes from the circulation into peripheral tissues.

Lymphocyte recirculation The continuous movement of naive lymphocytes from the blood to secondary lymphoid organs, and back into the blood.

Lymphocyte repertoire The complete collection of antigen receptors and therefore antigen specificities expressed by the B and T lymphocytes of an individual.

Lymphoid follicle A B cell–rich region of a lymph node or the spleen that is the site of antigen-induced B cell proliferation and differentiation. In T cell–dependent B cell responses to protein antigens, a germinal center forms within the follicles.

Lymphoid tissue inducer cells A type of hematopoietically derived innate lymphoid cell that stimulates the development of lymph nodes and other secondary lymphoid organs, in part through production of the cytokines lymphotoxin-α (LTα) and lymphotoxin-β (LTβ).

Lymphokine An old name for a cytokine (soluble protein mediator of immune responses) produced by lymphocytes.

Lymphokine-activated killer (LAK) cells NK cells with enhanced cytotoxic activity for tumor cells as a result of exposure to high doses of IL-2. LAK cells generated in vitro have been adoptively transferred back into patients with cancer to treat their tumors.

Lymphoma A malignant tumor of B or T lymphocytes usually arising in and spreading between lymphoid tissues but that may spread to other tissues. Lymphomas often express phenotypic characteristics of the normal lymphocytes from which they were derived.

Lymphotoxin (LT, TNF-β) A cytokine produced by T cells that is homologous to and binds to the same receptors as TNF. Like TNF, LT has proinflammatory effects, including endothelial and neutrophil activation. LT is also critical for the normal development of lymphoid organs.

Lysosome A membrane-bound, acidic organelle abundant in phagocytic cells that contains proteolytic enzymes that degrade proteins derived both from the extracellular environment and from within the cell. Lysosomes are involved in the class II MHC pathway of antigen processing.

M

M cells Specialized gastrointestinal mucosal epithelial cells overlying Peyer patches in the gut that play a role in delivery of antigens to Peyer patches.

M1 macrophages See **classical macrophage activation**.

M2 macrophages See **alternative macrophage activation**.

Macrophage A hematopoietically derived phagocytic cell that plays important roles in innate and adaptive immune responses. Macrophages are activated by microbial products such as endotoxin and by T cell cytokines such as IFN-γ. Activated macrophages phagocytose and kill microorganisms, secrete proinflammatory cytokines, and present antigens to helper T cells. Macrophages include cells derived from recently recruited blood monocytes at sites of inflammation and long-lived tissue-based cells derived from fetal hematopoietic organs. Tissue macrophages are given different names and may serve special functions; these include the microglia of the central nervous system, Kupffer cells in the liver, alveolar macrophages in the lung, and osteoclasts in bone.

Major histocompatibility complex (MHC) A large genetic locus (on human chromosome 6 and mouse chromosome 17) that includes the highly polymorphic genes encoding the peptide-binding molecules recognized by T lymphocytes. The MHC locus also includes genes encoding cytokines, molecules involved in antigen processing, and complement proteins.

Major histocompatibility complex (MHC) molecule A heterodimeric membrane protein encoded in the MHC locus that serves as a peptide display molecule for recognition by T lymphocytes. Two structurally distinct types of MHC molecules exist. Class I MHC molecules are present on most nucleated cells, bind peptides derived from cytosolic proteins, and are recognized by CD8+ T cells. Class II MHC molecules are restricted largely to dendritic cells, macrophages, and B lymphocytes, bind peptides derived from endocytosed proteins, and are recognized by CD4+ T cells.

Mannose-binding lectin (MBL) A plasma protein that binds to mannose residues on bacterial cell walls and acts as an opsonin by promoting phagocytosis of the bacteria by macrophages. Macrophages express a surface receptor for C1q that can also bind MBL and mediate uptake of the opsonized organisms.

Mannose receptor A carbohydrate-binding protein (lectin) expressed by macrophages that binds mannose and fucose residues on microbial cell walls and mediates phagocytosis of the organisms.

Marginal zone A peripheral region of splenic lymphoid follicles containing macrophages that are particularly efficient at trapping polysaccharide antigens. Such antigens may persist for prolonged periods on the surfaces of marginal zone macrophages, where they are recognized by specific B cells, or they may be transported into follicles.

Marginal zone B lymphocytes A subset of B lymphocytes, found exclusively in the marginal zone of the spleen, that respond rapidly to blood-borne microbial antigens by producing IgM antibodies with limited diversity.

Mass cytometry A method of simultaneous detection and analysis of many different molecules expressed in mixed cell populations, requiring a specialized instrument based on the single cell analysis of flow cytometer coupled with a time-of-flight mass spectrometer. This technique uses antibodies labeled with heavy metal ions, rather than fluorochromes used in flow cytometry.

Mast cell The major effector cell of immediate hypersensitivity (allergic) reactions. Mast cells are derived from the marrow, reside in most tissues adjacent to blood vessels, express a high-affinity Fc receptor for IgE, and contain numerous mediator-filled granules. Antigen-induced cross-linking of IgE bound to the mast cell Fcε receptors causes release of their granule contents as well as new synthesis and secretion of other mediators, leading to an immediate hypersensitivity reaction.

Mature B cell IgM- and IgD-expressing, functionally competent naive B cells that represent the final stage of B cell maturation in the spleen and that populate peripheral lymphoid organs.

Membrane attack complex (MAC) A lytic complex of the terminal components of the complement cascade, including complement proteins C5, C6, C7, C8, and multiple copies of C9, which forms in the membranes of target cells. The MAC causes lethal ionic and osmotic changes in cells.

Memory The property of the adaptive immune system to respond more rapidly, with greater magnitude, and more effectively to a repeated exposure to an antigen compared with the response to the first exposure.

Memory lymphocytes Memory B and T cells are produced by antigen stimulation of naive lymphocytes and survive in a functionally quiescent state for many years after the antigen is eliminated. Memory lymphocytes mediate rapid and enhanced (i.e., memory or recall) responses to second and subsequent exposures to antigens.

MHC restriction The characteristic of T lymphocytes that they recognize a foreign peptide antigen only when it is bound to a particular allelic form of an MHC molecule.

MHC tetramer A reagent used to identify and enumerate T cells that specifically recognize a particular MHC-peptide complex. The reagent consists of four recombinant, biotinylated MHC molecules (usually class I) loaded with a peptide and bound to a fluorochrome-labeled avidin molecule. T cells that bind the MHC tetramer can be detected by flow cytometry.

β2-Microglobulin The light chain of a class I MHC molecule. β2-Microglobulin is an extracellular protein encoded by a nonpolymorphic gene outside the MHC, is structurally homologous to an Ig domain, and is invariant among all class I molecules.

Mitogen-activated protein (MAP) kinase cascade A signal transduction cascade initiated by the active form of the Ras protein and involving the sequential activation of three serine/threonine kinases, the last one being MAP kinase. MAP kinase in turn phosphorylates and activates other enzymes and transcription factors. The MAP kinase pathway is one of several signal pathways activated by antigen binding to the TCR and BCR.

Mixed leukocyte reaction (MLR) An in vitro reaction of alloreactive T cells from one individual against MHC antigens on blood cells from another individual. The MLR involves proliferation of and cytokine secretion by both CD4+ and CD8+ T cells.

Molecular mimicry A postulated mechanism of autoimmunity triggered by infection with a microbe containing antigens that cross-react with self antigens. Immune responses to the microbe result in reactions against self-tissues.

Monoclonal antibody An antibody that is specific for one antigen and is produced by a B cell hybridoma (a cell line derived by the fusion of a single normal B cell and an immortal B cell tumor line). Monoclonal antibodies are widely used in research, clinical diagnosis, and therapy.

Monocyte A type of bone marrow–derived circulating blood cell that is the precursor of tissue macrophages. Monocytes are actively recruited into inflammatory sites, where they differentiate into macrophages.

Mononuclear phagocytes Cells with a common bone marrow lineage whose primary function is phagocytosis. These cells function as effector cells in innate and adaptive immunity. Mononuclear phagocytes circulate in the blood in an incompletely differentiated form called monocytes, and after they settle in tissues, they mature into macrophages.

Mucosa-associated lymphoid tissue (MALT) Collections of lymphocytes, dendritic cells, and other cell types within the mucosa of the gastrointestinal and respiratory tracts that are sites of adaptive immune responses to antigens. Mucosa-associated lymphoid tissues contain intraepithelial lymphocytes, mainly T cells, and organized collections of lymphocytes, often rich in B cells, below mucosal epithelia, such as Peyer patches in the gut or pharyngeal tonsils.

Mucosal-associated invariant T (MAIT) cells A subset of T cells that express an invariant αβ TCR specific for fungal and bacterial riboflavin metabolites presented by a nonpolymorphic class I MHC -related molecule. Most MAIT cells are CD8+, are activated either by microbial riboflavin derivatives or by cytokines, and may have inflammatory and cytotoxic functions. MAIT cells account for 20% to 40% of T cells in the human liver.

Mucosal immune system A part of the immune system that responds to and protects against microbes that enter the body through mucosal surfaces, such as the gastrointestinal and respiratory tracts, but also maintains tolerance to commensal organisms that live on the outside of the mucosal epithelium. The mucosal immune system is composed of organized mucosa-associated lymphoid tissues, such as Peyer patches, as well as diffusely distributed cells within the lamina propria.

Multiple myeloma A malignant tumor of antibody-producing plasma cells that often secretes Igs or parts of Ig molecules. The monoclonal antibodies produced by multiple myelomas were critical for early biochemical analyses of antibody structure.

Multiple sclerosis A chronic progressive autoimmune disease of the central nervous system characterized by inflammatory damage to the myelin sheath of neurons, mediated by autoreactive CD4+ T cells, leading to impairment of sensory and motor functions.

Multivalency See **polyvalency**.

Mycobacterium A genus of aerobic bacteria, many species of which can survive within phagocytes and cause disease. The principal host defense against mycobacteria such as *Mycobacterium tuberculosis* is cell-mediated immunity.

Myeloid cells   Cells derived from the myeloid lineage of hematopoietic precursors, including granulocytes, monocytes, and dendritic cells. Myeloid cells are distinct from lymphoid cells, which include B cells, T cells, innate lymphoid cells, and natural killer cells, all derived from a common lymphoid progenitor.

Myeloid-derived suppressor cells   A heterogeneous group of immature myeloid precursors that suppress antitumor immune responses and are found in lymphoid tissues, blood, or tumors of tumor-bearing animals and cancer patients. The cells express Ly6C or Ly6G and CD11b in mice and CD33, CD11b, and CD15 in humans.

N

N nucleotides   The name given to nucleotides randomly added to the junctions between V, D, and J gene segments in *Ig* or *TCR* genes during lymphocyte development. The addition of up to 20 of these nucleotides, which is mediated by the enzyme terminal deoxyribonucleotidyl transferase, contributes to the diversity of the antibody and TCR repertoires.

Naive lymphocyte   A mature B or T lymphocyte that has not previously encountered antigen. When naive lymphocytes are stimulated by antigen, they differentiate into effector lymphocytes, such as antibody-secreting B cells, cytokine-producing helper T cells, and CTLs capable of killing target cells. Naive lymphocytes have surface markers and recirculation patterns that are distinct from those of previously activated lymphocytes. ("Naive" also refers to an unimmunized individual.)

Natural antibodies   IgM antibodies, largely produced by B-1 cells, specific for bacteria that are common in the environment and gastrointestinal tract. Normal individuals contain natural antibodies without any evidence of infection or overt antigen exposure, and these antibodies serve as a preformed defense mechanism against microbes that succeed in penetrating epithelial barriers. Some of these antibodies cross-react with ABO blood group antigens and are responsible for transfusion reactions.

Natural killer (NK) cells   A subset of lymphoid cells, related to group 1 innate lymphoid cells, that function in innate immune responses to kill microbe-infected cells by direct lytic mechanisms and by

secreting IFN-γ. NK cells do not express clonally distributed antigen receptors like Ig receptors or TCRs, and their activation is regulated by a combination of cell surface stimulatory and inhibitory receptors, the latter recognizing self MHC molecules.

Natural killer T cells (NKT cells)   A numerically small subset of lymphocytes that express T cell receptors and some surface molecules characteristic of NK cells. Some NKT cells, called invariant NKT (iNKT), express αβ T cell antigen receptors with very little diversity and recognize lipid antigens presented by CD1 molecules. The physiologic functions of NKT cells are not well defined.

Negative selection   The process by which developing lymphocytes that express self-reactive antigen receptors are eliminated, thereby contributing to the maintenance of self tolerance. Negative selection of developing T lymphocytes (thymocytes) is best understood and involves high-avidity binding of a thymocyte to self MHC molecules with bound peptides on thymic APCs, leading to apoptotic death of the thymocyte.

Neoantigen   A macromolecule that is newly changed, either by chemical modification, or in the case of proteins, by mutation of the encoding gene, such that the new structure is recognized by antibodies or T cells. Neoantigens encoded by mutated proteins are the major inducers of tumor-specific T cell responses.

Neonatal Fc receptor (FcRn)   An IgG-specific Fc receptor that mediates the transport of maternal IgG across the placenta and the neonatal intestinal epithelium and, in adults, promotes the long half-life of IgG molecules in the blood by protecting them from catabolism by phagocytes and endothelial cells.

Neonatal immunity   Passive humoral immunity to infections in mammals in the first months of life, before full development of the immune system. Neonatal immunity is mediated by maternally produced antibodies transported across the placenta into the fetal circulation before birth or derived from ingested milk and transported across the gut epithelium.

Neutrophil (also polymorphonuclear leukocyte, PMN)   A phagocytic cell characterized by a segmented lobular nucleus and cytoplasmic granules filled with degradative enzymes. PMNs are the

most abundant type of circulating white blood cells and are the major cell type in acute inflammatory responses to bacterial infections.

Nitric oxide   A molecule with a broad range of activities that in macrophages functions as a potent microbicidal agent to kill ingested organisms.

Nitric oxide synthase   A member of a family of enzymes that synthesize the vasoactive and microbicidal compound nitric oxide from L-arginine. Macrophages express an inducible form of this enzyme on activation by various microbial or cytokine stimuli.

NOD-like receptors (NLRs)   A family of cytosolic multidomain proteins that sense cytoplasmic PAMPs and DAMPs and recruit other proteins to form signaling complexes that promote inflammation.

Notch 1   A cell surface signaling receptor that is proteolytically cleaved after ligand binding, and the cleaved intracellular portion translocates to the nucleus and regulates gene expression. Notch-1 signaling is required for commitment of developing T cell precursors to the αβ T cell lineage.

Nuclear factor κB (NF-κB)   A family of transcription factors composed of homodimers or heterodimers of proteins homologous to the c-Rel protein. NF-κB proteins are required for the inducible transcription of many genes important in both innate and adaptive immune responses.

Nuclear factor of activated T cells (NFAT)   A transcription factor required for the expression of IL-2, IL-4, and other cytokine genes. The four different NFATs are each encoded by separate genes; NFATp and NFATc are found in T cells. Cytoplasmic NFAT is activated by calcium/calmodulin-dependent, calcineurin-mediated dephosphorylation that permits NFAT to translocate into the nucleus and bind to consensus binding sequences in the regulatory regions of IL-2, IL-4, and other cytokine genes, usually in association with other transcription factors such as AP-1.

Nude mouse   A strain of mice that lacks development of the thymus, and therefore T lymphocytes, as well as hair follicles. Nude mice have been used experimentally to define the role of T lymphocytes in immunity and disease.

O

Oncofetal antigen Proteins that are expressed at high levels on some types of cancer cells and in normal developing fetal (but not adult) tissues. Antibodies specific for these proteins are often used in histopathologic identification of tumors or to monitor the progression of tumor growth in patients. CEA (CD66) and α-fetoprotein are two oncofetal antigens commonly expressed by certain carcinomas.

Opsonin A molecule that becomes attached to the surface of a microbe and can be recognized by surface receptors of neutrophils and macrophages and that increases the efficiency of phagocytosis of the microbe. Opsonins include IgG antibodies, which are recognized by the Fcγ receptor on phagocytes, and fragments of complement proteins, which are recognized by CR1 (CD35) and by the leukocyte integrin Mac-1.

Opsonization The process of attaching opsonins, such as IgG or complement fragments, to microbial surfaces to target the microbes for phagocytosis.

Oral tolerance The suppression of systemic humoral and cell-mediated immune responses to an antigen after the oral administration of that antigen as a result of anergy of antigen-specific T cells or the production of immunosuppressive cytokines such as transforming growth factor-β. Oral tolerance is a possible mechanism for prevention of immune responses to food antigens and to bacteria that normally reside as commensals in the intestinal lumen.

P

P nucleotides Short inverted repeat nucleotide sequences in the VDJ junctions of rearranged *Ig* and *TCR* genes that are generated by RAG-1- and RAG-2-mediated asymmetric cleavage of hairpin DNA intermediates during somatic recombination events. P nucleotides contribute to the junctional diversity of antigen receptors.

Paracrine factor A molecule that acts on cells in proximity to the cell that produces the factor. Most cytokines act in a paracrine fashion.

Passive immunity The form of immunity to an antigen that is established in one individual by transfer of antibodies or lymphocytes from another individual who is immune to that antigen. The recipient of such a transfer can become immune to the antigen without ever having been exposed to or having responded to the antigen. Examples of passive immunity are the transfer of human sera containing antibodies specific for certain microbial toxins or snake venom to a previously unimmunized individual, as well as maternal IgG that is delivered into the fetus through the placenta, which protects babies from infections for about 6 months.

Pathogen-associated molecular patterns (PAMPs) Structures produced by microorganisms but not mammalian (host) cells, which are recognized by and stimulate the innate immune system. Examples include bacterial lipopolysaccharide and viral double-stranded RNA.

Pathogenicity The ability of a microorganism to cause disease. Multiple mechanisms may contribute to pathogenicity, including production of toxins, stimulation of host inflammatory responses, and perturbation of host cell metabolism.

Pattern recognition receptors Signaling receptors of the innate immune system that recognize PAMPs and DAMPs, and thereby activate innate immune responses. Examples include Toll-like receptors (TLRs) and NOD-like receptors (NLRs).

PD-1 An inhibitory receptor homologous to CD28 that is expressed on activated T cells and binds to PD-L1 or PD-L2, members of the B7 protein family expressed on various cell types. PD-1 is upregulated on T cells following repeated or prolonged stimulation, e.g., in the setting of chronic infection or tumors, and blockade of PD-1 with monoclonal antibodies enhances antitumor immune responses.

Pentraxins A family of plasma proteins that contain five identical globular subunits; includes the acute-phase reactant C-reactive protein.

Peptide-binding cleft The portion of an MHC molecule that binds peptides for display to T cells. The cleft is composed of paired α helices resting on a floor made up of an eight-stranded β-pleated sheet. The polymorphic residues, which are the amino acids that vary among different MHC alleles, are located in and around this cleft.

Perforin A protein present in the granules of CTLs and NK cells. When perforin is released from the granules of activated CTLs or NK cells, it inserts into the plasma membrane of the adjacent infected or tumor cells and promotes entry of granzymes, leading to apoptotic death of the target cell.

Periarteriolar lymphoid sheath (PALS) A cuff of lymphocytes surrounding small arterioles in the spleen, adjacent to lymphoid follicles. A PALS contains mainly T lymphocytes, approximately two-thirds of which are CD4+ and one-third CD8+. In humoral immune responses to protein antigens, B lymphocytes are activated at the interface between the PALS and follicles and then migrate into the follicles to form germinal centers.

Peripheral lymphoid organs and tissues Organized collections of lymphocytes and accessory cells, including the spleen, lymph nodes, and mucosa-associated lymphoid tissues, in which adaptive immune responses are initiated. Synonymous with secondary lymphoid organs.

Peripheral tolerance Unresponsiveness to self antigens that are present in peripheral tissues and not usually in the generative lymphoid organs. Peripheral tolerance is induced by the recognition of antigens without adequate levels of the costimulators required for lymphocyte activation or by persistent and repeated stimulation by these self antigens.

Peyer patches Organized lymphoid tissue in the lamina propria of the small intestine in which immune responses to intestinal pathogens and other ingested antigens may be initiated. Peyer patches are composed mostly of B cells, with smaller numbers of T lymphocytes and other cells, all arranged in follicles similar to those found in lymph nodes, often with germinal centers.

Phagocytosis The process by which certain cells of the innate immune system, including macrophages and neutrophils, engulf large particles (>0.5 μm in diameter) such as intact microbes. The cell surrounds the particle with extensions of its plasma membrane by an energy- and cytoskeleton-dependent process; this process results in the formation of an intracellular vesicle called a phagosome, which contains the ingested particle.

Phagosome A membrane-bound intracellular vesicle that contains microbes or particulate material ingested from the extracellular environment. Phagosomes are formed during the process of phagocytosis. They fuse with other vesicles such as lysosomes, leading to enzymatic degradation of the ingested material.

Phosphatase (protein phosphatase) An enzyme that removes phosphate groups from the side chains of certain amino acid residues of proteins. Protein phosphatases in lymphocytes, such as SHP-1 and SHP-2, CD45 and calcineurin, regulate the activity of various signal transduction molecules and transcription factors. Some protein phosphatases may be specific for phosphotyrosine residues and others for phosphoserine and phosphothreonine residues.

Phospholipase Cγ (PLCγ) An enzyme that catalyzes hydrolysis of the plasma membrane phospholipid PIP_2 to generate two signaling molecules, IP3 and DAG. PLCγ becomes activated in lymphocytes by antigen binding to the antigen receptor.

Phytohemagglutinin (PHA) A carbohydrate-binding protein, or lectin, produced by plants that cross-links human T cell surface molecules, including the T cell receptor, thereby inducing polyclonal activation and agglutination of T cells. PHA has been used in experimental immunology to study T cell activation. In clinical medicine, PHA is used to assess whether a patient's T cells are functional or to induce T cell mitosis for the purpose of generating karyotypic data.

Plasmablast Circulating antibody-secreting cells that are precursors of the plasma cells that reside in the bone marrow and other tissues.

Plasma cell A terminally differentiated antibody-secreting B lymphocyte with a characteristic histologic appearance, including an oval shape, eccentric nucleus, and perinuclear halo.

Platelet-activating factor (PAF) A lipid mediator derived from membrane phospholipids in several cell types, including mast cells and endothelial cells. PAF can cause bronchoconstriction and vascular dilation and leak, and it may be an important mediator in asthma.

Polyclonal activators Agents that are capable of activating many clones of lymphocytes, regardless of their antigen specificities. Examples of polyclonal activators include anti-IgM antibodies for B cells and anti-CD3 antibodies, bacterial superantigens, and PHA for T cells.

Poly-Ig receptor An Fc receptor expressed by mucosal epithelial cells that mediates the transport of IgA and IgM through the epithelial cells into the intestinal lumen.

Polymerase chain reaction (PCR) A rapid method of copying and amplifying specific DNA sequences up to about 1 kb in length that is widely used as a preparative and analytical technique in all branches of molecular biology. The method relies on the use of short oligonucleotide primers complementary to the sequences at the ends of the DNA to be amplified and involves repetitive cycles of melting, annealing, and synthesis of DNA.

Polymorphism The existence of two or more alternative forms, or variants, of a gene that are present at stable frequencies in a population. Each common variant of a polymorphic gene is called an allele, and one individual may carry two different alleles of a gene, each inherited from a different parent. The MHC genes, some of which have thousands of alleles, are the most polymorphic genes in the mammalian genome.

Polyvalency The presence of multiple identical copies of an epitope on a single antigen molecule, cell surface, or particle. Polyvalent antigens, such as bacterial capsular polysaccharides, are often capable of activating B lymphocytes independent of helper T cells. Used synonymously with **multivalency**.

Positive selection The process by which developing T cells in the thymus (thymocytes) whose TCRs bind to self MHC molecules are rescued from programmed cell death, whereas thymocytes whose receptors do not recognize self MHC molecules die by default. Positive selection ensures that mature T cells are self MHC restricted and that CD8+ T cells are specific for complexes of peptides with class I MHC molecules and CD4+ T cells for complexes of peptides with class II MHC molecules.

Pre-B cell A developing B cell present only in hematopoietic tissues that is at a maturational stage characterized by expression of cytoplasmic Ig μ heavy chains and surrogate light chains but not Ig light chains. Pre-B cell receptors composed of μ chains and surrogate light chains deliver signals that stimulate further maturation of the pre-B cell into an immature B cell.

Pre-B cell receptor A receptor expressed on developing B lymphocytes at the pre-B cell stage that is composed of Ig μ heavy chains and invariant surrogate light chains. The pre-B cell receptor associates with the Igα and Igβ signal transduction proteins to form the pre-B cell receptor complex. Pre-B cell receptors are required for stimulating the proliferation and continued maturation of the developing B cell, serving as a checkpoint that ensures productive μ heavy chain VDJ rearrangement. It is not known whether the pre-B cell receptor binds a specific ligand.

Pre-T cell A developing T lymphocyte in the thymus at a maturational stage characterized by expression of the TCR β chain but not the α chain or CD4 or CD8. In pre-T cells, the TCR β chain is found on the cell surface as part of the pre-T cell receptor.

Pre-T cell receptor A receptor expressed on the surface of pre-T cells that is composed of the TCR β chain and an invariant pre-Tα protein. This receptor associates with CD3 and ζ molecules to form the pre-T cell receptor complex. The function of this complex is similar to that of the pre-B cell receptor in B cell development, namely, the delivery of signals that stimulate further proliferation, antigen receptor gene rearrangements, and other maturational events. It is not known whether the pre-T cell receptor binds a specific ligand.

Pre-Tα An invariant transmembrane protein with a single extracellular Ig-like domain that associates with the TCR β chain in pre-T cells to form the pre-T cell receptor.

Primary immune response An adaptive immune response that occurs after the first exposure of an individual to a foreign antigen. Primary responses are characterized by relatively slow kinetics and small magnitude compared with the responses after a second or subsequent exposure.

Primary immunodeficiency See **congenital immunodeficiency**.

Pro-B cell A developing B cell in the bone marrow that is the earliest cell committed to the B lymphocyte lineage. Pro-B cells do not produce Ig, but they can be distinguished from other immature cells by the expression of B lineage-restricted surface molecules such as CD19 and CD10.

Pro-T cell A developing T cell in the thymic cortex that is a recent arrival from the bone marrow and does not express TCRs, CD3, ζ chains, or CD4 or CD8 molecules. Pro-T cells are also called double-negative thymocytes.

Professional antigen-presenting cells (professional APCs) A term sometimes used to refer to APCs that activate T lymphocytes; includes dendritic cells, mononuclear phagocytes, and B lymphocytes, all of which are capable of expressing class II MHC molecules and costimulators. The most important professional APCs for initiating primary T cell responses are dendritic cells.

Programmed cell death See **apoptosis**.

Promoter A DNA sequence immediately 5′ to the transcription start site of a gene where the proteins that initiate transcription bind. The term *promoter* is often used to mean the entire 5′ regulatory region of a gene, including enhancers, that are additional sequences that bind transcription factors and interact with the basal transcription complex to increase the rate of transcriptional initiation. Other enhancers may be located at a significant distance from the promoter, either 5′ of the gene, in introns, or 3′ of the gene.

Prostaglandins A class of lipid inflammatory mediators that are derived from arachidonic acid in many cell types through the cyclooxygenase pathway and that have vasodilator, bronchoconstrictor, and chemotactic activities. Prostaglandins made by mast cells are important mediators of allergic reactions.

Proteasome A large multiprotein enzyme complex with a broad range of proteolytic activity that is found in the cytoplasm of most cells and generates from cytosolic proteins the peptides that bind to class I MHC molecules. Proteins are targeted for proteasomal degradation by covalent linkage of ubiquitin molecules.

Protein kinase C (PKC) Any of several isoforms of an enzyme that mediates the phosphorylation of serine and threonine residues in many different protein substrates and thereby serves to propagate various signal transduction pathways leading to transcription factor activation. In T and B lymphocytes, PKC is activated by diacyl glycerol (DAG), which is generated in response to antigen receptor ligation.

Protein tyrosine kinases (PTKs) Enzymes that mediate the phosphorylation of tyrosine residues in proteins and thereby promote phosphotyrosine-dependent protein-protein interactions. PTKs are involved in numerous signal transduction pathways in cells of the immune system.

Protozoa Single-celled eukaryotic organisms, many of which are human parasites and cause diseases. Examples of pathogenic protozoa include *Entamoeba histolytica*, which causes amebic dysentery; *Plasmodium*, which causes malaria; and *Leishmania*, which causes leishmaniasis. Protozoa stimulate both innate and adaptive immune responses.

Provirus A DNA copy of the genome of a retrovirus that is integrated into the host cell genome and from which viral genes are transcribed and the viral genome is reproduced. HIV proviruses can remain inactive for long periods and thereby represent a latent form of HIV infection that is not accessible to immune defense.

Purified antigen (subunit) vaccine A vaccine composed of purified antigens or subunits of microbes. Examples of this type of vaccine include diphtheria and tetanus toxoids, pneumococcus and *Haemophilus influenzae* polysaccharide vaccines, and purified polypeptide vaccines against hepatitis B and influenza virus. Purified antigen vaccines may stimulate antibody and helper T cell responses, but they typically do not generate CTL responses.

Pyogenic bacteria Bacteria, such as gram-positive staphylococci and streptococci, that induce inflammatory responses rich in polymorphonuclear leukocytes (giving rise to pus).

Pyroptosis A form of programmed cell death of macrophages and DCs induced by inflammasome activation of caspase-1, characterized by cell swelling, loss of plasma membrane integrity, and release of inflammatory mediators, such as IL-1α. Pyroptosis results in the death of certain microbes that gain access to the cytosol, enhances inflammatory clearance of bacteria, but also contributes to septic shock.

R

Radioimmunoassay A highly sensitive and specific immunologic method of quantifying the concentration of an antigen in a solution that relies on a radioactively labeled antibody specific for the antigen. Usually, two antibodies specific for the antigen are used. The first antibody is unlabeled but attached to a solid support, where it binds and immobilizes the antigen whose concentration is being determined. The amount of the second, labeled antibody that binds to the immobilized antigen, as determined by radioactive decay detectors, is proportional to the concentration of antigen in the test solution.

Rapamycin An immunosuppressive drug (also called sirolimus) used clinically to prevent allograft rejection. Rapamycin inhibits the activation of a protein called mammalian target of rapamycin (mTOR), which is a key signaling molecule in a variety of metabolic and cell growth pathways including the pathway required for interleukin-2–mediated T cell proliferation.

Ras A member of a family of 21-kD guanine nucleotide-binding proteins with intrinsic GTPase activity that are involved in many different signal transduction pathways in diverse cell types. Mutated *ras* genes are associated with neoplastic transformation. In T cell activation, Ras is recruited to the plasma membrane by tyrosine-phosphorylated adaptor proteins, where it is activated by GDP-GTP exchange factors. GTP·Ras then initiates the MAP kinase cascade, which leads to expression of the *fos* gene and assembly of the AP-1 transcription factor.

Reactive oxygen species (ROS) Highly reactive metabolites of oxygen, including superoxide anion, hydroxyl radical, and hydrogen peroxide, that are produced by activated phagocytes, particularly neutrophils. Reactive oxygen species are used by the phagocytes to form oxyhalides that damage ingested bacteria. They may also be released from cells and promote inflammatory responses or cause tissue damage.

Reagin IgE antibody that mediates an immediate hypersensitivity reaction.

Receptor editing A process by which some immature B cells that recognize self antigens in the bone marrow may be induced to change their Ig specificities. Receptor editing involves reactivation of the *RAG* genes, additional light chain VJ recombinations, and new Ig light chain production, which allows the cell to express a different Ig receptor that is not self-reactive.

Recombination-activating genes 1 and 2 (*RAG1* and *RAG2*)   The genes encoding RAG-1 and RAG-2 proteins, which make up the V(D)J recombinase and are expressed in developing B and T cells. RAG proteins bind to recombination signal sequences and are critical for DNA recombination events that form functional *Ig* and *TCR* genes. Therefore, RAG proteins are required for expression of antigen receptors and for the maturation of B and T lymphocytes.

Recombination signal sequences   Specific DNA sequences found adjacent to the V, D, and J segments in the antigen receptor loci and recognized by the RAG-1/RAG-2 complex during V(D)J recombination. The recognition sequences consist of a highly conserved stretch of 7 nucleotides, called the heptamer, located adjacent to the V, D, or J coding sequence, followed by a spacer of exactly 12 or 23 nonconserved nucleotides and a highly conserved stretch of 9 nucleotides, called the nonamer.

Red pulp   An anatomic and functional compartment of the spleen composed of vascular sinusoids, scattered among which are large numbers of erythrocytes, macrophages, dendritic cells, sparse lymphocytes, and plasma cells. Red pulp macrophages clear the blood of microbes, other foreign particles, and damaged red blood cells.

Regulatory T cells   A population of T cells that inhibits the activation of other T cells and is necessary to maintain peripheral tolerance to self-antigens. Most regulatory T cells are CD4+ and express the α chain of the IL-2 receptor (CD25), CTLA-4, and the transcription factor FoxP3.

Respiratory burst   The process by which reactive oxygen intermediates such as superoxide anion, hydroxyl radical, and hydrogen peroxide are produced in neutrophils and macrophages. The respiratory burst is mediated by the enzyme phagocyte oxidase and is usually triggered by inflammatory mediators, such as the cytokines IFN-γ and TNF, or by bacterial products, such as LPS.

Reverse transcriptase   An enzyme encoded by retroviruses, such as HIV, that synthesizes a DNA copy of the viral genome from the RNA genomic template. Purified reverse transcriptase is used widely in molecular biology research for purposes of cloning complementary DNAs encoding a gene of interest from messenger RNA. Reverse transcriptase inhibitors are used as drugs to treat HIV-1 infection.

Rh blood group antigens   A complex system of protein alloantigens expressed on red blood cell membranes that are the cause of transfusion reactions and hemolytic disease of the newborn. The most clinically important Rh antigen is designated D.

Rheumatoid arthritis   An autoimmune disease characterized primarily by inflammatory damage to joints and sometimes inflammation of blood vessels, lungs, and other tissues. CD4+ T cells, activated B lymphocytes, and plasma cells are found in the inflamed joint lining (synovium), and numerous proinflammatory cytokines, including IL-1 and TNF, are present in the synovial (joint) fluid.

RIG-like receptors (RLRs)   Cytosolic receptors of the innate immune system that recognize viral RNA and induce production of type I interferons. The two best characterized RLRs are RIG-I (retinoic acid–inducible gene I) and MDA5 (melanoma differentiation-associated gene 5).

RORγT (retinoid-related orphan receptor γ T)   A transcription factor expressed in and required for differentiation of Th17 cells and group 3 innate lymphoid cells.

S

Scavenger receptors   A family of cell surface receptors expressed on macrophages, originally defined as receptors that mediate endocytosis of oxidized or acetylated low-density lipoprotein particles but that also bind and mediate the phagocytosis of a variety of microbes.

SCID   See **severe combined immunodeficiency**.

SCID mouse   A mouse strain in which B and T cells are absent because of an early block in maturation from bone marrow precursors. SCID mice carry a mutation in a component of the enzyme DNA-dependent protein kinase, which is required for double-stranded DNA break repair. Deficiency of this enzyme results in abnormal joining of Ig and TCR gene segments during recombination and therefore failure to express antigen receptors.

Secondary immune response   An adaptive immune response that occurs on second exposure to an antigen. A secondary response is characterized by more rapid kinetics and greater magnitude relative to the primary immune response, which occurs on first exposure.

Secondary immunodeficiency   See **acquired immunodeficiency**.

Second-set rejection   Allograft rejection in an individual who has previously been sensitized to the donor's tissue alloantigens by having received another graft or transfusion from that donor. In contrast to first-set rejection, which occurs in an individual who has not previously been sensitized to the donor alloantigens, second-set rejection is rapid and occurs in 3 to 7 days as a result of immunologic memory.

Secondary lymphoid organ   See **peripheral lymphoid organ**.

Secretory component   The proteolytically cleaved portion of the extracellular domain of the poly-Ig receptor that remains bound to an IgA molecule in mucosal secretions.

Selectin   Any one of three separate but closely related carbohydrate-binding proteins that mediate adhesion of leukocytes to endothelial cells. Each of the selectin molecules is a single-chain transmembrane glycoprotein with a similar modular structure, including an extracellular calcium-dependent lectin domain. The selectins include L-selectin (CD62L), expressed on leukocytes; P-selectin (CD62P), expressed on platelets and activated endothelium; and E-selectin (CD62E), expressed on activated endothelium.

Selective immunoglobulin deficiency   Immunodeficiencies characterized by a lack of only one or a few Ig classes or subclasses. IgA deficiency is the most common selective Ig deficiency, followed by IgG3 and IgG2 deficiencies. Patients with these disorders may be at increased risk for bacterial infections, but many are normal.

Self MHC restriction   The limitation (or restriction) of T cells to recognize antigens displayed by MHC molecules that the T cell encountered during maturation in the thymus (and thus sees as self MHC).

Self tolerance   Unresponsiveness of the adaptive immune system to self antigens, largely as a result of inactivation or death of self-reactive lymphocytes induced by exposure to these antigens. Self tolerance is a cardinal feature of the normal immune system, and failure of self tolerance leads to autoimmune diseases.

Septic shock A severe complication of bacterial infections that spread to the blood stream (sepsis), and is characterized by vascular collapse, disseminated intravascular coagulation, and metabolic disturbances. This syndrome is most often due to the effects of bacterial cell wall components, such as LPS or peptidoglycan, that bind to TLRs on various cell types and induce expression of inflammatory cytokines, including TNF and IL-12.

Seroconversion The production of detectable antibodies in the serum specific for a microorganism during the course of an infection or in response to immunization.

Serology The study of blood (serum) antibodies and their reactions with antigens. The term *serology* is often used to refer to the diagnosis of infectious diseases by detection of microbe-specific antibodies in the serum.

Serotype An antigenically distinct subset of a species of an infectious organism that is distinguished from other subsets by serologic (i.e., serum antibody) tests. Humoral immune responses to one serotype of microbes (e.g., influenza virus) may not be protective against another serotype.

Serum The cell-free fluid that remains when blood or plasma forms a clot. Blood antibodies are found in the serum fraction.

Serum amyloid A (SAA) An acute-phase protein whose serum concentration rises significantly in the setting of infection and inflammation, mainly because of IL-1- and TNF-induced synthesis by the liver. SAA activates leukocyte chemotaxis, phagocytosis, and adhesion to endothelial cells.

Serum sickness A disease caused by the injection of large doses of a protein antigen into the blood and characterized by the deposition of antigen–antibody (immune) complexes in blood vessel walls, especially in the kidneys and joints. Immune complex deposition leads to complement fixation and leukocyte recruitment and subsequently to glomerulonephritis and arthritis. Serum sickness

was originally described as a disorder that occurred in patients receiving injections of animal (horse or goat) serum containing antitoxin antibodies to prevent diphtheria.

Severe combined immunodeficiency (SCID) Immunodeficiency diseases in which both B and T lymphocytes do not develop or do not function properly, and therefore both humoral immunity and cell-mediated immunity are impaired. Children with SCID usually have infections during the first year of life and succumb to these infections unless the immunodeficiency is treated. SCID has several different genetic causes.

Shwartzman reaction An experimental model of the pathologic effects of bacterial LPS and TNF in which two intravenous injections of LPS are administered to a rabbit 24 hours apart. After the second injection, the rabbit suffers disseminated intravascular coagulation and neutrophil and platelet plugging of small blood vessels.

Signal transducer and activator of transcription (STAT) A member of a family of proteins that function as transcription factors in response to binding of cytokines to type I and type II cytokine receptors. STATs are present as inactive monomers in the cytosol of cells and are recruited to the cytoplasmic tails of cross-linked cytokine receptors, where they are tyrosine phosphorylated by JAKs. The phosphorylated STAT proteins dimerize and move to the nucleus, where they bind to specific sequences in the promoter regions of various genes and stimulate their transcription. Different STATs are activated by different cytokines.

Single-chain variable fragment (single chain Fv) A genetically engineered polypeptide that includes both Ig heavy chain and light chain V domains that fold to form an antibody binding site of known specificity, used as a research reagent, or as the tumor antigen-binding part of chimeric antigen receptors.

Single-positive thymocyte A maturing T cell precursor in the thymus that expresses CD4 or CD8 molecules but not both. Single-positive thymocytes are found mainly in the medulla and have matured from the double-positive stage, during which thymocytes express both CD4 and CD8 molecules.

Smallpox A disease caused by variola virus. Smallpox was the first infectious disease shown to be preventable by vaccination and the first disease to be completely eradicated by a worldwide vaccination program.

Somatic hypermutation High-frequency point mutations in Ig heavy and light chains that occur in germinal center B cells in response to signals from Tfh cells. Mutations that result in increased affinity of antibodies for antigen impart a selective survival advantage to the B cells producing those antibodies and lead to affinity maturation of a humoral immune response.

Somatic recombination The process of DNA recombination by which the functional genes encoding the variable regions of antigen receptors are formed during lymphocyte development. A relatively limited set of inherited, or germline, DNA sequences that are initially separated from one another are brought together by enzymatic deletion of intervening sequences and re-ligation. This process occurs only in developing B or T lymphocytes and is mediated by RAG-1 and RAG-2 proteins. This process is also called **V(D)J recombination**.

Specificity A cardinal feature of the adaptive immune system, namely, that immune responses are directed toward and able to distinguish between distinct antigens or small parts of macromolecular antigens. This fine specificity is attributed to lymphocyte antigen receptors that may bind to one molecule but not to another, even closely related, molecule.

Spleen A secondary lymphoid organ in the left upper quadrant of the abdomen. The spleen is the major site of adaptive immune responses to blood-borne antigens. The red pulp of the spleen is composed of blood-filled vascular sinusoids lined by active phagocytes that ingest opsonized antigens and damaged red blood cells. The white pulp of the spleen contains lymphocytes and lymphoid follicles where B cells are activated.

Src family kinases A family of protein tyrosine kinases, homologous to the Src tyrosine kinase, which initiate signaling downstream of immune receptors by phosphorylating tyrosine residues on ITAM motifs. Lck is a prominent Src-family kinase in T cells and Lyn in B cells.

Src homology 2 (SH2) domain A three-dimensional domain structure of approximately 100 amino acid residues present in many signaling proteins that permits specific noncovalent interactions with other proteins by binding to phosphotyrosines. Each SH2 domain has a unique binding specificity that is determined by the amino acid residues adjacent to the phosphotyrosine on the target protein. Several proteins involved in early signaling events in T and B lymphocytes interact with one another through SH2 domains.

Src homology 3 (SH3) domain A three-dimensional domain structure of approximately 60 amino acid residues present in many signaling proteins that mediates protein-protein binding. SH3 domains bind to proline residues and function cooperatively with the SH2 domains of the same protein. For instance, SOS, the guanine nucleotide exchange factor for Ras, contains both SH2 and SH3 domains, and both are involved in SOS binding to the adaptor protein Grb-2.

Stem cell An undifferentiated cell that divides continuously and gives rise to additional stem cells and to cells of multiple different lineages. For example, all blood cells arise from a common hematopoietic stem cell.

STING (Stimulator of IFN Genes) An adaptor protein located in the endoplasmic reticulum membrane, which is utilized by several cytoplasmic DNA sensor molecules to transduce signals that activate the IRF3 transcription factor, leading to type 1 IFN gene expression.

Superantigens Proteins that bind to and activate all of the T cells in an individual that express a particular set or family of Vβ *TCR* genes. Superantigens are presented to T cells by binding to nonpolymorphic regions of class II MHC molecules on APCs, and they interact with conserved regions of TCR Vβ domains. Several staphylococcal enterotoxins are superantigens. Their importance lies in their ability to activate many T cells, which results in production of large amounts of cytokine and a clinical syndrome that is similar to septic shock.

Suppressor T cells T cells that block the activation and function of other T lymphocytes. It has been difficult to clearly identify suppressor T cells, and the term is not widely used at this time. The much better defined T cells that function to control immune responses are **regulatory T cells**.

Surrogate light chains Two nonvariable proteins that associate with Ig μ heavy chains in pre-B cells to form the pre-B cell receptor. The two surrogate light chain proteins include the V pre-B protein, which is homologous to a light-chain V domain, and λ5, which is covalently attached to the μ heavy chain by a disulfide bond.

Switch recombination The molecular mechanism underlying Ig isotype switching in which a rearranged VDJ gene segment in an antibody-producing B cell recombines with a downstream C gene and the intervening C gene or genes are deleted. DNA recombination events in switch recombination are triggered by CD40 and cytokines, as well as activation-induced cytidine deaminase, and involve nucleotide sequences called switch regions located in the introns at the 5′ end of each C_H locus.

Syk A cytoplasmic protein tyrosine kinase, similar to ZAP-70 in T cells, that is critical for early signaling steps in antigen-induced B cell activation. Syk binds to phosphorylated tyrosines in the cytoplasmic tails of the Igα and Igβ chains of the BCR complex and in turn phosphorylates adaptor proteins that recruit other components of the signaling cascade.

Syngeneic Genetically identical. All animals of an inbred strain and monozygotic twins are syngeneic.

Syngeneic graft A graft from a donor who is genetically identical to the recipient. Syngeneic grafts are not rejected.

Synthetic vaccine Vaccines composed of recombinant DNA-derived antigens. Synthetic vaccines for hepatitis B virus and herpes simplex virus are now in use.

Systemic inflammatory response syndrome (SIRS) The systemic changes observed in patients who have disseminated bacterial infections and other conditions that induce widespread inflammation, such as burns. In its mild form, SIRS consists of neutrophilia, fever, and a rise in acute-phase reactants in the plasma. These changes are stimulated by bacterial products such as LPS and are mediated by cytokines of the innate immune system. In severe cases, SIRS may include disseminated intravascular coagulation, adult respiratory distress syndrome, and shock.

Systemic lupus erythematosus (SLE) A chronic systemic autoimmune disease that affects predominantly women and is characterized by rashes, arthritis, glomerulonephritis, hemolytic anemia, thrombocytopenia, and central nervous system involvement. Many different autoantibodies are found in patients with SLE, particularly anti-DNA antibodies. Many of the manifestations of SLE are due to the formation of immune complexes composed of autoantibodies and their specific antigens, with deposition of these complexes in small blood vessels in various tissues. The underlying mechanism for the breakdown of self-tolerance in SLE is not understood.

T

T cell receptor (TCR) The clonally distributed antigen receptor on T lymphocytes. The most common form of TCR is composed of a heterodimer of two disulfide-linked transmembrane polypeptide chains, designated α and β, each containing one N-terminal Ig-like variable (V) domain, one Ig-like constant (C) domain, a hydrophobic transmembrane region, and a short cytoplasmic region. The αβ TCR is expressed on CD4+ and CD8+ T cells and recognizes complexes of foreign peptides bound to self MHC molecules on the surface of APCs. (Another less common type of TCR, composed of γ and δ chains, is found on a small subset of T cells and recognizes different forms of antigen.)

T cell receptor (TCR) transgenic mouse A genetically engineered strain of mouse that expresses transgenically encoded TCR α and β genes encoding a TCR of a single defined specificity. Because of allelic exclusion of endogenous TCR genes, most or all of the T cells in a TCR transgenic mouse have the same antigen specificity, which is a useful property for various research purposes.

T follicular helper (Tfh) cells A subset of CD4+ helper T cells present within lymphoid follicles that are critical in providing signals to B cells in the germinal center reaction that stimulate somatic hypermutation, isotype switching, and the generation of memory B cells and long-lived plasma cells. Tfh cells express CXCR5, ICOS, IL-21, and Bcl-6.

T lymphocyte The key component of cell-mediated immune responses in the adaptive immune system. T lymphocytes mature in the thymus, circulate in the blood, populate secondary lymphoid tissues, and are recruited to peripheral sites of antigen exposure. They express antigen receptors (TCRs) that recognize peptide fragments of foreign proteins bound to self MHC molecules. Functional subsets of T lymphocytes include CD4+ helper T cells and CD8+ CTLs.

T-bet A T-box family transcription factor that promotes the differentiation of Th1 cells from naive T cells.

T-dependent antigen An antigen that requires both B cells and helper T cells to stimulate an antibody response. T-dependent antigens are protein antigens that contain some epitopes recognized by T cells and other epitopes recognized by B cells. Helper T cells produce cytokines and cell surface molecules that stimulate B cell growth and differentiation into antibody-secreting cells. Humoral immune responses to T-dependent antigens are characterized by isotype switching, affinity maturation, and memory.

Tacrolimus An immunosuppressive drug (also known as FK506) of the calcineurin inhibitor class, used to prevent allograft rejection, that blocks T cell cytokine gene transcription, similar to cyclosporine. Tacrolimus binds to a cytosolic protein called FK506-binding protein, and the resulting complex binds to the phosphatase calcineurin, thereby inhibiting activation and nuclear translocation of the transcription factor NFAT.

Tertiary lymphoid organ A collection of lymphocytes and antigen-presenting cells organized into B cell follicles and T cell zones that develop in sites of chronic immune-mediated inflammation, such as the joint synovium of rheumatoid arthritis patients.

Th1 cells A subset of CD4+ helper T cells that secrete a particular set of cytokines, including IFN-γ, and whose principal function is to stimulate phagocyte-mediated defense against infections, especially with intracellular microbes.

Th2 cells A subset of CD4+ helper T cells that secrete a particular set of cytokines, including IL-4, IL-5, and IL-13, and whose principal function is to stimulate IgE and eosinophil/mast cell–mediated immune reactions.

Th17 cells A subset of CD4+ helper T cells that secrete a particular set of inflammatory cytokines, including IL-17 and IL-22, that are protective against bacterial and fungal infections and also mediate inflammatory reactions in autoimmune and other inflammatory diseases.

Thymic epithelial cells Epithelial cells abundant in the cortical and medullary stroma of the thymus that play a critical role in T cell development. In the process of positive selection, maturing T cells that weakly recognize self peptides bound to MHC molecules on the surface of thymic epithelial cells are rescued from programmed cell death.

Thymocyte A precursor of a mature T lymphocyte present in the thymus.

Thymus A bilobed organ situated in the anterior mediastinum that is the site of maturation of T lymphocytes from bone marrow-derived precursors. Thymic tissue is divided into an outer cortex and an inner medulla and contains stromal thymic epithelial cells, macrophages, dendritic cells, and numerous T cell precursors (thymocytes) at various stages of maturation.

T-independent antigen Nonprotein antigens, such as polysaccharides and lipids, which can stimulate antibody responses without a requirement for antigen-specific helper T lymphocytes. T-independent antigens usually contain multiple identical epitopes that can cross-link membrane Ig on B cells and thereby activate them. Humoral immune responses to T-independent antigens show relatively little heavy-chain isotype switching or affinity maturation, two processes that require signals from helper T cells.

Tissue typing The determination of the particular MHC alleles expressed by an individual for the purpose of matching allograft donors and recipients. Tissue typing, also called HLA typing, is usually done by molecular (PCR-based) sequencing of HLA alleles or by serologic methods (lysis of an individual's cells by panels of anti-HLA antibodies).

TNF receptor-associated factors (TRAFs) A family of adaptor molecules that interact with the cytoplasmic domains of various receptors in the TNF receptor family, including TNF-RII, lymphotoxin (LT)-β receptor, and CD40. Each of these receptors contains a cytoplasmic motif that binds different TRAFs, which in turn engage other signaling molecules, leading to activation of the transcription factors AP-1 and NF-κB.

Tolerance Unresponsiveness of the adaptive immune system to antigens, as a result of inactivation or death of antigen-specific lymphocytes, induced by exposure to the antigens. Tolerance to self antigens is a normal feature of the adaptive immune system, but tolerance to foreign antigens may be induced under certain conditions of antigen exposure.

Tolerogen An antigen that induces immunologic tolerance, in contrast to an immunogen, which induces an immune response. Many antigens can be either tolerogens or immunogens, depending on how they are administered. All self antigens are tolerogenic. Tolerogenic forms of foreign antigens include large doses of proteins administered without adjuvants and orally administered antigens.

Toll-like receptors A family of pattern recognition receptors of the innate immune system that are expressed on the surface and in endosomes of many cell types and that recognize microbial structures, such as endotoxin and viral RNA, and transduce signals that lead to the expression of inflammatory and antiviral genes.

Tonsils Partially encapsulated secondary lymphoid tissues located beneath barrier epithelium in the nasopharynx and oropharynx, including adenoids (pharyngeal tonsils), palatine tonsils, and lingual tonsils. Tonsils are sites of initiation of adaptive immune responses to microbes in the upper respiratory tract.

Toxic shock syndrome An acute complication of *Staphylococcus aureus* infection characterized by shock, skin exfoliation, conjunctivitis, and diarrhea that is associated with tampon use and post-surgical infections. It is caused by bacterial exotoxins, called superantigens, that are able to activate many clones of T cells, leading to excessive cytokine release.

Transfusion Transplantation of circulating blood cells, platelets, or plasma from one individual to another. Transfusions are performed to treat blood loss from hemorrhage or to treat a deficiency in one or more blood cell types resulting from inadequate production or excess destruction.

Transfusion reactions An immunologic reaction against transfused blood products, usually mediated by preformed antibodies in the recipient that bind to donor blood cell antigens, such as ABO blood group antigens or histocompatibility antigens. Transfusion reactions can lead to intravascular lysis of red blood cells and, in severe cases, kidney damage, fever, shock, and disseminated intravascular coagulation.

Transgenic mouse A mouse that expresses an exogenous gene that has been introduced into the genome by injection of a specific DNA sequence into the pronuclei of fertilized mouse eggs. Transgenes insert randomly at chromosomal break points and are subsequently inherited as simple Mendelian traits. By the design of transgenes with tissue-specific regulatory sequences, mice can be produced that express a particular gene only in certain tissues. Transgenic mice are used extensively in immunology research to study the functions of various cytokines, cell surface molecules, and intracellular signaling molecules.

Transplantation The process of transferring cells, tissues, or organs (i.e., grafts) from one individual to another or from one site to another in the same individual. Transplantation is used to treat a variety of diseases in which there is a functional disorder of a tissue or organ. The major barrier to successful transplantation between individuals is immunologic reaction to the transplanted graft (rejection).

Transporter associated with antigen processing (TAP) An ATP-dependent peptide transporter that mediates the active transport of peptides from the cytosol to the site of assembly of class I MHC molecules inside the endoplasmic reticulum. TAP is a heterodimeric molecule composed of TAP-1 and TAP-2 polypeptides, both encoded by genes in the MHC. Because antigenic peptides are required for stable assembly of class I MHC molecules, TAP-deficient animals express few cell surface class I MHC molecules, which results in diminished development and activation of CD8$^+$ T cells.

Tumor immunity Protection against the development or progression of tumors by the immune system. Although immune responses to naturally occurring tumors can frequently be demonstrated, tumors often escape these responses. New therapies that target T cell inhibitory molecules, such as PD-1, are proving effective in enhancing T cell–mediated antitumor immunity.

Tumor-infiltrating lymphocytes (TILs) Lymphocytes isolated from the inflammatory infiltrates present in and around surgical resection samples of solid tumors that are enriched with tumor-specific CTLs and NK cells. In an experimental mode of cancer treatment, TILs are grown in vitro in the presence of high doses of IL-2 and are then adoptively transferred back into patients with the tumor.

Tumor necrosis factor receptor superfamily (TNFRSF) A large family of structurally homologous transmembrane proteins that bind TNF superfamily proteins and generate signals that regulate proliferation, differentiation, apoptosis, and inflammatory gene expression (see Appendix II).

Tumor necrosis factor superfamily (TNFSF) A large family of structurally homologous transmembrane proteins that regulate diverse functions in responding cells, including proliferation, differentiation, apoptosis, and inflammatory gene expression. TNFSF members typically form homotrimers, either within the plasma membrane or after proteolytic release from the membrane, and bind to homotrimeric TNF receptor superfamily (TNFRSF) molecules, which then initiate a variety of signaling pathways (see Appendix II).

Tumor-specific antigen An antigen whose expression is restricted to a particular tumor and is not expressed by normal cells. Tumor-specific antigens may serve as target antigens for antitumor immune responses.

Tumor-specific transplantation antigen (TSTA) An antigen expressed on experimental animal tumor cells that can be detected by induction of immunologic rejection of tumor transplants. TSTAs were originally defined on chemically induced rodent sarcomas and shown to stimulate CTL-mediated rejection of transplanted tumors.

Two-signal hypothesis A now-proven hypothesis that states that the activation of lymphocytes requires two distinct signals, the first being antigen and the second either microbial products or components of innate immune responses to microbes. The requirement for antigen (so-called signal 1) ensures that the ensuing immune response is specific. The requirement for additional

stimuli triggered by microbes or innate immune reactions (signal 2) ensures that immune responses are induced when they are needed, that is, against microbes and other noxious substances and not against harmless substances, including self antigens. Signal 2 is referred to as costimulation and is often mediated by membrane molecules on APCs, such as B7 proteins.

Type 1 diabetes mellitus A disease characterized by a lack of insulin that leads to various metabolic and vascular abnormalities. The insulin deficiency results from autoimmune destruction of the insulin-producing β cells of the islets of Langerhans in the pancreas, usually during childhood. CD4$^+$ and CD8$^+$ T cells, antibodies, and cytokines have been implicated in the islet cell damage.

U

Ubiquitination Covalent linkage of one or several copies of a small polypeptide called ubiquitin to a protein. Ubiquitination frequently serves to target proteins for proteolytic degradation by proteasomes, a critical step in the class I MHC pathway of antigen processing and presentation.

Uracil N-glycosylase (UNG) An enzyme that removes uracil residues from DNA, leaving an abasic site. UNG is a key participant in isotype switching, and homozygous UNG mutations result in a hyper-IgM syndrome.

Urticaria Localized transient swelling and redness of the skin caused by leakage of fluid and plasma proteins from small vessels into the dermis during an immediate hypersensitivity reaction.

V

V gene segments A DNA sequence that encodes the variable domain of an Ig heavy chain or light chain or a TCR α, β, γ, or δ chain. Each antigen receptor locus contains many different V gene segments, any one of which may recombine with downstream D or J segments during lymphocyte maturation to form functional antigen receptor genes.

V(D)J recombinase The complex of RAG1 and RAG2 proteins that catalyzes lymphocyte antigen receptor gene recombination.

Vaccine A preparation of microbial antigen, often combined with adjuvants, which is administered to individuals to induce protective immunity against microbial infections. The antigen may be in the form of live but avirulent microorganisms, killed microorganisms, purified macromolecular components of a microorganism, or a plasmid that contains a complementary DNA encoding a microbial antigen.

Variable region The extracellular, N-terminal region of an Ig heavy or light chain or a TCR α, β, γ, or δ chain that contains variable amino acid sequences that differ between every clone of lymphocytes and that are responsible for the specificity for antigen. The antigen-binding variable sequences are localized to extended loop structures or hypervariable segments.

Vasoactive amines Low–molecular-weight nonlipid compounds, such as histamine, that all have an amine group, are stored in and released from the cytoplasmic granules of mast cells, and mediate many of the biologic effects of immediate hypersensitivity (allergic) reactions. (Also called biogenic amines.)

Virus A primitive obligate intracellular parasitic organism or infectious particle that consists of a simple nucleic acid genome packaged in a protein capsid, sometimes surrounded by a membrane envelope. Many pathogenic animal viruses cause a wide range of diseases. Humoral immune responses to viruses can be effective in blocking infection of cells, and NK cells and CTLs are necessary to kill cells already infected.

W

Western blot An immunologic technique to determine the presence of a protein in a biologic sample. The method involves separation of proteins in the sample by electrophoresis, transfer of the protein array from the electrophoresis gel to a support membrane by capillary action (blotting), and finally detection of the protein by binding of an enzymatically or radioactively labeled antibody specific for that protein.

Wheal-and-flare reaction Local swelling and redness in the skin at a site of an immediate hypersensitivity reaction. The wheal reflects increased vascular permeability, and the flare results from increased local blood flow, both changes resulting from mediators such as histamine released from activated dermal mast cells.

White pulp The part of the spleen that is composed predominantly of lymphocytes, arranged in periarteriolar lymphoid sheaths, and follicles and other leukocytes. The remainder of the spleen contains sinusoids lined with phagocytic cells and filled with blood, called the **red pulp**.

Wiskott-Aldrich syndrome An X-linked disease characterized by eczema, thrombocytopenia (reduced blood platelets), and immunodeficiency manifested as susceptibility to bacterial infections. The defective gene encodes a cytosolic protein involved in signaling cascades and regulation of the actin cytoskeleton.

X

XBP-1 A transcription factor that is required for the unfolded protein response and plasma cell development.

Xenoantigen An antigen on a graft from another species.

Xenograft (xenogeneic graft) An organ or tissue graft derived from a species different from the recipient. Transplantation of xenogeneic grafts (e.g., from a pig) to humans is not yet practical because of special problems related to immunologic rejection.

Xenoreactive Describing a T cell or antibody that recognizes and responds to an antigen on a graft from another species (a xenoantigen). The T cell may recognize an intact xenogeneic MHC molecule or a peptide derived from a xenogeneic protein bound to a self MHC molecule.

X-linked agammaglobulinemia An immunodeficiency disease, also called Bruton agammaglobulinemia, characterized by a block in early B cell maturation and an absence of serum Ig. Patients suffer from pyogenic bacterial infections. The disease is caused by mutations or deletions in the gene encoding Btk, an enzyme involved in signal transduction in developing B cells.

Z

ζ Chain A transmembrane protein expressed in T cells as part of the TCR complex that contains ITAMs in its cytoplasmic tail and binds the ZAP-70 protein tyrosine kinase during T cell activation.

Zeta-associated protein of 70 kD (ZAP-70) A cytoplasmic protein tyrosine kinase, similar to Syk in B cells, that is critical for early signaling steps in antigen-induced T cell activation. ZAP-70 binds to phosphorylated tyrosines in the cytoplasmic tails of the ζ chain and CD3 chains of the TCR complex and in turn phosphorylates adaptor proteins that recruit other components of the signaling cascade.

Principal Features of Selected CD Molecules

The following list includes selected CD molecules that are referred to in the text. Many cytokines and cytokine receptors have been assigned CD numbers, but we refer to these by the more descriptive cytokine designation, and these are listed in Appendix II. A complete and up-to-date listing of CD molecules may be found at http://www.hcdm.org.

CD Number (Other Names)	Molecular Structure, Family	Main Cellular Expression	Known or Proposed Function(s)
CD1a–d	49 kD; class I MHC-like Ig superfamily; β_2-microglobulin associated	Thymocytes, dendritic cells (including Langerhans cells)	Presentation of nonpeptide (lipid and glycolipid) antigens to some T cells
CD1e	28 kD; class I MHC-like; $\beta2$-microglobulin associated	Dendritic cells	Same as CD1a
CD2 (LFA-2)	50 kD; Ig superfamily	T cells, NK cells	Adhesion molecule (binds CD58); T cell activation; cytotoxic T lymphocyte (CTL)– and natural killer (NK) cell–mediated lysis
CD3g (CD3γ)	25–28 kD; associated with CD3δ and CD3ε in TCR complex; Ig superfamily; ITAM in cytoplasmic tail	T cells	Cell surface expression of and signal transduction by the T cell antigen receptor
CD3d (CD3δ)	20 kD; associated with CD3γ and CD3ε in TCR complex; Ig superfamily; ITAM in cytoplasmic tail	T cells	Cell surface expression of and signal transduction by the T cell antigen receptor
CD3e (CD3ε)	20 kD; associated with CD3δ and CD3γ in TCR complex; Ig superfamily; ITAM in cytoplasmic tail	T cells	Cell surface expression of and signal transduction by the T cell antigen receptor
CD4	55 kD; Ig superfamily	Class II MHC-restricted T cells; some macrophages	Coreceptor in class II MHC-restricted antigen-induced T cell activation (binds to class II MHC molecules); thymocyte development; receptor for HIV
CD5	67 kD; scavenger receptor family	T cells; B-1 B cell subset	Signaling molecule; binds CD72
CD8a	34 kD; expressed as a homodimer or heterodimer with CD8b chain	Class I MHC-restricted T cells; subset of dendritic cells	Coreceptor in class I MHC-restricted antigen-induced T cell activation (binds to class I MHC molecules); thymocyte development

CD Number (Other Names)	Molecular Structure, Family	Main Cellular Expression	Known or Proposed Function(s)
CD8b	34 kD; expressed as a heterodimer with CD8a chain Ig superfamily	Class I MHC-restricted T cells	Same as CD8α
CD10	100 kD; type II membrane protein	Immature and some mature B cells; lymphoid progenitors, granulocytes	Metalloproteinase; unknown function in the immune system
CD11a (LFA-1 α chain)	180 kD; noncovalently linked to CD18 to form LFA-1 integrin	Leukocytes	Cell-cell adhesion; binds to ICAM-1 (CD54), ICAM-2 (CD102), and ICAM-3 (CD50)
CD11b (Mac-1; CR3)	165 kD; noncovalently linked to CD18 to form Mac-1 integrin	Granulocytes, monocytes, macrophages, dendritic cells, NK cells	Phagocytosis of iC3b-coated particles; neutrophil and monocyte adhesion to endothelium (binds CD54) and extracellular matrix proteins
CD11c (p150,95; CR4α chain)	145 kD; noncovalently linked to CD18 to form p150,95 integrin	Monocytes, macrophages, granulocytes, NK cells	Similar functions as CD11b
CD14	53 kD; GPI linked	Dendritic cells, monocytes, macrophages, granulocytes	Binds complex of LPS and LPS-binding protein and displays LPS to TLR4; required for LPS-induced macrophage activation
CD16a (FcγRIIIA)	50–70 kD; transmembrane protein; Ig superfamily	NK cells, macrophages	Binds Fc region of IgG; phagocytosis and antibody-dependent cellular cytotoxicity
CD16b (FcγRIIIB)	50–70 kD; GPI linked; Ig superfamily	Neutrophils	Binds Fc region of IgG; synergy with Fcγ RII in immune complex–mediated neutrophil activation
CD18	95 kD; noncovalently linked to CD11a, CD11b, or CD11c to form β2 integrins	Leukocytes	See CD11a, CD11b, CD11c
CD19	95 kD; Ig superfamily	Most B cells	B cell activation; forms a coreceptor complex with CD21 and CD81 that delivers signals that synergize with signals from B cell antigen receptor complex
CD20	35–37 kD; tetraspan (TM4SF) family	B cells	Possible role in B cell activation or regulation; calcium ion channel
CD21 (CR2; C3d receptor)	145 kD; regulators of complement activation	Mature B cells, follicular dendritic cells	Receptor for complement fragment C3d; forms a coreceptor complex with CD19 and CD81 that delivers activating signals in B cells; receptor for Epstein-Barr virus
CD22 (Siglec-2)	130–140 kD; Ig superfamily; Siglec family; ITIM in cytoplasmic tail	B cells	Regulation of B cell activation; adhesion molecule
CD23 (FcεRIIB)	45 kD; C-type lectin	Activated B cells, monocytes, macrophages	Low-affinity Fcε receptor, induced by IL-4; function is not clear

Continued

CD Number (Other Names)	Molecular Structure, Family	Main Cellular Expression	Known or Proposed Function(s)
CD25 (IL-2 receptor α chain)	55 kD; noncovalently associated with IL-2Rββ (CD122) and IL-2Rγ (CD132) chains to form a high-affinity IL-2 receptor	Activated T and B cells, regulatory T cells (Treg)	Binds IL-2 and promotes responses to low concentrations of IL-2
CD28	Homodimer of 44-kD chains; Ig superfamily	T cells (all CD4+ and >50% of CD8+ cells in humans; all mature T cells in mice)	T cell receptor for costimulatory molecules CD80 (B7-1) and CD86 (B7-2)
CD29	130 kD; noncovalently linked to CD49a–d chains to form VLA (β_1) integrins	T cells, B cells, monocytes, granulocytes	Leukocyte adhesion to extracellular matrix proteins and endothelium (see CD49)
CD30 (TNF receptor superfamily 8 [TNFRSF8])	120 kD; TNFR superfamily	Activated T and B cells; NK cells, monocytes, Reed-Sternberg cells in Hodgkin disease	Not established
CD31 (platelet/endothelial cell adhesion molecule 1 [PECAM-1])	130–140 kD; Ig superfamily	Platelets, monocytes, granulocytes, B cells, endothelial cells	Adhesion molecule involved in leukocyte transmigration through endothelium
CD32 (FcγRII)	40 kD; Ig superfamily; A, B, and C forms are products of different but homologous genes; ITAM in cytoplasmic tail of A form; ITIM in cytoplasmic tail of B form.	B cells, macrophages, dendritic cells, granulocytes	Fc receptor for aggregated IgG; B form acts as inhibitory receptor that blocks activation signals in B cells and other cells
CD34	105–120 kD; sialomucin	Precursors of hematopoietic cells; endothelial cells in high endothelial venules	? Role in cell–cell adhesion
CD35 (type 1 complement receptor, CR1)	190–285 kD (four products of polymorphic alleles); regulator of complement activation family	Granulocytes, monocytes, erythrocytes, B cells, follicular dendritic cells, some T cells	Binds C3b and C4b; promotes phagocytosis of C3b- or C4b-coated particles and immune complexes; regulates complement activation
CD36	85–90 kD	Platelets, monocytes, macrophages, endothelial cells	Scavenger receptor for oxidized low-density lipoprotein; platelet adhesion; phagocytosis of apoptotic cells
CD40	Homodimer of 44- to 48-kD chains; TNFR superfamily	B cells, macrophages, dendritic cells, endothelial cells	Binds CD154 (CD40L); role in T cell-mediated activation of B cells, macrophages, and dendritic cells
CD43	95–135 kD; sialomucin	Leukocytes (except circulating B cells)	? Role in cell–cell adhesion
CD44	80–>100 kD, highly glycosylated	Leukocytes, erythrocytes	Binds hyaluronan; involved in leukocyte adhesion to endothelial cells and extracellular matrix

CD Number (Other Names)	Molecular Structure, Family	Main Cellular Expression	Known or Proposed Function(s)
CD45 (Leukocyte common antigen [LCA])	Multiple isoforms, 180–220 kD (see CD45R); protein tyrosine phosphatase receptor family; fibronectin type III family	Hematopoietic cells	Tyrosine phosphatase that regulates T and B cell activation
CD45R	CD45RO:180 kDCD45RA: 220 kDCD45RB: 190-, 205-, and 220-kD isoforms	CD45RO: memory T cells; subset of B cells, monocytes, macrophages CD45RA: naive T cells, B cells, monocytes CD45RB: B cells, subset of T cells	See CD45
CD46 (Membrane cofactor protein [MCP])	52–58 kD; regulators of complement activation family	Leukocytes, epithelial cells, fibroblasts	Regulation of complement activation
CD47	47–52 kD; Ig superfamily	All hematopoietic cells, epithelial cells, endothelial cells, fibroblasts	Leukocyte adhesion, migration, activation; ligand for signal regulatory protein α (SIRPα); "don't eat me" signal to phagocytes
CD49d	150 kD; noncovalently linked to CD29 to form VLA-4 ($\alpha_4\beta_1$ integrin)	T cells, monocytes, B cells, NK cells, eosinophils, dendritic cells, thymocytes	Leukocyte adhesion to endothelium and extracellular matrix; binds to VCAM-1 and Mad-CAM-1; binds fibronectin and collagens
CD54 (ICAM-1)	75–114 kD; Ig superfamily	T cells, B cells, monocytes, endothelial cells (cytokine inducible)	Cell-cell adhesion; ligand for CD11aCD18 (LFA-1) and CD11bCD18 (Mac-1); receptor for rhinovirus
CD55 (Decay-accelerating factor [DAF])	55–70 kD; GPI linked; regulators of complement activation family	Broad	Regulation of complement activation
CD58 (Leukocyte function–associated antigen 3 [LFA-3])	55–70 kD; GPI-linked or integral membrane protein	Broad	Leukocyte adhesion; binds CD2
CD59	18–20 kD; GPI linked	Broad	Binds C9; inhibits formation of complement membrane attack complex
CD62E (E-selectin)	115 kD; selectin family	Endothelial cells	Leukocyte-endothelial adhesion
CD62L (L-selectin)	74–95 kD; selectin family	B cells, T cells, monocytes, granulocytes, some NK cells	Leukocyte-endothelial adhesion; homing of naive T cells to peripheral lymph nodes
CD62P (P-selectin)	140 kD; selectin family	Platelets, endothelial cells (present in granules, translocated to cell surface on activation)	Leukocyte adhesion to endothelium, platelets; binds CD162 (PSGL-1)
CD64 (FcγRI)	72 kD; Ig superfamily; noncovalently associated with the FcR common γ chain	Monocytes, macrophages, activated neutrophils	High-affinity Fcγ receptor; role in phagocytosis, ADCC, macrophage activation

Continued

CD Number (Other Names)	Molecular Structure, Family	Main Cellular Expression	Known or Proposed Function(s)
CD66e (Carcinoembryonic antigen [CEA])	180–220 kD; Ig superfamily; CEA family	Colonic and other epithelial cells	? Adhesion; clinical marker of carcinoma burden
CD69	23 kD; C-type lectin	Activated B cells, T cells, NK cells, neutrophils	Binds to and impairs surface expression of S1PR1, thereby promoting retention of recently activated lymphocytes in lymphoid tissues
CD74 (Class II MHC invariant chain [Ii])	33-, 35-, and 41-kD isoforms	B cells, dendritic cells, monocytes, macrophages; other class II MHC-expressing cells	Binds to and directs intracellular sorting of newly synthesized class II MHC molecules
CD79a (Igα)	33, 45 kD; forms dimer with CD79b; Ig superfamily; ITAM in cytoplasmic tail	Mature B cells	Required for cell surface expression of and signal transduction by the B cell antigen receptor complex
CD79b (Igβ)	37–39 kD; forms dimer with CD79α; Ig superfamily; ITAM in cytoplasmic tail	Mature B cells	Required for cell surface expression of and signal transduction by the B cell antigen receptor complex
CD80 (B7-1)	60 kD; Ig superfamily	Dendritic cells, activated B cells and macrophages	Costimulator for T lymphocyte activation; ligand for CD28 and CD152 (CTLA-4)
CD81 (Target for antiproliferative antigen 1 [TAPA-1])	26 kD; tetraspan (TM4SF)	T cells, B cells, NK cells, dendritic cells, thymocytes, endothelial cells	B cell activation; forms a coreceptor complex with CD19 and CD21 that delivers signals that synergize with signals from the B cell antigen receptor complex
CD86 (B7-2)	80 kD; Ig superfamily	B cells, monocytes; dendritic cells; some T cells	Costimulator for T lymphocyte activation; ligand for CD28 and CD152 (CTLA-4)
CD88 (C5a receptor)	43 kD; G protein–coupled, seven membrane-spanning receptor family	Granulocytes, monocytes, dendritic cells, mast cells	Receptor for C5a complement fragment; role in complement-induced inflammation
CD89 (Fcα receptor [FcαR]Facer)	55–75 kD; Ig superfamily; non-covalently associated with the common FcR γ chain	Granulocytes, monocytes, macrophages, T cell subset, B cell subset	Binds IgA; mediates IgA-dependent cellular cytotoxicity
CD90 (Thy-1)	25–35 kD; GPI linked; Ig superfamily	Thymocytes, peripheral T cells (mice), CD34+ hematopoietic progenitor cells, neurons	Marker for T cells; unknown function
CD94	43 kD; C-type lectin; on NK cells, covalently assembles with other C-type lectin molecules (NKG2)	NK cells; subset of CD8+ T cells	CD94/NKG2 complex functions as an NK cell inhibitory receptor; binds human leukocyte antigen E (HLA-E) class I MHC molecules
CD95 (Fas)	Homotrimer of 45-kD chains; TNFR superfamily	Broad	Binds Fas ligand; delivers signals leading to apoptotic death

CD Number (Other Names)	Molecular Structure, Family	Main Cellular Expression	Known or Proposed Function(s)
CD102 (ICAM-2)	55–65 kD; Ig superfamily	Endothelial cells, lymphocytes, monocytes, platelets	Ligand for CD11aCD18 (LFA-1); cell–cell adhesion
CD103 (α_E integrin subunit)	Dimer of 150- and 25-kD subunits; noncovalently linked to β_7 integrin subunit to form $\alpha_E\beta_7$ integrin	Intraepithelial lymphocytes, other cell types	Role in T cell homing to and retention in mucosa; binds E-cadherin
CD106 (VCAM-1)	100–110 kD; Ig superfamily	Endothelial cells, macrophages, follicular dendritic cells, marrow stromal cells	Adhesion of cells to endothelium; receptor for CD49dCD29 (VLA-4) integrin; role in lymphocyte trafficking, activation
CD134 (OX40, TNFRSF4)	29 kD; TNFR superfamily	Activated T cells	Receptor for T cell CD252; T cell costimulation
CD141 (BDCA-3, thrombomodulin)	60 kD; EGF-like domains	Cross-presenting dendritic cells, monocytes, endothelial cells	Binds thrombin and prevents blood coagulation
CD150 (Signaling lymphocyte activation molecule [SLAM])	37 kD; Ig superfamily	Thymocytes, activated lymphocytes, dendritic cells, endothelial cells	Regulation of B cell–T cell interactions and lymphocyte activation
CD152 (Cytotoxic T lymphocyte–associated protein 4 [CTLA-4])	33, 50 kD; Ig superfamily	Activated T lymphocytes, regulatory T cells	Mediates suppressive function of regulatory T cells; inhibits T cell responses; binds CD80 (B7-1) and CD86 (B7-2) on antigen-presenting cells
CD154 (CD40 ligand [CD40L])	Homotrimer of 32- to 39-kD chains; TNFR superfamily	Activated CD4+ T cells	Activation of B cells, macrophages, and endothelial cells; ligand for CD40
CD158 (Killer Ig-like receptor [KIR])	50, 58 kD; Ig superfamily; KIR family; ITIMs or ITAMs in cytoplasmic tail	NK cells, T cell subset	Inhibition or activation of NK cells on interaction with appropriate class I HLA molecules
CD159a (NKG2A)	43 kD; C-type lectin; forms heterodimer with CD94	NK cells, T cell subset	Inhibition or activation of NK cells on interaction with class I HLA molecules
CD159c (NKG2C)	40 kD; C-type lectin; forms heterodimer with CD94	NK cells	Activation of NK cells on interaction with the appropriate class I HLA molecules
CD162 (P-selectin glycoprotein ligand 1 [PSGL-1])	Homodimer of 120-kD chains; sialomucin	T cells, monocytes, granulocytes, some B cells	Ligand for selectins (CD62P, CD62L); adhesion of leukocytes to endothelium
CD178 (Fas ligand [FasL])	Homotrimer of 31-kD subunits; TNF superfamily	Activated T cells	Ligand for CD95 (Fas); triggers apoptotic death
CD206 (Mannose receptor)	166 kD; C-type lectin	Macrophages	Binds high-mannose-containing glycoproteins on pathogens; mediates macrophage endocytosis of glycoproteins and phagocytosis of bacteria, fungi, and other pathogens

Continued

CD Number (Other Names)	Molecular Structure, Family	Main Cellular Expression	Known or Proposed Function(s)
CD223 (Lympho-cyte-activation gene 3 [LAG3])	57.4 kD; Ig superfamily;	T cells, NK cells, B cells, plasmacytoid DCs	Binds class II MHC; inhibits T cell activation
CD244 (2B4)	41 kD; Ig superfamily; CD2/CD48/CD58 family; SLAM family	NK cells, CD8 T cells, γδ T cells	Receptor for CD148; modulates NK cell cytotoxic activity
CD247 (TCR ζ chain)	18 kD; ITAMs in cytoplasmic tail	T cells; NK cells	Signaling chain of TCR complex– and NK cell–activating receptors
CD252 (OX40 ligand)	21 kD; TNF superfamily	Dendritic cells, macro-phages, B cells	Ligand for CD134 (OX40, TNFRSF4); costimulates T cells
CD267 (TACI)	31 kD; TNFR superfamily	B cells	Receptor for cytokines BAFF and APRIL; mediates T-independent B cell responses and B cell survival
CD268 (BAFF receptor)	19 kD; TNFR superfamily	B cells	Receptor for BAFF; mediates B cell survival
CD269 (B cell mat-uration antigen [BCMA])	20 kD; TNFR superfamily	B cells	Receptor for BAFF and APRIL; mediates plasma cell survival
CD273 (PD-L2)	25 kD; Ig superfamily; structur-ally homologous to B7	Dendritic cells, mono-cytes, macrophages	Ligand for PD-1; inhibits T cell activation
CD274 (PD-L1)	33 kD; Ig superfamily; structur-ally homologous to B7	Leukocytes, other cells	Ligand for PD-1; inhibits T cell activation
CD275 (ICOS ligand)	60 kD; Ig superfamily; structur-ally homologous to B7	B cells, dendritic cells, monocytes	Binds ICOS (CD278); T cell costimulation
CD278 (inducible costimulator [ICOS])	55–60 kD; Ig superfamily; structurally homologous to CD28	Activated T cells	Binds ICOS-L (CD275); T cell costimulation and Tfh differentiation
CD279 (PD1)	55 kD; Ig superfamily; structur-ally homologous to CD28; ITIM and ITSM in cytoplasmic tail	Activated T and B cells	Binds PD-L1 and PD-L2; inhibits T cell activation
CD303 (BDCA2, C-type lectin domain family 4 member C [CLEC4C])	25 kD; C-type lectin superfamily	Plasmacytoid dendritic cells	Binds to microbial carbohydrates; inhibits dendritic cell (DC) activation
CD304 (BDCA4, Neuropilin)	103 kD; complement-binding, coagulation factor V/VIII, and meprin domains	Plasmacytoid dendritic cells, many other cell types	Vascular endothelial growth factor A receptor
CD314 (NKG2D)	42 kD; C-type lectin	NK cells, activated CD8+ T cells, NK-T cells, some myeloid cells	Binds MHC class I, and the class I–like molecules MIC-A, MIC-B, Rae1, and ULBP4; role in NK cell and CTL activation
CD357 (GITR, TNFRSF18)	26 kD; TNFR superfamily	CD4+ and CD8+ T cells, Treg	? Role in T cell/Treg function
CD363 (type 1 sphin-gosine-1-phos-phate receptor 1 [S1PR1])	42.8 kD; G protein–coupled, seven membrane-spanning receptor family	Lymphocytes, endothe-lial cells	Binds sphingosine 1-phosphate and mediates chemotaxis of lymphocytes out of lymphoid organs

CD Number (Other Names)	Molecular Structure, Family	Main Cellular Expression	Known or Proposed Function(s)
CD365 (hepatitis A virus cellular receptor 1 [HAVCR1], TIM-1)	38.7 kD; Ig superfamily, T cell transmembrane, immunoglobulin, and mucin family, T cell transmembrane, immunoglobulin, and mucin family	T cells, kidney and testis	Receptor for several viruses
CD366 (hepatitis A virus cellular receptor 2 [HAVCR2], TIM-3)	33.4 kD; Ig superfamily, Ig superfamily, T cell transmembrane, immunoglobulin, and mucin family, T cell transmembrane, immunoglobulin, and mucin family	T cells, macrophages, dendritic cells, NK cells	Receptor for several viruses; binds phosphatidylserine on apoptotic cells; inhibits T cell responses
CD369 (CLEC7A, DECTIN 1)	27.6 kD; C-type lectin	Dendritic cells, monocytes, macrophages, B cells	Pattern recognition receptor specific for fungal and bacterial cell wall glucans

The lowercase letters affixed to some CD numbers refer to CD molecules that are encoded by multiple genes or that belong to families of structurally related proteins.

ADCC, Antibody-dependent cell-mediated cytotoxicity; *APRIL,* a proliferation-inducing ligand; *BAFF,* B cell–activating factor belonging to the TNF family; *CTL,* cytotoxic T lymphocyte; *gp,* glycoprotein; *GITR,* glucocorticoid-induced TNFR-related; *GPI,* glycophosphatidylinositol; *ICAM,* intercellular adhesion molecule; *Ig,* immunoglobulin; *IL,* interleukin; *ITAM,* immunoreceptor tyrosine-based activation motif; *ITIM,* immunoreceptor tyrosine-based inhibition motif; *LFA,* lymphocyte function-associated antigen; *LPS,* lipopolysaccharide; *MadCAM,* mucosal addressin cell adhesion molecule; *MHC,* major histocompatibility complex; *NK cells,* natural killer cells; *TACI,* transmembrane activator and CAML interactor; *TCR,* T cell receptor; *TLR,* Toll-like receptor; *TNF,* tumor necrosis factor; *TNFR,* TNF receptor; *VCAM,* vascular cell adhesion molecule; *VLA,* very late activation.

Cytokines

Cytokine and Subunits	Principal Cell Source	Cytokine Receptor and Subunits*	Principal Cellular Targets and Biologic Effects
Type I Cytokine Family Members			
Interleukin-2 (IL-2)	T cells	CD25 (IL-2Rα) CD122 (IL-2Rβ) CD132 (γc)	T cells: proliferation and differentiation into effector and memory cells; promotes regulatory T cell development, survival, and function NK cells: proliferation, activation
Interleukin-3 (IL-3)	T cells	CD123 (IL-3Rα) CD131 (βc)	Immature hematopoietic progenitors: maturation of all hematopoietic lineages
Interleukin-4 (IL-4)	CD4+ T cells (Th2, Tfh), mast cells	CD124 (IL-4Rα) CD132 (γc)	B cells: isotype switching to IgE, IgG4 (in humans; IgG1 in mice) T cells: Th2 differentiation, proliferation Macrophages: alternative activation and inhibition of IFN-γ–mediated classical activation
Interleukin-5 (IL-5)	CD4+ T cells (Th2), group 2 ILCs	CD125 (IL-5Rα) CD131 (βc)	Eosinophils: activation, increased generation
Interleukin-6 (IL-6)	Macrophages, endothelial cells, T cells	CD126 (IL-6Rα) CD130 (gp130)	Liver: synthesis of acute phase protein B cells: proliferation of antibody-producing cells T cells: Th17 differentiation
Interleukin-7 (IL-7)	Fibroblasts, bone marrow stromal cells	CD127 (IL-7R) CD132 (γc)	Immature lymphoid progenitors: proliferation of early T and B cell progenitors T lymphocytes: survival of naive and memory cells
Interleukin-9 (IL-9)	CD4+ T cells	CD129 (IL-9R) CD132 (γc)	Mast cells, B cells, T cells, and epithelial cells: survival and activation
Interleukin-11 (IL-11)	Bone marrow stromal cells	IL-11Rα CD130 (gp130)	Production of platelets
Interleukin-12 (IL-12): IL-12A (p35) IL-12B (p40)	Macrophages, dendritic cells	CD212 (IL-12Rβ1) IL-12Rβ2	T cells: Th1 differentiation NK cells and T cells: IFN-γ synthesis, increased cytotoxic activity
Interleukin-13 (IL-13)	CD4+ T cells (Th2), NKT cells, group 2 ILCs, mast cells	CD213a1 (IL-13Rα1) CD213a2 (IL-13Rα2) CD132 (γc)	B cells: isotype switching to IgE Epithelial cells: increased mucus production Macrophages: alternative activation

Cytokine and Subunits	Principal Cell Source	Cytokine Receptor and Subunits*	Principal Cellular Targets and Biologic Effects
Interleukin-15 (IL-15)	Macrophages, other cell types	IL-15Rα CD122 (IL-2Rβ) CD132 (γc)	NK cells: proliferation T cells: survival and proliferation of memory CD8+ cells
Interleukin-17A (IL-17A) Interleukin-17F (IL-17F)	CD4+ T cells (Th17), group 3 ILCs	CD217 (IL-17RA) IL-17RC	Epithelial cells, macrophages and other cell types: increased chemokine and cytokine production; GM-CSF and G-CSF production
Interleukin-21 (IL-21)	Tfh cells	CD360 (IL-21R) CD132 (γc)	B cells: activation, proliferation, differentiation
Interleukin-23 (IL-23): IL-23A (p19) IL-12B (p40)	Macrophages, dendritic cells	IL-23R CD212 (IL-12Rβ1)	T cells: differentiation and proliferation of Th17 cells
Interleukin-25 (IL-25; IL-17E)	T cells, mast cells, eosinophils, macrophages, mucosal epithelial cells	IL-17RB	T cells and various other cell types: expression of IL-4, IL-5, IL-13
Interleukin-27 (IL-27): IL-27 (p28), EBI-3	Macrophages, dendritic cells	IL-27Rα CD130 (gp130)	T cells: enhancement of Th1 differentiation; inhibition of Th17 differentiation NK cells: IFN-γ synthesis?
Interleukin 35 (IL-35)	Treg	IL-12Rβ2 CD130 (gp130)	T cells: inhibits proliferation
Stem cell factor (c-Kit ligand)	Bone marrow stromal cells	CD117 (KIT)	Pluripotent hematopoietic stem cells: maturation of all hematopoietic lineages
Granulocyte-monocyte CSF (GM-CSF)	T cells, macrophages, endothelial cells, fibroblasts	CD116 (GM-CSFRα) CD131 (βc)	Immature and committed progenitors, mature macrophages: maturation of granulocytes and monocytes, macrophage activation
Monocyte CSF (M-CSF, CSF1)	Macrophages, endothelial cells, bone marrow cells, fibroblasts	CD115 (CSF1R)	Committed hematopoietic progenitors: maturation of monocytes
Granulocyte CSF (G-CSF, CSF3)	Macrophages, fibroblasts, endothelial cells	CD114 (CSF3R)	Committed hematopoietic progenitors: maturation of granulocytes
Thymic stromal lymphopoietin (TSLP)	Keratinocytes, bronchial epithelial cells, fibroblasts, smooth muscle cells, endothelial cells, mast cells, macrophages, granulocytes and dendritic cells	TSLP-receptor CD127 (IL-7R)	Dendritic cells: activation Eosinophils: activation Mast cells: cytokine production T cells: Th2 differentiation
Type II Cytokine Family Members			
Interferon-α (IFN-α) (multiple proteins)	Plasmacytoid dendritic cells, macrophages	IFNAR1 CD118 (IFNAR2)	All cells: antiviral state, increased class I MHC expression NK cells: activation
Interferon-β (IFN-β)	Fibroblasts, plasmacytoid dendritic cells	IFNAR1 CD118 (IFNAR2)	All cells: antiviral state, increased class I MHC expression NK cells: activation

Continued

Cytokine and Subunits	Principal Cell Source	Cytokine Receptor and Subunits*	Principal Cellular Targets and Biologic Effects
Interferon-γ (IFN-γ)	T cells (Th1, CD8+ T cells), NK cells, group 1 ILCs	CD119 (IFNGR1) IFNGR2	Macrophages: classical activation (increased microbicidal functions) B cells: isotype switching to opsonizing and complement-fixing IgG subclasses (established in mice, not humans) T cells: Th1 differentiation Various cells: increased expression of class I and class II MHC molecules, increased antigen processing and presentation to T cells
Interleukin-10 (IL-10)	Macrophages, T cells (mainly regulatory T cells)	CD210 (IL-10Rα) IL-10Rβ	Macrophages, dendritic cells: inhibition of expression of IL-12, costimulators, and class II MHC
Interleukin-22 (IL-22)	Th17 cells	IL-22Rα1 or IL-22Rα2 IL-10Rβ2	Epithelial cells: production of defensins, increased barrier function Hepatocytes: survival
Interleukin-26 (IL-26)	T cells, monocytes	IL-20R1 IL-10R2	Not established
Interferon-λs (type III interferons)	Dendritic cells	IFNLR1 (IL-28Rα) CD210B (IL-10Rβ2)	Epithelial cells: antiviral state
Leukemia inhibitory factor (LIF)	Embryonic trophectoderm, bone marrow stromal cells	CD118 (LIFR) CD130 (gp130)	Stem cells: block in differentiation
Oncostatin M	Bone marrow stromal cells	OSMR CD130 (gp130)	Endothelial cells: regulation of hematopoietic cytokine production Cancer cells: inhibition of proliferation

TNF Superfamily Cytokines[†]

APRIL (CD256, TNFSF13)	T cells, dendritic cells, monocytes, follicular dendritic cells	TACI (TNFRSF13B) or BCMA (TNFRSF17)	B cells: survival, proliferation
BAFF (CD257, TNFSF13B)	Dendritic cells, monocytes, follicular dendritic cells, B cells	BAFF-R (TNFRSF13C) or TACI (TNFRSF13B) or BCMA (TNFRSF17)	B cells: survival, proliferation
Lymphotoxin-α (LTα, TNFSF1)	T cells, B cells	CD120a (TNFRSF1) or CD120b (TNFRSF2)	Same as TNF
Lymphotoxin-αβ (LTαβ)	T cells, NK cells, follicular B cells, lymphoid inducer cells	LTβR	Lymphoid tissue stromal cells and follicular dendritic cells: chemokine expression and lymphoid organogenesis
Tumor necrosis factor (TNF, TNFSF1)	Macrophages, NK cells, T cells	CD120a (TNFRSF1) or CD120b (TNFRSF2)	Endothelial cells: activation (inflammation, coagulation) Neutrophils: activation Hypothalamus: fever Muscle, fat: catabolism (cachexia)
Osteoprotegerin (OPG, TNFRSF11B)	Osteoblasts	RANKL	Osteoclast precursor cells: inhibits osteoclast differentiation

Cytokine and Subunits	Principal Cell Source	Cytokine Receptor and Subunits*	Principal Cellular Targets and Biologic Effects
IL-1 Family Cytokines			
Interleukin-1α (IL-1α)	Macrophages, dendritic cells, fibroblasts, endothelial cells, keratinocytes, hepatocytes	CD121a (IL-1R1) IL-1RAP *or* CD121b (IL-1R2)	Endothelial cells: activation (inflammation, coagulation) Hypothalamus: fever
Interleukin-1β (IL-1β)	Macrophages, dendritic cells, fibroblasts, endothelial cells, keratinocytes	CD121a (IL-1R1) IL-1RAP *or* CD121b (IL-1R2)	Endothelial cells: activation (inflammation, coagulation) Hypothalamus: fever Liver: synthesis of acute-phase proteins T cells: Th17 differentiation
Interleukin-1 receptor antagonist (IL-1RA)	Macrophages	CD121a (IL-1R1) IL-1RAP	Various cells: competitive antagonist of IL-1
Interleukin-18 (IL-18)	Monocytes, macrophages, dendritic cells, Kupffer cells, keratinocytes, chondrocytes, synovial fibroblasts, osteoblasts	CD218a (IL-18Rα) CD218b (IL-18Rβ)	NK cells and T cells: IFN-γ synthesis Monocytes: expression of GM-CSF, TNF, IL-1β Neutrophils: activation, cytokine release
Interleukin-33 (IL-33)	Endothelial cells, smooth muscle cells, keratinocytes, fibroblasts	ST2 (IL1RL1) IL-1 Receptor Accessory Protein (IL1RAP)	T cells: Th2 development ILCs: activation of group 2 ILCs
Other Cytokines			
Transforming growth factor-β (TGF-β)	T cells (mainly Tregs), macrophages, other cell types	TGF-β R1 TGF-β R2 TGF-β R3	T cells: inhibition of proliferation and effector functions; differentiation of Th17 and Treg B cells: inhibition of proliferation; IgA production Macrophages: inhibition of activation; stimulation of angiogenic factors Fibroblasts: increased collagen synthesis

*Most cytokine receptors are dimers or trimers composed of different polypeptide chains, some of which are shared between receptors for different cytokines. The set of polypeptides that compose a functional receptor (cytokine binding plus signaling) for each cytokine is listed. The functions of each subunit polypeptide are not listed.

†All TNF superfamily (TNFSF) members are expressed as cell surface transmembrane proteins, but only the subsets that are predominantly active as proteolytically released soluble cytokines are listed in the table. Other TNFSF members that function predominantly in the membrane-bound form and are not, strictly speaking, cytokines are not listed in the table. These membrane-bound proteins and the TNFRSF receptors they bind to include OX40L (CD252, TNFSF4):OX40 (CD134, TNFSF4); CD40L (CD154, TNFSF5):CD40 (TNFRSF5); FasL (CD178, TNFSF6):Fas (CD95, TNFRSF6); CD70 (TNFSF7):CD27 (TNFRSF27); CD153 (TNFSF8):CD30 (TNFRSF8); TRAIL (CD253, TNFSF10):TRAIL-R (TNFRSF10A-D); RANKL (TNFSF11):RANK (TNFRSF11); TWEAK (CD257, TNFSF12):TWEAKR (CD266, TNFRSF12); LIGHT (CD258, TNFSF14):HVEM (TNFRSF14); GITRL (TNFSF18):GITR (CD357 TNFRSF18); and 4-IBBL:4-IBB (CD137). *APRIL,* A proliferation-inducing ligand; *BAFF,* B cell–activating factor belonging to the TNF family; *BCMA,* B cell maturation protein; *CSF,* colony-stimulating factor; *IFN,* interferon; *IgE,* immunoglobulin E; *ILCs,* innate lymphoid cells; *MHC,* major histocompatibility complex; *NK cell,* natural killer cell; *NKT cell,* natural killer T cell; *OSMR,* oncostatin M receptor; *RANK,* receptor activator for nuclear factor κB ligand; *RANKL,* RANK ligand; *TACI,* transmembrane activator and calcium modulator and cyclophilin ligand interactor; *Th,* T helper; *Tfh,* T follicular helper; *TNF,* tumor necrosis factor; *TNFSF,* TNF superfamily; *TNFRSF,* TNF receptor superfamily; *Treg,* regulatory T cell.

Clinical Cases

This appendix presents five clinical cases illustrating various diseases involving the immune system. These cases are not meant to teach clinical skills but rather to show how the basic science of immunology contributes to our understanding of human diseases. Each case illustrates typical ways in which a disease manifests, what tests are used in diagnosis, and common modes of treatment. The appendix was compiled with the assistance of Dr. Richard Mitchell and Dr. Jon Aster, Department of Pathology, Brigham and Women's Hospital, Boston; Dr. Robin Colgrove, Harvard Medical School, Boston; Dr. George Tsokos, Department of Medicine, Beth Israel-Deaconess Hospital, Boston; Dr. David Erle and Dr. Laurence Cheng, Department of Medicine, University of California San Francisco; and Dr. James Faix, Department of Pathology, Stanford University School of Medicine, Palo Alto.

CASE 1: LYMPHOMA

E.B. was a 58-year-old chemical engineer who had been well all his life. One morning, he noticed a lump in his left groin while showering. It was not tender, and the overlying skin appeared normal. After a few weeks, he began to worry about it because it did not go away, and he finally made an appointment with a physician after 2 months. On physical examination, the physician noted a subcutaneous firm, movable nodule, approximately 3 cm in diameter, in the left inguinal region. The physician asked E.B. if he had recently noticed any infections of his left foot or leg; E.B. had not. E.B. did complain that he had been waking up frequently at night drenched in perspiration. The physician also found some slightly enlarged lymph nodes in E.B.'s right neck. Otherwise, the physical examination findings were normal. The physician explained that the inguinal mass probably was a lymph node that was

enlarged as a result of a reaction to some infection. However, he drew blood for tests and referred E.B. to a surgeon, who performed a fine-needle aspiration of cells from the lymph node. Examination of smears prepared from aspirated cells revealed mainly small, irregular lymphocytes. Flow cytometric evaluation of these cells showed a 10-fold excess of B cells expressing λ immunoglobulin (Ig) light chain compared with B cells expressing κ Ig light chain.

Because of the suspicion of B cell lymphoma, a malignant tumor of cells of the B lymphocyte lineage, the surgeon elected to remove the entire lymph node. Histologic examination revealed an expansion of the node by follicular structures composed of mainly small- to intermediate-sized lymphocytes with irregular or "cleaved" nuclear contours mixed with smaller numbers of large lymphocytes with prominent nucleoli (Fig. A.1). Flow cytometric analysis of these cells showed a predominant population of B cells expressing IgM, λ light chain, CD10, and CD20, and immunohistochemical stains performed on slides showed strong cytoplasmic staining for BCL-2. On this basis, the diagnosis of follicular lymphoma of low histologic grade was made.

1. Why does the presence of a B cell population in which a large majority of the cells express λ light chain indicate a neoplasm rather than a response to an infection?
2. If the lymph node cells were analyzed by polymerase chain reaction (PCR) to assess Ig heavy-chain rearrangements, what abnormal finding would you expect?
3. Normal follicular center B cells fail to express the BCL-2 protein. Why might the tumor cells express BCL-2?

E.B.'s blood tests indicated that he was anemic (low red blood cell count). He underwent staging tests to

Fig. A.1 Lymph node biopsy with follicular lymphoma. The microscopic appearance of the patient's inguinal lymph node is shown. The follicular structures are abnormal, composed of a monotonous collection of neoplastic cells. By contrast, a lymph node with reactive hyperplasia would have follicles with germinal center formation, containing a heterogeneous mixture of cells.

determine the extent of his lymphoma. Positron emission tomography (PET) and computed tomography (CT) scanning showed enlarged hilar and mediastinal lymph nodes, an enlarged spleen, and lesions in the liver. A bone marrow biopsy also showed presence of lymphoma. E.B. was treated with injections of a mouse/human chimeric monoclonal IgG antibody called rituximab, which is specific for human CD20. Imaging studies performed 6 months after the rituximab treatment was begun showed regression in the size of lesions, and E.B. felt well enough to continue working.

4. By what mechanisms would the anti-CD20 antibody help this patient?
5. What are the advantages of using a "humanized" antibody, such as rituximab, as a drug instead of a mouse antibody?

Answers to Questions for Case 1

1. During the maturation of B cells, the cells first express a rearranged μ heavy chain gene, which associates with the surrogate light chain to produce the pre–B cell receptor (see Chapter 4). The cells then rearrange a light chain gene: first κ, then λ. If the κ protein is produced, the λ gene does not rearrange; λ rearrangement occurs only if the κ rearrangement is unsuccessful or if the assembled Ig molecule is strongly self-reactive. So, any B cell can produce only one of the two light chains. In humans, about 50% to 60% of the mature B cells express κ and 40% to 50% express λ. In a polyclonal response to an infection or other stimulus, many B cells respond and this ratio is maintained. However, if there is a marked over-representation of one light chain (in this case, λ), it indicates that a λ-producing B cell has proliferated massively. This is characteristic of a B cell tumor (lymphoma), which arises from a single B cell.

2. Each clone of B cells has a unique rearrangement of V, (D) and J gene segments, forming the gene that encodes V regions of heavy and light chains. B cell lymphomas are monoclonal, being composed of cells that all contain the same Ig heavy-chain and light-chain gene rearrangements. Such tumors can be reliably distinguished by the use of PCR amplification of rearranged Ig heavy-chain (IgH) gene segments. This method uses consensus PCR primers that hybridize with virtually all IgH variable (V) gene segments and joining (J) gene segments. These primers are used in the PCR to amplify essentially all the heavy-chain gene rearrangements in a sample (e.g., DNA prepared from enlarged lymph node). The size of the amplified products is then analyzed by capillary electrophoresis, which can separate PCR products that differ in size by as little as a single nucleotide. When the V, D, and J segments of IgH genes (as well as other antigen receptor genes) are joined during antigen receptor rearrangement in pre–B cells, the rearranged segments are of differing length due to the action of enzymes that remove nucleotides (nucleases) and add bases (a specialized DNA polymerase called terminal deoxyribonucleotide transferase [TdT]). Within a normal population of B cells, many PCR products of different sizes are generated, and these appear as a broad distribution of fragments of differing size. In the case of a B cell lymphoma, all the B cells have the same VDJ rearrangement, and the PCR product is of one size, appearing as a single, sharp peak.

3. Many lymphomas have characteristic underlying acquired chromosomal translocations or mutations that dysregulate specific oncogenes. More than 90% of follicular lymphomas have an acquired 14;18 chromosomal translocation that fuses the coding sequence of *BCL2*, a gene on chromosome 18 encoding a protein that inhibits programmed cell death (apoptosis),

to enhance elements within the Ig heavy chain locus located on chromosome 14. As a result, BCL-2 is over-expressed in follicular lymphoma cells. Parenthetically, in most instances the chromosomal breakpoint in the IgH gene involved in the translocation is located precisely at the point where RAG proteins normally cut the DNA of B cells that are undergoing Ig gene rearrangement, suggesting that the translocation stems from a mistake that occurs during normal antigen receptor gene rearrangement. Clinically, the presence of a BCL-2/IgH fusion gene, the consequence of the t(14;18), may be determined by fluorescent in situ hybridization using probes of different colors that are specific for IgH and BCL-2. These probes are hybridized to sections prepared of tissues involved by follicular lymphoma, and spatial superimposition of the probes within the nuclei of tumor cells indicates the existence of an IgH/BCL-2 fusion gene. Alternatively, it is possible to perform PCR on DNA isolated from the tumor with primer pairs in which one primer is specific for IgH and the other specific for BCL-2. These primers will produce a product only when the IgH and BCL-2 genes are joined to one another, which is taken as indirect evidence of a t(14;18).

4. CD20 is expressed on most mature B cells and is also uniformly expressed by all the tumor cells in follicular lymphomas. Injected rituximab (Rituxan) will therefore bind to the lymphoma cells and facilitate their destruction, likely through similar mechanisms by which antibodies normally destroy microbes. These mechanisms involve binding of the Fc portion of rituximab to different proteins in the patient, including Fc receptors on macrophages leading to phagocytic clearance of the lymphoma cells, and to complement proteins leading to complement-mediated killing of the lymphoma cells (see Chapter 8). Many normal B cells will also be destroyed by rituximab, although antibody-secreting plasma cells, which do not express CD20, are not affected. The immune deficiency caused by loss of normal B cells can be corrected by administration of pooled IgG from healthy donors, a form of passive immunity.

5. Monoclonal antibodies (mAbs) derived from non-human B cells (e.g., mouse) will appear foreign to the human immune system. When injected multiple times with these mAbs, humans will mount humoral immune responses and produce antibodies specific for the injected foreign mAb. These anti-antibody responses will promote clearance of the mAb from the circulation and therefore reduce the therapeutic benefits of the mAb. Furthermore, the Fc regions of human IgG bind better than mouse IgG to human Fc receptors and complement proteins, both of which are important for the effectiveness of mAb drugs (see Answer 3). For these reasons, most recently developed mAbs used as drugs have been genetically engineered to contain mainly or all human Ig amino acid sequences. Patients will generally not react against these drugs, just as they do not respond to their own antibodies. Rituximab is a chimeric mAb, with the CD20-binding variable regions originating from mouse IgG, and the remainder of the antibody including the Fc region from human IgG. The small amount of mouse sequences in rituximab do not appear to induce anti-antibody responses in patients, perhaps because potentially responding B cells are destroyed by the drug.

CASE 2: HEART TRANSPLANTATION COMPLICATED BY ALLOGRAFT REJECTION

C.M., a computer software salesman, was 48 years old when he came to his primary care physician because of fatigue and shortness of breath. He had not seen a doctor on a regular basis before this visit and felt well until 1 year ago, when he began experiencing difficulty climbing stairs or playing basketball with his children. Over the past 6 months he has had trouble breathing when he was recumbent. He did not remember ever experiencing significant chest pain and had no family history of heart disease. He did recall that approximately 18 months ago he had to take 2 days off from work because of a severe flu-like illness.

On examination, he had a pulse of 105 beats per minute, a respiratory rate of 32 breaths per minute, and a blood pressure of 100/60 mm Hg and was afebrile. His physician heard rales (evidence of abnormal fluid accumulation) in the bases of both lungs. His feet and ankles were swollen. A chest x-ray showed pulmonary edema and pleural effusions and a significantly enlarged left ventricle. These findings were consistent with right and left ventricular congestive heart failure, which is a reduced capacity of the heart to pump normal volumes of blood, resulting in fluid accumulation in various tissues. C.M. was admitted to the cardiology service of the University Hospital. On the basis of further tests, including coronary angiography and echocardiography, C.M. was given the diagnosis of dilated cardiomyopathy (a progressive and fatal form of heart failure in which the heart chambers become dilated and inefficient at pumping blood). His physicians told him he may benefit from aggressive medical management, including drugs that enhance heart muscle contraction, reduce the workload of the heart, and enhance excretion of accumulated fluid, but if his underlying heart disease continued to progress, the best long-term option would be to receive a heart transplant. Unfortunately, despite optimal medical management, his symptoms of congestive heart failure continued to worsen until he was no longer able to manage even routine activities of daily living, and he was listed for heart transplantation.

A panel-reactive antibody (PRA) test was performed on C.M.'s serum to determine whether he had been previously sensitized to alloantigens. This test (performed monthly) showed the patient had no circulating antibodies against human leukocyte antigens (HLAs), and there was no further immunologic testing done at that time. Two weeks later in a nearby city, a donor heart was removed from a victim of a construction site accident. The donor had the same ABO blood group type as C.M. The transplant surgery, performed 4 hours after the donor heart was removed, went well, and the allograft was functioning properly postoperatively.

1. What problems might arise if the transplant recipient and the donor have different blood types or if the recipient has high levels of anti-HLA antibodies?

C.M. was placed on immunosuppressive therapy the day after transplantation, which included daily doses of tacrolimus, mycophenolic acid, and prednisone. Endomyocardial biopsy was performed 1 week after surgery and showed no evidence of myocardial injury or inflammatory cells. He was sent home 10 days after surgery, and within a month he was able to do light exercise without problems. A routinely scheduled endomyocardial biopsy performed within the first 3 months after transplantation was normal, but a biopsy performed 14 weeks after surgery showed the presence of numerous lymphocytes within the myocardium and a few necrotic muscle fibers (Fig. A.2). The findings were interpreted as evidence of acute allograft rejection.

2. What was the patient's immune system responding to, and what were the effector mechanisms in the acute rejection episode?

Fig. A.2 Endomyocardial biopsy showing acute cellular rejection. The heart muscle is infiltrated by lymphocytes, and necrotic muscle fibers are present. (Courtesy Dr. Richard Mitchell, Department of Pathology, Brigham and Women's Hospital, Boston.)

C.M.'s serum creatinine level, an indicator of renal function, was high (2.2 mg/dL; normal, <1.5 mg/dL). His physicians therefore did not want to increase his tacrolimus dose because this drug can be toxic to the kidneys. He was given three additional doses of methyl prednisolone (a steroid drug) over 18 hours, and a repeat endomyocardial biopsy 1 week later showed only a few scattered macrophages and a small focus of healing tissue. C.M. went home feeling well, and he was able to live a relatively normal life, taking tacrolimus, mycophenolic acid, and prednisone daily.

3. What is the goal of the immunosuppressive drug therapy?

Coronary angiograms performed yearly since the transplant showed a gradual diffuse narrowing of the lumens of the coronary arteries. In the sixth year after transplantation, C.M. began experiencing shortness of breath after mild exercise and showed left ventricular dilation on radiographic examination. An intravascular ultrasound examination demonstrated significant diffuse thickening of the coronary arterial walls with luminal narrowing (Fig. A.3). An endomyocardial biopsy showed areas of microscopic subendocardial infarction, as well as evidence of sublethal ischemia (myocyte vacuolization). C.M. and his physicians are now considering the possibility of a second cardiac transplant.

4. What process has led to failure of the graft after 6 years?

Fig. A.3 Coronary artery with transplant-associated arteriosclerosis. This histologic section was taken from a coronary artery of a cardiac allograft that was removed from a patient 5 years after transplantation because of graft failure. The lumen is greatly narrowed by the presence of intimal smooth muscle cells. (Courtesy Dr. Richard Mitchell, Department of Pathology, Brigham and Women's Hospital, Boston.)

Answers to Questions for Case 2

1. If the recipient and the heart donor had different blood types, or if the recipient had high levels of anti-HLA antibodies, hyperacute rejection might occur after transplantation (see Chapter 10). People with type A, B, or O blood groups have preformed circulating IgM antibodies against the antigens they do not possess (B, A, or both, respectively). People who have received previous blood transfusions or transplants or were previously pregnant may have circulating anti-HLA antibodies. Blood group and HLA antigens are present on endothelial cells. If the antibodies are already present in the recipient at the time of transplantation, they can bind to the antigens on graft endothelial cells, causing complement activation, leukocyte recruitment, and thrombosis. As a result, the graft blood supply becomes impaired and the organ can rapidly undergo ischemic necrosis. The PRA test typically is performed to determine whether a patient needing a transplant has preexisting antibodies specific for a broad panel of HLA antigens. The test is performed by mixing the patient's serum with a collection of HLA-coated microbeads; antibody binding is detected by flow cytometry of the beads, after addition of fluorescence-labeled antibodies directed against human Ig. The results are expressed as a percentage (0%–100%) of the various HLA-coated beads that have bound to the patient's serum antibodies.

The higher the PRA value obtained, the greater the chance that the recipient will have an antibody that can potentially react with a graft and cause hyperacute rejection. The test is typically performed on a monthly basis as the patient is awaiting a heart. This is because many events can induce new anti-HLA antibodies, including a blood transfusion, or new exposures to microbes or drugs, which can potentially elicit antibodies that by chance cross-react with donor HLA.

2. In the acute rejection episode, the patient's immune system is responding to alloantigens in the graft. The main antigens are donor major histocompatibility complex (MHC) molecules encoded by alleles not shared by the recipient; milder reactions may also occur against unshared allelic variants of other proteins (minor histocompatibility antigens). These alloantigens may be expressed on the donor endothelial cells, leukocytes, and parenchymal cells within the donor heart. The effector mechanisms in the acute rejection episode include both cell-mediated and antibody-mediated reactions. Recipient CD4+ T cells secrete cytokines that promote macrophage activation and inflammation and can cause myocyte or endothelial cell injury and dysfunction, and CD8+ cytotoxic T lymphocytes can directly kill graft cells. Recipient antibodies, produced in response to graft antigens, can bind to graft cells (particularly endothelium), leading to complement activation and leukocyte recruitment.

3. The goal of immunosuppressive drug therapy is to suppress the recipient's immune response to alloantigens present in the graft, thereby preventing rejection. The drugs work by depleting T cells (antithymocyte globulin) and by blocking T cell activation (tacrolimus, cyclosporine, and rapamycin), lymphocyte proliferation (mycophenolic acid), and/or inflammatory cytokine production (prednisone). An attempt is made to preserve some immune function to combat infections.

4. The graft has failed because of thickening of the walls and narrowing of the lumens of the graft arteries (see Chapter 10). This vascular change, called graft arteriosclerosis or transplant-associated arteriosclerosis, diffusely involves the coronary vasculature and leads to downstream ischemic damage to the heart; it is the most frequent reason for long-term graft failure. It may be caused by a T cell–mediated inflammatory reaction directed against

vessel wall alloantigens, which subsequently smolders as a chronic macrophage-mediated injury that results in cytokine-stimulated smooth muscle cell migration into the intima, with smooth muscle cell proliferation and increased matrix synthesis.

CASE 3: ALLERGIC ASTHMA

Ten-year-old I.E. was brought to her pediatrician's office in November because of frequent coughing for the past 2 days, audible wheezing, and a feeling of tightness in her chest. Her symptoms had been especially severe at night. In addition to her routine checkups, she had visited the physician in the past for occasional ear and upper respiratory tract infections but had not previously experienced wheezing or chest tightness. She had eczema, but otherwise she was in good health and was developmentally normal. Her immunizations were up to date. She lived at home with her mother, father, two sisters aged 12 and 4, and a pet cat. Both of her parents smoked cigarettes, and her father suffered from allergic rhinitis.

At the time of her physical examination, I.E. had a temperature of 37° C (98.6° F), blood pressure of 105/65 mm Hg, and a respiratory rate of 40 breaths per minute. She did not appear short of breath but had mild subcostal retractions. There were no signs of ear infection or pharyngitis. Auscultation of the chest revealed diffuse wheezing in both lungs. There was no evidence of pneumonia. The physician made a presumptive diagnosis of bronchospasm and referred I.E. to a pediatric allergist-immunologist. In the meantime, she was given a prescription for a short-acting β2-adrenergic agonist bronchodilator inhaler and was instructed to administer the drug every 4 hours to relieve symptoms. This drug binds to β2-adrenergic receptors on bronchial smooth muscle cells and causes them to relax, resulting in dilation of the bronchioles. The family was also prescribed a spacer, a device to optimize delivery of the medication, and taught to administer the inhaler using the spacer.

1. Asthma is often an *atopic* disease, particularly in patients older than 6 to 8 years of age. What are the different ways in which atopy may manifest clinically?

One week later, I.E. was seen again by the allergist. He auscultated her lungs and confirmed the presence of wheezing. I.E. was instructed to blow into a spirometer, and the physician determined that her forced expiratory volume in 1 second (FEV1) was 65% of the total amount of air exhaled or forced vital capacity (FVC), indicating airway obstruction. The physician then administered a nebulized

bronchodilator and 10 minutes later performed the test again. The repeat FEV1 was 85% of FVC indicating reversibility of the airway obstruction. Blood was drawn and sent for total and differential blood cell count and determination of IgE levels. In addition, a skin test was performed to determine hypersensitivity to various antigens and showed a positive result for cat dander and house dust (Fig. A.4). The patient was instructed to begin using an inhaled corticosteroid and to use her bronchodilator only as needed for respiratory symptoms. Her parents were instructed to make a return appointment 2 weeks later for reevaluation of I.E. and discussion of blood test results.

2. What is the immunologic basis for a positive skin test?

At I.E.'s return appointment 2 weeks later, laboratory tests revealed that she had a serum IgE level of 1200 IU/mL (normal range, 0 to 180) and a total white blood cell count of 7000/mm³ (normal, 4300 to 10,800/mm³), with an absolute eosinophil count of 700/mm³ (normal, <500). When she returned to the allergist's office 1 week later, her respiratory status on physical examination was significantly improved, with no audible wheezing. I.E.'s FEV1 had improved to 75% of FVC. The family was told that I.E. had reversible airway obstruction, possibly triggered by a viral illness and possibly related to cat and dust allergies. The physician advised that, although rehoming the cat is ideal, at the very least the cat should be kept out of I.E.'s bedroom. The mother was told that smoking in the house probably was contributing to I.E.'s symptoms. The physician recommended that I.E. continue to use the short-acting inhaler for acute episodes of

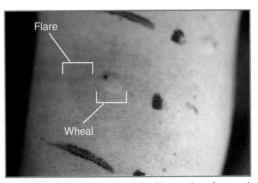

Fig. A.4 Positive result on prick skin testing for environmental antigens. Small amounts of the antigens are applied into the superficial layers of the skin using a short needle to prick the skin. If mast cells are present with bound immunoglobulin E specific for the test antigen, the antigen will crosslink the Fc receptors to which the IgE is bound. This induces degranulation of the mast cells and the release of mediators that cause the wheal and flare reaction.

wheezing or shortness of breath. She was asked to return in 3 months, or sooner if she used the inhaler more than twice per month, particularly for nighttime symptoms.

3. What is the mechanism for the increased IgE levels seen in patients who have allergic symptoms?

The family cat was given to a neighbor, and I.E. did well on the therapy for approximately 6 months, experiencing only mild wheezing a few times. The next spring, she began to have more frequent episodes of coughing and wheezing. During a soccer game one Saturday, she became very short of breath, and her parents brought her to the emergency department (ED) of the local hospital. After confirming that she was wheezing and showed signs of accessory respiratory muscle use, the ED physician treated her with a nebulized β2-agonist bronchodilator and an oral corticosteroid. After 6 hours, her symptoms resolved, and she was sent home. The following week, I.E. was brought to her allergist, who increased her maintenance dose of the inhaled corticosteroid. She has subsequently been well, with occasional mild attacks that are cleared by the bronchodilator inhaler.

4. What are the therapeutic approaches to allergic asthma?

Answers to Questions for Case 3

1. Atopic reactions to harmless environmental antigens (allergens) are mediated by IgE on mast cells but may manifest in a variety of ways (see Chapter 11). The signs and symptoms usually reflect the site of entry of the allergen. Hay fever (allergic rhinitis) and asthma usually are responses to inhaled allergens, whereas urticaria and eczema more often occur with skin exposure or ingestion. Food allergies may also cause gastrointestinal or respiratory symptoms. The most dramatic presentation of allergies to insect venom, foods, or drugs is anaphylaxis, a reaction characterized by systemic vasodilation, increased vascular permeability, and airway obstruction (laryngeal edema or bronchoconstriction). Without intervention, patients with anaphylaxis may progress to asphyxia and cardiovascular collapse.

2. If an individual with an allergy is challenged with a small dose of the allergen injected into the skin, there is immediate release of histamine from triggered mast cells, which produces a central wheal of edema (from leakage of plasma) and the surrounding flare of vascular congestion (from vessel dilation). The injected allergen binds to previously produced IgE antibodies, which coat mast cells by attaching to Fcε receptors. The allergy

skin test should not be confused with the skin test used to assess prior sensitization to certain infectious agents, such as *Mycobacterium tuberculosis*. A positive tuberculosis skin test is an example of a delayed-type hypersensitivity (DTH) reaction, mediated by antigen-stimulated helper T cells, which release cytokines such as interferon-γ, leading to macrophage activation and inflammation (see Chapter 6). Serum allergen-specific IgE tests are also routinely performed and give complementary information to traditional allergy prick skin testing.

3. For unknown reasons, patients with atopy mount type 2 helper T cell responses to a variety of essentially harmless protein antigens, in which Th2 cells produce interleukin-4 (IL-4), IL-5, and IL-13 and Tfh cells produce IL-4. IL-4 induces IgE synthesis by B cells, IL-5 activates eosinophils, and IL-13 stimulates mucus production (see Chapter 11). Atopy appears to run in families, and genetic susceptibility is clearly involved. Attention has been focused especially on genes on the long arm of chromosome 5 (5q) that encode several Th2 cytokines; on 11q, where the gene for the α chain of the IgE receptor is located; and on genes on chromosomes 2 and 9, which encode the IL-33 receptor (ST2) and IL-33, respectively. IL-33 is a cytokine secreted by epithelial cells that is believed to activate group 2 innate lymphoid cells (ILC2), which may play a role in inducing strong Th2 responses.

4. A major therapeutic approach for allergies is prevention by avoidance of precipitating allergens, identified through either allergy skin testing or serum IgE measurement. Although pharmacologic therapy previously has been focused on treating the symptoms of bronchoconstriction by elevating intracellular cyclic adenosine monophosphate (cAMP) levels (using β2-adrenergic agents and inhibitors of cAMP degradation), the balance of therapy has shifted to the use of antiinflammatory agents. These include corticosteroids (which block cytokine release) and receptor antagonists for lipid mediators (e.g., leukotrienes). Newer treatments that have been developed for treatment of asthma and other allergies include mAbs targeting IgE, IL-5, or IL-4/IL-13 receptors. The most effective treatment for anaphylaxis is the administration of epinephrine through intramuscular injection. Epinephrine causes blood vessel constriction, dilation of bronchioles, and increased cardiac output, thereby reversing the fall in blood pressure and airway obstruction.

CASE 4: SYSTEMIC LUPUS ERYTHEMATOSUS

N.Z., a 25-year-old woman, presented to her primary care physician with complaints of joint pain involving her wrists, fingers, and ankles. When seen in the physician's office, N.Z. had normal body temperature, heart rate, blood pressure, and respiratory rate. There was a noticeable red rash on her cheeks, most marked around her nose, sparing the nasolabial folds, and on questioning she said the redness worsened after being in the sun for 1 or 2 hours. The joints of her hands and her wrists were swollen and tender. The other physical examination findings were unremarkable.

Her physician took a blood sample for various tests. Her hematocrit was 35% (normal, 37%–48%). The total white blood cell count was 9800/mm³ (within normal range), with a normal differential count. The erythrocyte sedimentation rate (ESR) was 40 mm per hour (normal, 1 to 20). Her serum antinuclear antibody (ANA) test was positive at 1:2560 dilution (normally, negative at 1:40 dilution). Other laboratory findings were unremarkable. On the basis of these findings, a diagnosis of systemic lupus erythematosus (SLE) was made. N.Z.'s physician prescribed oral prednisone, a corticosteroid, and with this treatment, her joint pain subsided.

1. What is the significance of the positive result for the ANA test?

Three months later, N.Z. began feeling unusually tired and thought she had the flu. For approximately a week she had noticed that her ankles were swollen, and she had difficulty putting on her shoes. She returned to her primary care physician. Her ankles and feet showed severe edema (swollen as a result of extra fluid in the tissue). Her abdomen appeared slightly distended, with a mild shifting dullness to percussion (a sign of an abnormally large amount of fluid in the peritoneal cavity). Her physician ordered several laboratory tests. Her ANA test result was still positive, with a titer of 1:256, and her ESR was 120 mm/hour. Serum albumin was 0.8 g/dL (normal, 3.5 to 5.0). Measurement of serum complement proteins revealed a C3 of 42 mg/dL (normal, 80 to 180) and a C4 of 5 mg/dL (normal, 15 to 45). Urinalysis showed 4+ proteinuria, both red and white blood cells, and numerous hyaline and granular casts. A 24-hour urine sample contained 4 g of protein.

2. What is the likely reason for the decreased complement levels and the abnormalities in blood and urinary proteins?

Because of the abnormal urinalysis findings, the physician recommended a renal biopsy, which was performed 1 week later. The biopsy specimen was examined by routine histologic methods, immunofluorescence, and electron microscopy (Fig. A.5).

Granular deposits of immunoglobulin
and complement in the basement membrane

Fig. A.5 Glomerulonephritis with immune complex deposition in systemic lupus erythematosus. A, Light micrograph of a renal biopsy specimen in which neutrophilic infiltration in a glomerulus can be seen. B, Immunofluorescence micrograph showing granular deposits of immunoglobulin G (IgG) along the basement membrane. (In this technique, called immunofluorescence microscopy, a frozen section of the kidney is incubated with a fluorescein-conjugated antibody against IgG, and the site of deposition of the IgG is defined by determining where the fluorescence is located.) C, Electron micrograph of the same tissue revealing immune complex deposition. (Courtesy Dr. Helmut Rennke, Department of Pathology, Brigham and Women's Hospital, Boston.)

3. What is the explanation for the pathologic changes seen in the kidney?

The physician made the diagnosis of proliferative lupus glomerulonephritis, prescribed a higher dose of prednisone, and recommended treatment with a cyto-toxic drug (mycophenolate). N.Z.'s proteinuria and edema subsided over a 2-week period, and serum C3 levels returned to normal. Her corticosteroid dose was tapered to a lower amount. Over the next few years, she has had intermittent flare-ups of her disease, with joint pain and tissue swelling and laboratory tests indicating depressed C3 levels and proteinuria. These have been effectively managed with corticosteroids, and N.Z. has been able to lead an active life.

Answers to Questions for Case 4

1. A positive ANA test reveals the presence of serum antibodies that bind to components of cellular nuclei. The test is performed by placing different dilutions of the patient's serum on top of a monolayer of human cells on a glass slide. A second fluorescently labeled anti-Ig antibody is then added, and the cells are examined with a fluorescent microscope to detect if any serum antibodies bound to the nuclei. The ANA titer is the maximum dilution of the serum that still produces detectable nuclear staining. Almost all patients with SLE have ANAs, which may be specific for histones, other nuclear proteins, or double-stranded DNA. These are autoantibodies, and their production is evidence of autoimmunity. ANAs are not specific for SLE, and this test is gradually being replaced or supplemented with a more specific test for antibodies against double-stranded DNA, which are considered diagnostic for SLE. Autoantibodies may also be produced against various cell membrane protein antigens. The development of autoantibodies generally precedes the clinical onset of SLE by as much as 9 to 10 years. Titers of autoantibodies do not reflect disease activity and should not be used to adjust treatment.

2. Some of the autoantibodies form circulating immune complexes by binding to antigens in the blood. Nuclear antigens may be increased in the circulation of patients with SLE because of increased apoptosis of several cell types (e.g., white blood cells, keratinocytes) and defective clearance of apoptotic cells. When these immune complexes deposit in the basement membranes of vessel walls, they may activate the classical pathway of complement, leading to inflammation and depletion of complement proteins through consumption. Inflammation caused by the immune complexes in the kidney leads to leakage of protein and red blood cells into the urine. The loss of protein in the urine results in reduced plasma albumin, reduction of osmotic pressure of the plasma, and fluid loss into the tissues. This explains the edema of the feet and abdominal distention.

3. The pathologic changes in the kidney result from the deposition of circulating immune complexes in the basement membranes of renal glomeruli. In addition, autoantibodies may bind directly to tissue antigens and form in situ immune complexes. These deposits can be seen by immunofluorescence (indicating type of antibody deposited) and electron microscopy (showing exact localization). The immune complexes activate complement, and leukocytes are recruited by complement by-products (C3a, C5a) and by binding of leukocyte Fc receptors to the IgG molecules in the complexes. These leukocytes become activated, and they produce reactive oxygen species and lysosomal enzymes that damage the glomerular basement membrane. These findings are characteristic of immune complex–mediated tissue injury, and complexes may deposit in joints and small blood vessels anywhere in the body, as well as in the kidney. SLE is a prototype of an immune complex disease (see Chapter 11).

CASE 5: HUMAN IMMUNODEFICIENCY VIRUS INFECTION: ACQUIRED IMMUNODEFICIENCY SYNDROME

On first presentation to a clinic physician, J.C. was a 28-year-old assistant carpenter with 3 weeks of low-grade fevers, sore throat, and lymphadenopathy. Physical examination revealed "track marks," and when asked, the patient stated that 2 months earlier, he had begun using heroin with shared needles because he could no longer afford the cost of escalating doses of street oxycodone. Other findings on physical examination included lymphadenopathy, thrush (fungal infection of the oropharynx), and a faint, diffuse rash. Point-of-care tests for Epstein-Barr virus infection (monospot) and oropharyngeal streptococcal infection (rapid strep) were negative, as were blood cultures for bacteria and fungi. He was discharged with a presumed viral syndrome and given topical nystatin, an oral antifungal for his thrush.

1. What is the significance of 3 weeks of low-grade fevers and lymphadenopathy?

J.C. was seen the next week in the infectious diseases clinic, where enzyme-linked immunosorbent assays (ELISAs) performed on his blood were found to be negative for anti–human immunodeficiency virus (HIV) antibody but positive for HIV nucleocapsid p24. The concentration of HIV viral genomes in his blood (viral load) was determined to be 700,000/mL, and his blood CD4$^+$ T cell count was 300/mm^3 (Fig. A.6). Hepatitis B virus (HBV) ELISAs were negative for anti-HBV surface antigen and HBV surface antigen. HIV genotyping showed a lysine-to-asparagine mutation at codon 103 (K103N) of the HIV reverse transcriptase gene. Antiretroviral therapy (ART) was recommended, but the patient was lost to follow-up.

2. What was this patient's major risk factor for acquiring HIV infection? What are other risk factors for HIV infection?

3. Why do the HIV tests include testing for the presence of both HIV antibodies and p24 protein?

Six months later, J.C. was seen at a community hospital for an abscess at an injection site. After incision and drainage, he left against medical advice. A CD4$^+$ T cell count obtained at that time was 200, and viral load was 15,000. He still refused ART therapy. Six years later, J.C. was admitted to the hospital after a week of fevers and shortness of breath. A chest x-ray showed faint, diffuse infiltrates, and oxygen saturation was 90%. Initial microscopic examination of sputum stained for fungi (silver stain) was unrevealing, but he was started on antibiotics plus prednisone. PCR testing of sputum was positive for *Pneumocystis jirovecii*. J.C.'s condition initially worsened, but eventually he recovered fully. A repeat CD4$^+$ T cell count was now 150, with a viral load of 50,000/mL. At this point, J.C. was amenable to ART and was started on elvitegravir/cobicistat (an HIV integrase inhibitor with a boosting codrug), plus two nucleoside/nucleotide analog inhibitors of the HIV reverse transcriptase (nucleoside/nucleotide analog reverse transcriptase inhibitors [NRTIs]), tenofovir/emtricitabine. He was also continued on trimethoprim/sulfa antibiotics. He was advised to stop smoking.

4. Why does ART therapy for HIV typically include three different antiviral drugs?

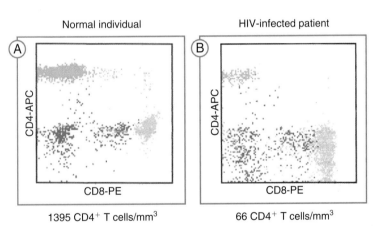

Fig. A.6 Flow cytometry analysis of CD4$^+$ and CD8$^+$ T cells in blood of patient with human immunodeficiency virus *(HIV)* infection. A suspension of the patient's white blood cells was incubated with monoclonal antibodies specific for CD4 and CD8. The anti-CD4 antibody was labeled with the fluorochrome allophycocyanin *(APC)*, and the anti-CD8 antibody was labeled with the fluorochrome phycoerythrin *(PE)*. These two fluorochromes emit light of different colors when excited by the appropriate wavelengths. The cell suspensions were analyzed in a flow cytometer, which can enumerate the number of cells stained by each of the differently labeled antibodies. In this way, the number of CD4$^+$ and CD8$^+$ T cells can be determined. Shown here are two-color plots of a control blood sample **(A)** and that of the patient **(B)**. The CD4$^+$ T cells are shown in orange *(upper left quadrant)*, and the CD8$^+$ T cells are shown in green *(lower right quadrant)*. (Note that these are not the colors of light emitted by the APC and PE fluorochromes.)

5. What caused the gradual decline in J.C.'s CD4+ T cell count?

6. Why were antibiotics and prednisone started in the patient before a diagnosis of *P. jirovecii* infection was established by PCR?

One year later, his CD4 count was 800 and his viral load was undetectable, but he developed methicillin-resistant *Staphylococcus aureus* (MRSA) infection of his mitral valve (staph endocarditis), requiring surgical replacement with a bioprosthetic valve. Preoperative cardiac catheterization showed significant coronary artery disease. Postoperatively, he was able to discontinue heroin use with methadone maintenance. His antiretroviral drugs were continued, but the trimethoprim sulfa was stopped. He has remained in good health since. His long-term partner remains HIV negative.

7. What are the main risks to J.C.'s life at this point?

Answers to Questions for Case 5

1. This pattern is referred to as acute HIV syndrome. Although a very large number of infectious agents can cause an acute viral syndrome for a few days, the persistence in this case suggests one of a relatively small number of causes in a young, previously healthy person, including HIV infection.

2. Intravenous drug use is the major risk factor for HIV infection in this patient. Shared needles among drug addicts transmit blood-borne viral particles from one infected person to others. Other major risk factors for HIV infection include sexual intercourse with an infected person, transfusion of contaminated blood products, and birth from an infected mother (see Chapter 12). Intravenous drug users account for only less than 10% of HIV cases in the United States. Most (70%) are men who have sex with other men and the rest are heterosexuals (~25%). Globally, greater than 90% of new infections occur in heterosexuals. The demographics of the epidemic have changed over the past few decades.

3. In acute infection, there has often been insufficient time to develop an antibody response, but levels of virus are high, so viral proteins can readily be detected. This is a screening test that, to be deployed widely, must be highly sensitive but also simple and inexpensive. New, so-called fourth-generation tests were approved in the United States in 2010, several years later than in other

countries. If the screening test was positive, it would be followed up with more specific (but more complex) assays for levels and genotype of viral nucleic acid.

4. HIV has a very high mutation rate. Mutations in the reverse-transcriptase gene that render the enzyme resistant to nucleoside inhibitors occur frequently in patients receiving these drugs. Resistance to protease inhibitors may come about by similar mechanisms. Triple-drug therapy greatly reduces the chances of viral drug resistance, but poor compliance permits the emergence of mutant strains resistant to several drugs. Nonnucleoside analog reverse transcriptase inhibitors (NNRTIs) are also effective anti-HIV drugs, but the lysine-to-asparagine mutation at codon 103 (K103N) of the HIV reverse transcriptase gene, discovered at the time of diagnosis, would make this patent resistant to NNRTIs. Integrase inhibitors are another major class of anti-HIV drugs used in combination therapy. Other drugs include inhibitors of HIV entry into and fusion with cells.

5. After initial infection, which often starts in mucosal tissues, HIV rapidly enters various types of cells in the body, mainly CD4+ T lymphocytes, but also dendritic cells and mononuclear phagocytes. The gradual decline in CD4+ T cells in this patient was caused by repetitive cycles of HIV infection of CD4+ T cells in lymphoid organs, leading to death of the cells. The symptoms of acquired immunodeficiency syndrome (AIDS) do not usually occur until the blood count of CD4+ T cells is less than 200/mm³, reflecting a severe depletion of T cells in the lymphoid organs.

6. This presentation in a person with known HIV infection is so highly suggestive of *P. jirovecii* pneumonia (PJP) that there was no need to wait for confirmatory diagnosis. The deficiencies in T cell–mediated immunity in patients with AIDS lead to impaired immunity to viruses, fungi, and protozoa, which otherwise are easily controlled by a normal immune system and are therefore called opportunistic infections. *P. jirovecii* is a fungal organism that can live within phagocytes, but usually it is eradicated by the action of activated CD4+ T cells. In the first days of antifungal treatment, a potent inflammatory response to the dying microorganisms can cause dangerous clinical worsening, so steroid antiinflammatories are started immediately for severe cases.

7. With well-controlled HIV infection, patients can have a near-normal life expectancy, and most deaths are from causes not directly related to HIV infection. Both HIV infection itself and some of the antiretroviral drugs accelerate coronary artery disease; hence infected persons who are effectively treated with antiretrovirals tend to die more frequently of disorders not directly related to the viral infection. The highest risk to this patient was active intravenous drug use, now discontinued. In addition, people with well-suppressed HIV infection very rarely transmit the virus to others, so treatment can both prevent and control infection.

INDEX

Page numbers followed by "f" indicate figures, "t" indicate tables, and "b" indicate boxes